PUBLIC HEALTH IN THE 21ST CENTURY

SMOKING RESTRICTIONS, RISK PERCEPTIONS AND ITS HEALTH AND ENVIRONMENTAL IMPACTS

PUBLIC HEALTH IN THE 21ST CENTURY

Additional books in this series can be found on Nova's website under the Series tab.

Additional e-books in this series can be found on Nova's website under the e-book tab.

PUBLIC HEALTH IN THE 21ST CENTURY

SMOKING RESTRICTIONS, RISK PERCEPTIONS AND ITS HEALTH AND ENVIRONMENTAL IMPACTS

NAZMI SARI, PH.D.
EDITOR

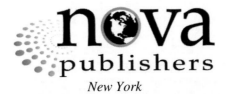

Copyright © 2014 by Nova Science Publishers, Inc.

All rights reserved. No part of this book may be reproduced, stored in a retrieval system or transmitted in any form or by any means: electronic, electrostatic, magnetic, tape, mechanical photocopying, recording or otherwise without the written permission of the Publisher.

For permission to use material from this book please contact us:
Telephone 631-231-7269; Fax 631-231-8175
Web Site: http://www.novapublishers.com

NOTICE TO THE READER

The Publisher has taken reasonable care in the preparation of this book, but makes no expressed or implied warranty of any kind and assumes no responsibility for any errors or omissions. No liability is assumed for incidental or consequential damages in connection with or arising out of information contained in this book. The Publisher shall not be liable for any special, consequential, or exemplary damages resulting, in whole or in part, from the readers' use of, or reliance upon, this material. Any parts of this book based on government reports are so indicated and copyright is claimed for those parts to the extent applicable to compilations of such works.

Independent verification should be sought for any data, advice or recommendations contained in this book. In addition, no responsibility is assumed by the publisher for any injury and/or damage to persons or property arising from any methods, products, instructions, ideas or otherwise contained in this publication.

This publication is designed to provide accurate and authoritative information with regard to the subject matter covered herein. It is sold with the clear understanding that the Publisher is not engaged in rendering legal or any other professional services. If legal or any other expert assistance is required, the services of a competent person should be sought. FROM A DECLARATION OF PARTICIPANTS JOINTLY ADOPTED BY A COMMITTEE OF THE AMERICAN BAR ASSOCIATION AND A COMMITTEE OF PUBLISHERS.

Additional color graphics may be available in the e-book version of this book.

Library of Congress Cataloging-in-Publication Data

ISBN: 978-1-63321-148-3

Library of Congress Control Number: 2014941043

Published by Nova Science Publishers, Inc. † New York

CONTENTS

Preface vii

About the Editor ix

PART I: Smoking Restrictions and Anti-Smoking Policies 1

Chapter 1 Anti-Smoking Policies and Their Effects on Smoking Prevalence and Behavior: Lessons from OECD Countries 3
Alper Altinanahtar, Ph.D. and Nazmi Sari, Ph.D.

Chapter 2 Smoking Behaviour and Tobacco Policy in the Rural Context: The Australian Experience 21
Margaret Stebbing, Ph.D.

PART II: Socio-Economic and Behavioral Determinants 33

Chapter 3 Smoking, Socioeconomic Status and Health 35
Lori J. Curtis, Ph.D.

Chapter 4 Youth Smoking in Canada and the Review of Related Literature 65
Hideki Ariizumi, Ph.D.

Chapter 5 How Long Do Japanese Mothers Stop Smoking When They Start Raising Children? New Evidence from a Very Large National Survey 79
Seiritsu Ogura, Ph.D, and Sanae Nakazono

PART III: Health and Environmental Hazards of Smoking 115

Chapter 6 Potential Health Hazards of Ignoring Submicron Particles in Low-Tar and Nicotine Cigarettes 117
W. D. van Dijk, M.D., Ph.D.

Chapter 7 Psychopathological Disorders, Tobacco Smoking, Smoking Cessation and Reduction 127
P. Caponnetto, G. Minutolo, R. Auditore, M. Maglia, A. Alamo, F. Benfatto, M. D'Alessandro, G. Nasca, V. Palumbo, C. Russo and R. Polosa

Chapter 8	Impacts of Smoking on Periodontal and Peri-Implant Health *Mirella Lindoso Gomes Campos, Mônica Grazieli Corrêa* *and Antonio Wilson Sallum*	**135**
Chapter 9	Health and Environmental Pitfalls and Fallacies of Smoking *Dr. Sona B. Nair*	**173**
Chapter 10	Assessment of Cigarette Smoking Toxicity Using Cancer Stem Cells *Kanda Yasunari*	**185**
Index		**197**

PREFACE

Smoking behavior and its health and environmental consequences have been one of the topics of interest for policy makers and academic audiences during the last decades. The prevalence of smoking was relatively low at the beginning of last century, and it started to escalate especially after the Great Depression. In 1960s and 1970s, smoking prevalence has reached to almost 50% of the population in many OECD countries. Since then smoking rates have been steadily declining in these countries, but it is still too high in many developing countries.

Starting from the second half of the 20th century, a growing literature has emphasized harmful health and environmental effects of smoking with specific reference to its direct link to the major non-communicable chronic diseases. 1964 US Surgeon General Report claimed that smoking is the primary cause of chronic bronchitis and correlated with emphysema, heart disease, and lung cancer. Following this landmark report, negative health consequences of smoking for not only smokers but also non-smokers due to second hand smoking, has been studied extensively. As scientific evidence on negative health effects has been established, and public awareness on harmful effects of smoking has started to increase, policy makers as an attempt to reduce smoking prevalence have started to implement wide range of anti-smoking policies including indoor smoking restrictions and bans, advertising bans for tobacco products, excise taxes, and smoking restrictions to protect the children against second hand smoke.

In this edited volume, a number of renowned scholars contribute to this literature with specific emphasis on anti-smoking policies, smoking behaviour and its socio-economic determinants, and impacts on health. The first section of the book includes chapters on anti-smoking policies and their impacts on smoking prevalence. This section provides an overview of the policies and their impacts in OECD countries, as well as their effects within rural setting for specific populations in Australian context. The second section of the book consists of chapters focusing on socio-economic and behavioral determinants of smoking with examples drawn from Canada and Japan. The authors examine socio-economic and behavioral aspects of smoking for various population groups including Canadian youth and adults, and Japanese pregnant mothers during and after the pregnancy. The third section includes chapters studying health and environmental hazards of smoking. This section focuses on specific health effects of smoking that are not widely examined elsewhere, the role of nicotine in cancer stem cells, and potential harmful effects of ignoring submicron particles in low-tar and nicotine cigarettes.

This book which provides a collection of papers reviewing most recent literature and offering new evidence in this body of literature has been primarily written for general public and policy makers. However, it also serves as a reference book for researchers, advanced level undergraduate and graduate students studying related aspects of smoking. With its focus on public policy, I hope that the book would help the policy makers in developing and designing health and public policies aimed at reducing smoking, and its harmful effects.

Nazmi Sari, Ph.D.
March 2014
Saskatoon, Canada

ABOUT THE EDITOR

Dr. Sari earned Ph.D. in economics at Boston University in 2001. Currently he is an associate professor in the Department of Economics at the University of Saskatchewan. Before joining the University of Saskatchewan in 2004, he worked as an assistant professor at the School of Policy and Management, Florida International University, USA. He is health economist with research interests covering wide range of topics in health economics and economics of health behaviour. His research has been published in academic journals in economics, health economics, public health, health policy and health sciences.

Tel: +1(306) 966-5216
Fax: +1(306) 966-5232
Email: nas961@mail.usask.ca

PART I: SMOKING RESTRICTIONS AND ANTI-SMOKING POLICIES

Chapter 1

ANTI-SMOKING POLICIES AND THEIR EFFECTS ON SMOKING PREVALENCE AND BEHAVIOR: LESSONS FROM OECD COUNTRIES

Alper Altinanahtar, Ph.D.[1*] *and Nazmi Sari, Ph.D.*[2]
[1]Yeditepe University, Department of Economics
[2]University of Saskatchewan, Department of Economics

ABSTRACT

As shown in recent literature, tobacco consumption is responsible for a substantial number of deaths in the world. As it is widely acknowledged after the release of 1964 US Surgeon General Report, smoking is accepted as the primary cause of chronic bronchitis and correlated with emphysema, heart disease, and lung cancer. The report encouraged many government agencies and health organizations to investigate further active and passive smoking-related health problems. Following the realization of its adverse health effects and its link with cancer, there were wide spread initiatives aimed to restrict tobacco consumption and campaigns against smoking. These were later followed by government regulations and bans on tobacco consumption. In this chapter, our aim is to provide a review of literature on smoking trends and anti-smoking policies in OECD countries. We discuss the impacts of advertising bans and smoking regulations in indoor and public places.

Keywords: Smoking, tobacco, OECD, smoking ban in public places, advertising and sponsorhip bans, social norm, displacement effect

---

[*] Correspondence: *Alper Altinanahtar* - Yeditepe University, Department of Economics, 26 Agustos Yerleskesi, Kayisdagi, Istanbul, Turkey; Tel.: +90(216) 578-0789; Fax: +90(216) 578-0797; Email: aaltinanahtar@yeditepe.edu.tr.
Nazmi Sari – University of Saskatchewan, Department of Economics, Saskatoon, Canada; Tel.: +1(306) 966-5216; Email: nazmi.sari@usask.ca.

1. INTRODUCTION

Smoking is a habit that goes back more than several millenniums. After the Europeans' arrival in Asia in the 16th century, tobacco became major merchandise and the modernization of production technology and distribution methods later followed by global advertisements increased its consumption over the years. The tobacco industry expanded notably. Currently, annual revenues from the global tobacco industry are almost half a trillion dollars. However, until a few decades ago, no one actually thought about banning its use or even restricting its consumption. However, with the realization of its adverse health effects and especially medical evidence linking cancer and smoking, a global opposition to smoking has started. Roughly after the Second World War, more and more studies showed that smoking is one of the major causes of serious health problems leading to death.

As shown in the recent body of literature, globally tobacco is responsible for 16% of deaths among men and 7% of deaths among women. It is described as the only risk factor that is common to all four (cancer, cardiovascular disease, diabetes, and chronic respiratory diseases) of the major non-communicable chronic diseases (Eriksen et al. 2012). As indicated in CDC (2013), smoking among pregnant women can also lead to low birth weight and illnesses among new born babies.

The Surgeon General's Report in 1964 was the first of 28 reports on the health consequences of smoking. The report claimed smoking to be the primary cause of chronic bronchitis and correlated with emphysema, and heart disease. It also pointed out the proven relationship between cigarette smoking and lung cancer. This report encouraged many government agencies and health organizations to investigate further active and passive smoking-related health problems. During the decades following the report issued by the US Surgeon General, several national and international agencies have followed the footsteps of the Surgeon General. The US Environmental Protection Agency declared tobacco as *class A carcinogen* in 1992. In 1997, the World Bank and the World Health Organization (WHO) initiated a global partnership to provide a strong base for designing effective tobacco control policies (see Jha and Chaloupka 2000). A decade after the US Environmental Protection Agency, the International Agency for Research on Cancer also declared Environmental Tobacco Smoke (ETS) - one of the leading causes of preventable deaths - a *class A carcinogen*. In May 2003, at the 56th World Health Assembly, WHO has initiated a process to ban smoking globally with 168 member states adopting the world's first public health treaty (Rivero et al. 2006). As of September 2013, 177 member states adopted the treaty. In 2007, the European Commission emphasized the importance of comprehensive smoking bans in its 2007 Green Paper (European Commission, 2007). When the word started to spread, civilians were also involved in the restriction of tobacco consumption and campaigns against smoking. These were later followed by government regulations and bans on tobacco consumption. First, pilot programs were conducted and later, nationwide bans were put in place.

In this chapter, our aim is to provide a review of this body of literature. We will present an overview of smoking trends across the world, and OECD countries in the next section. In section 3, we present an overview of the anti-smoking policies implemented in OECD countries. In section 4, we summarize the impact of advertising and sponsorship bans on smoking. Section 5 will focus on the smoking regulations in indoor and public places in which we present an overview of the policies implemented in OECD countries and review the evidence from literature on the effectiveness of indoor smoking bans on smoking prevalence. The final section is devoted to a summary and discussions.

2. OVERVIEW OF SMOKING TREND AROUND THE WORLD

By the beginning of the 20th century, smoking prevalence was relatively low, but started to grow in the first decade of the century. While the mass production of cigarettes has started to pick up, smoking rates also increased accordingly. Especially after the great depression, the increase in smoking rates was quite steep and reached its peak around the 1960s and 1970s. During these decades, smoking prevalence reached almost 50% of the population in many OECD countries including Japan, Netherlands, Denmark, and the UK. Since then, smoking rates have been steadily declining (OECD 2010).

With known negative health consequences, smoking has started to decline during the second half of the 20th century. In 1964, the US Surgeon General issued the first comprehensive report reviewing the evidence from literature in terms of its negative health effects. This report identified policies such as health campaigns, bans, and restrictions of smoking in indoor places that would be effective in reducing tobacco consumption. These anti-smoking policies initiated by the US Surgeon General created a downward trend in tobacco use (Unites States Department of Health 1964). During this period, both adult female and male smoking rates decreased substantially. For instance, adult male smoking prevalence from 1960 to 2010 decreased from 81% to 38% in Japan, 61% to 22% in the UK, and 52% to 22% in the US. Adult female smoking prevalence on the other hand decreased from 13% to 11 % in Japan, 42% to 21% in the UK, and 34% to 17% in the US (Eriksen et al. 2012).

The weighted average adult prevalence rates for smoking in 2010, for males and females in WHO regions are as follows: Africa 18%-3%, America 26%-13%, South-East Asia 28%-3%, Europe 41%-19%, Eastern Mediterranean 35%-3%, Western Pacific 48%-4% (WHO 2012). Given these estimates, the global average for smoking prevalence for males is 36% and for females it is 7%. In terms of income levels, the highest smoking prevalence for males exists in middle-income countries at 37%. For females, the highest prevalence is observed in high-income countries with 14%. In low income countries, smoking prevalence is at its lowest for both males and females.

Table 1. Smoking Prevalence in OECD Countries in 2009

Country	Per Capita Consumption (numbers of cigarettes)	Daily Smoker (% of population aged 15 and over)	Age Standardized Smoking rate (%) Male	Age Standardized Smoking rate (%) Female
Australia	1,034	16.6	15	18
Austria	1,650	23.2	19	27
Belgium	1,455	20.5	18	24
Brazil[1]	504	15.5	13	19
Canada	809	16.2	14	18
Chile	860	29.8	26	33
Czech Republic	2,125	24.6	19	30

Table 1. (Continued)

Country	Per Capita Consumption (numbers of cigarettes)	Daily Smoker (% of population aged 15 and over)	Age Standardized Smoking rate (%) Male	Age Standardized Smoking rate (%) Female
Denmark	1,413	19.0	17	22
Estonia	1,523	26.2	17	39
Finland	671	18.6	16	22
France	854	26.2	22	31
Germany	1,045	21.9	18	26
Greece	2,795	39.7	34	45
Hungary	1,518	26.5	22	32
Iceland	477	15.8	16	16
Ireland	1,006	29.0	27	31
Israel	1,037	20.3	13	28
Italy	1,475	23.3	17	30
Japan	1,841	24.9	12	39
Korea	1,958	25.6	7	44
Luxembourg	928	19.0	17	22
Mexico	371	13.3	7	22
Netherlands	801	22.6	20	26
New Zealand	579	18.1	17	19
Norway	534	21.0	20	21
Poland	1,586	27.0	21	34
Portugal	1,114	18.6	11	27
Russian Federation[1]	2,786	33.8	16	55
Slovak Republic	1,403	19.4	12	27
Slovenia	2,369	18.9	16	22
Spain	1,757	26.2	21	31
Sweden	715	14.3	15	14
Switzerland	1,722	20.4	18	23
Turkey	1,399	27.4	12	44
United Kingdom	750	21.5	21	22
United States	1,028	16.1	14	18

Source : Eriksen et al. (2012) and OECD (2011).

Note: [1] We included Brazil and Russian Federation in the table even though they are not part of OECD countries. These are the two countries closely work with OECD in aligning their policies to follow the OECD guidelines. The figures show the data from 2009 or the closest year for each country.

Table 1 presents the smoking rates for males and females, and the *per capita* consumption of tobacco products in numbers of cigarettes in OECD countries. The first column shows the variation in numbers of cigarettes smoked per person. Some countries such as Greece, Czech Republic, Slovenia and Korea are the countries with highest per capita smoking. We also reported smoking prevalence for males and females as well as proportions of daily smokers in each country. The data for the table is gathered from OECD (2011) and

Eriksen et al. (2012). As a result, the comparability of these rates among countries is limited due to different measurement techniques used in data gathering. However, it is safe to say that Sweden is the only OECD country where smoking prevalence among females is higher than males. In Iceland, the UK, Norway, New Zealand and Ireland, the rates are nearly equal. In Korea, smoking prevalence among males is 6.3 times that of females. It is 3.7 in Turkey, 3.4 in the Russian Federation, 3.3 in Japan, and 3.1 in Mexico. The average smoking prevalence among men in OECD countries is 27% whereas among women it is 17%.

While the smoking rate shows a substantial decrease in OECD countries, it increased in other parts of the world. As we observe a decrease in Western Europe by 26% from 1990 to 2009, smoking has increased by 57% during the same period in the Middle East and Africa. This increase was large enough to offset the decrease in cigarette consumption in high-income countries. Nearly 20% of the world's adult population smoked cigarettes and consumed approximately 5.9 trillion cigarettes in 2009 (Eriksen et al. 2012).

In the 20th century, tobacco caused 100 million deaths. This trend suggests that the total number of deaths is expected to reach 1 billion by the end of the 21st century. According to recent estimates, the consumption of smoking leads to about 6 million deaths each year, including more than 600,000 individuals who die from exposure to second-hand smoke (Shafey et al. 2009).

In 2004, 47% of secondhand smoke deaths occurred among women, 28% among children, and almost 26% among men. The total deaths related to secondhand smoking in 2004 was a little over 600,000. Europe has the highest death rates in secondhand smoking (28.6%), followed by South-East Asia, (26.9%), and Americans have the lowest rates among 6 WHO regions with 5.6% (Eriksen et al. 2012). In Table 2, we present a snapshot of smoking and its economic implications, as well as smoking-related death in OECD countries.

Table 2 presents the nation-wide direct cost of smoking, 7-year average population (2003 to 2010), per capita direct cost of smoking, and proportion of deaths attributable to smoking in OECD countries. Costs provided here reflect the estimates of both private and medical costs of treating tobacco-related illnesses in various years. We do not include indirect costs related to smoking. Due to inconsistency across countries in reporting tobacco related data, we report 7-year population averages in each column. We used these population averages to compute *per capita* costs. These are reported in column 4 of the table. Finally, the last two columns in Table 2 present the percentage of deaths associated with smoking for males and females in 2004. The figures in the table provide an overall picture as a summary measure but they are not directly useful to make comparisons among countries. Especially, the cost *per capita* may not be compared given that they are not corrected for differences in purchasing power. However, the deaths which are attributable to smoking suggest that smoking is a major cause of deaths in all OECD countries. These numbers imply that about one fifth of deaths among males are attributable to tobacco consumption in most of OECD countries. It is somewhat lower but not insignificant for females. The range of estimates for this group is around 10-15% in many countries.

Table 2. Cost of Smoking and Percentage of Deaths due to smoking in OECD Countries

Country	Direct cost of tobacco use (million USD)	Population (million)	Per capita cost (USD)	Deaths due to tobacco (% estimates in 2004) Male	Deaths due to tobacco (% estimates in 2004) Female
Australia	8,860	20.9	424	17	14
Austria		8.2		19	10
Belgium		10.6		31	8
Brazil[1]	185	186.4	1	15	6
Canada	2,803	32.8	85	23	20
Chile	1,140	16.5	69	11	8
Czech Republic	367	10.3	36		
Denmark	1,390	5.4	257	23	21
Estonia	14	1.3	11	26	7
Finland	309	5.3	58	16	6
France	16,650	61.7	270	22	5
Germany	8,490	82.2	103	22	9
Greece		11.1		25	7
Hungary	1,715	10	172	30	18
Iceland	67	0.3	223	16	20
Ireland		4.2		22	22
Israel	469	7.1	66	14	8
Italy		59.1		24	7
Japan	12,021	127.7	94	22	12
Korea	194	48.6	4		
Luxembourg		0.47			
Mexico	5,700	105.3	54	7	6
Netherlands	325	16.4	20	28	14
New Zealand	166	4.2	40	18	16
Norway		4.7		17	13
Poland	5	38.2	0.13	31	12
Portugal		10.5		17	3
Russian Federation[1]		143.3		28	4
Slovak Republic		5.4		26	6
Slovenia		2		27	11
Spain	221	44.3	5	25	2
Sweden	341	9.1	37	10	9
Switzerland	1,445	7.6	190	17	8
Turkey		69.9		38	6
United Kingdom	9,584	60.1	159	22	20
United States	96,000	299.8	320	23	23

Source: Eriksen et al. (2012), and authors' calculations.

Note: The direct costs for each country show the most recent avaiable data. For most of the countries, it is calculated for 2008, and 2009. However for some countries such as New Zeland, it shows the data from 2004. [1] We include Brazil and Russian Federation in the table even though they are not part of OECD countries. These are the two countries closely work with the OECD in aligning their policies to follow the OECD guidelines.

3. OVERVIEW OF THE ANTI-SMOKING POLICIES IMPLEMENTED IN THE OECD COUNTRIES

In this section, we outline anti-smoking policies taken place in OECD countries including advertising and sponsorship bans as well as smoking restrictions and bans in public places. Table 3 presents a summary of the anti-smoking policies implemented in OECD countries. There has been an extensive level of advertising tobacco products. For instance in the US, there were almost $10 billion spent on cigarette advertising and promotion in 2008, about $8.2 billion of which comes from price discounts, coupons and retail value-added promotions (Eriksen et al. 2012).

In an attempt to curtail smoking, the policy makers started to implement wide spread advertising bans on tobacco products. As stated in one of the most recent studies, tobacco consumption could decrease between 7% and 16% if there is a comprehensive ban on all tobacco advertising, promotion and sponsorship. This study indicates that advertising bans are one of the most cost effective ways to reduce tobacco use (WHO 2013a).

Advertising bans have been implemented in various media. They include advertising bans on television, radio, cinema, outdoor billboards, newspaper and magazines, shop advertising, and sponsorships. Indirect advertising such as brand names on non-tobacco products were also banned by these policies (Nelson 2003). In May 1996, WHO initiated a road map for tobacco control policies followed by the countries around the globe. For this purpose, WHO has created the Framework Convention on Tobacco Control (FCTC) which is *"an evidence-based set of legally binding provisions that establish a roadmap for successful global tobacco control"* (WHO 2013b p.16). The framework was finalized and adopted in 2003 after the realization of the critical nature of tobacco crises by the members of the WHO. Table 3 presents the date of entry for each country to the WHO FCTC.

The WHO FCTC, also referred to as *the force*, provides member states with provisions focusing on both demand and supply side concerns. There are eight articles concentrating on demand reduction and three articles focusing on the supply reduction, each with various numbers of guidelines within them. Although there are some variations across countries, most of OECD countries adopted the FCTC in 2005. In addition to the date of entry to the force, we present the numbers of guidelines met for two of the important Articles (Articles 11 and 13) of the force. These are presented in columns 3 and 4.

Article 11 defines the health warning signs placed on all tobacco product packages. It requires member states to place health warnings that should cover a minimum of 30% but a preferred 50% of the visible area, on all forms of smoking and smokeless tobacco product packages. There are a total of 8 guidelines related to Article 11 that need to be met before the 3 year deadline of the implementation of the article. In column 5, we present the number of guidelines met before the deadline for each country. As shown in the table, most of the countries have met 6 or more guidelines by the deadline set by the WHO for the implementation of Article 11.

Table 3. Smoking bans and regulations in OECD countries

Country	Date of entry to the FCTC	Guidelines met for Article 11[1]	Advertising ban met for Article 13[2]	Date of smoking restrictions in work and public places Weak	Date of smoking restrictions in work and public places Strong
Australia	02/2005	8	2		
Austria	12/2005	6	2	2009	2010
Belgium	01/2006	7	2	2006	2011
Brazil[3]	02/2006	8	2		2011
Canada	02/2005	8		1989	2010
Chile	09/2005	7			2013
Czech Republic	08/2012			2009	
Denmark	03/2005	7	1	2007	
Estonia	10/2005	6	1	2007	
Finland	04/2005	6	2	2007	
France	02/2005	6	2	2008	
Germany	03/2005	6	2	2007-2009	
Greece	04/2006	6	2	2009	2010
Hungary	02/2005	7	2		2012
Iceland	02/2005	7	1	2006	
Ireland	02/2006	6	2	1988	2004
Israel	11/2005	6		1983	2007
Italy	09/2008	6	2	2005	
Japan	02/2005	6		2010	
Korea				2013	
Luxembourg	09/2005			2006	
Mexico	02/2005	8		2004	2008
Netherlands	04/2005	6		2008	
New Zealand	02/2005	8	2		2004
Norway	02/2005	7	1	1988	2004
Poland	12/2006			2011	
Portugal	02/2006	6	2	2008	
Russian Federation[3]	09/2008	4		2013	2014
Slovak Republic	02/2005			2004	2010
Slovenia	06/2005	6	2	2007	
Spain	04/2005	7	2	2006	2011
Sweden	10/2005	5	2	2005	
Switzerland				2010	
Turkey	03/2005	7	1	1997	2009
United Kingdom	03/2005	7	2	2006	2007
United States[4]	05/2004				

Source: WHO (2012; 2013c), For Korea see The Jeju Weekly (2013).

Note: [1] The value in the column shows the number of guidelines met before the 3 year deadline. There are 8 guidelines for implementation of Article 11. [2] The value in this column denotes the types of advertising bans met by the member country before the 5-year deadline. [3] We included Brazil and Russian Federation in the table even though they are not part of OECD countries. These are the two countries closely work with the OECD in aligning their policies to follow the OECD guidelines. [4] The US signed the FCTC and expressed interest to become a part of the Convention but we cannot reach to additional information from the WHO sources mentioned above if it became a full member.

Column 4 in the table indicates the guidelines related to banning tobacco advertising and promotion. The FCTC sets out rules in Article 13 which refers to the banning of tobacco advertising, promotion and sponsorship within the country as well as cross-border. The number in the corresponding column indicates the types of ban on advertising and promotion met before the 5 year deadline of the implementation of the article. For instance, if the value in this column is 1, that means that the country has imposed a comprehensive ban on tobacco advertising, promotion and sponsorship. However, the definition of a comprehensive ban does not always cover all the procedures suggested by the guidelines. On the other hand, the value of 2 means that the ban also covers cross-border advertising, promotion and sponsorship which originates from the country's territory.

Another anti-smoking policy is the restriction or bans on smoking in indoor places. Area bans have been implemented in health care and educational facilities, governmental working places, restaurants, pubs and bars, indoor working places, and theatres and cinemas. The most recent restrictions and bans on smoking in indoor places have become effective in work places and restaurants and bars. In the last column of Table 3, we show the restrictions and/or bans on smoking in work places and restaurants/bars implemented in various countries. We identify the policies as weak or strong, based on the degree of strictness. However, there are substantial variations in the implementation of the policies across OECD countries.

The type of smoking regulations as weak or strong is determined based on whether the smoking is completely banned regardless of the place (workplace, restaurant or bar), size and the seating capacity of the place (strong), or it is relaxed depending on the seating capacity of restaurants (weak). For instance in Austria, smoking is not prohibited for places with one guest room and size less than 50 square meters (In Denmark, it is less than 40 square meters). There is some flexibility if the restaurants or work places have designated smoking rooms. For places bigger than 50 square meters, the restaurant can be divided into multiple sections with designated smoking and non-smoking sections (Reichmann and Reichmann 2012). In Poland on the other hand, smoking is completely prohibited in places less than 100 square meters whereas smoking is permitted in larger restaurants with a separate and properly ventilated room (WBJ 2010). In the table, we categorize the countries with *weak* policies, and present the date for the start of the discussion and weak implementations of smoking bans in public places. In the last column, we show the date when the country moved to more stringent smoking bans in public places, including restaurants and bars.

In countries like Australia, Canada and the U.S., with many states, tobacco control programs are not unified among states. Lacking a nationwide federal smoking ban, each state has its own regulations and restrictions on smoking. Some states may implement much stronger policies while others implement weaker policies. For instance, Massachusetts banned smoking in workplaces, restaurants, bars and in gambling places in 2004. At the same time, in

Idaho smoking was restricted only in restaurants. Indiana waited until 2012 to ban smoking in restaurants and workplaces. California's smoking ban was effective by 1998 and covered restaurants, bars and gambling places. In Utah, smoking was banned in restaurants in 1995, in bars in 1999, and in workplaces in 2006 (ANRF 2013). Meanwhile, Needham, MA and New York City increased the smoking age to 21 while in other states, the minimum age to buy any tobacco products is either 18 or 19 (Hartocollis 2013).

Norway implemented weak smoking regulation in 1988 which restricted smoking in all public indoor places unless they provide a separate, well ventilated smoking room. After 2004 however, smoking was prohibited in every public areas. Similarly, until 2011, Spain had weak smoking regulations, and restaurants and bars could create a smoking section within the facility. However, in 2011 Spanish smoking regulations became much stronger and smoking has been restricted in every indoor public places, regardless of their seating capacity.

4. IMPACT OF ADVERTISING AND SPONSORSHIP BANS ON SMOKING

Tobacco products have been one of the most heavily advertised products. We have observed high advertisement of tobacco products around the world. For instance, the US tobacco industry spent $5.1 billion on advertising and promotion activities in 1996 (Chaloupka and Warner, 2000). This corresponds to about 1% of the total healthcare expenditure in the corresponding year. As the industry spends extensively for promotion and advertising of tobacco products, there is ongoing controversy around the influence of advertising on demand for tobacco products. Public health agencies argue that advertising tobacco products encourages smoking while tobacco companies argue that the purpose of advertising campaigns is not to increase the aggregate consumption of tobacco but to increase the market shares of individual brands (Blecher 2008). These companies also claim that advertisements only provide information to the consumers about tar and nicotine content, and are not an attempt to change individuals' preferences. This empirical question has been tackled by many researchers who used data from various countries such as Australia, and Spain, and OECD countries. These studies reached mixed results (Bardsley and Olekalns 1999; Hamilton 1972; Laugesen and Meads 1991; Stewart 1993; Saffer and Chaloupka 2000; Sari 2013).

Laugesen and Meads (1991), for instance, use data from 22 OECD countries between 1960 and 1986 and conclude that tobacco advertising restrictions have increasingly been associated with lower tobacco consumption since 1973. However, the impact was positive until 1973. As a response to Laugesen and Meads (1991), Stewart (1992) emphasizes the role of country-specific factors that would explain the differences in consumption. He argues that the omission of these factors leads to biased estimates for the advertising restriction coefficients.

While Sargent (2006) claims that the increase in smoking prevalence can be attributable to the misleading messages through advertising campaigns, implying that smoking is socially desirable normal behavior, subsequent studies reveal that advertisements have insignificant impact on tobacco consumption (Hamilton 1972; Laugesen and Meads 1991; Nelson 2003; Sari 2013; Stewart 1993). As also stated in Nelson (2003), the advertisements have had insignificant impact on tobacco consumption due to the fact that tobacco users were already aware of the adverse health effects of tobacco consumption.

In an interesting work, Saffer and Chaloupka (2000) points out the importance of the degree of bans, and they argue that a comprehensive ban on tobacco advertising reduces consumption. Their study uses data from the OECD and argues that the marginal gain of advertising declines with an increase in advertising bans for tobacco products. Therefore, advertising bans in more and more media push tobacco companies to a point where marginal gain from spending more for advertising in non-banned media is lower than marginal costs. Their empirical results from fixed effect models support their conclusion that a comprehensive ban on tobacco advertising reduces the smoking. As an attempt to review the literature, Eriksen et al. (2012) suggests that a comprehensive ban on all tobacco advertising, promotion and sponsorship could decrease tobacco consumption by about 7%. This is consistent with the conclusions of Blecher (2008) under the weak policy regime, which corresponds to a 6.7% decline in *per capita* consumption. The imposition of limited advertising bans does not have a significant impact on consumption because tobacco companies are substituting the media with no bans in place of the media that is banned to air their advertisements of their products (Saffer and Chaloupka 2000). However, using a recent data set from OECD countries, Sari (2013) suggests that advertising bans, even a more comprehensive one, do not have significant impacts on demand.

As stated in Sari (2013), promotion and advertising bans have an immediate impact but their marginal effect disappears over time after they have been implemented. These bans may be useful in eliminating any potential increase in smoking that would have been created through advertising tobacco products. However, they may have decreasing returns in discouraging smoking over time. It is likely that we have already achieved what we can achieve in terms of reduction in smoking; therefore, further reduction due to these policies could not be possible as they have been in place for a long time. However, the advertising bans, especially comprehensive bans, are important due to their influence on changing social norms related to smoking behavior. Therefore, there might be an indirect prolonged effect through their effects on social norms of smoking behavior.

5. IMPACT OF SMOKING RESTRICTIONS IN PUBLIC PLACES ON SMOKING

In addition to advertising bans in tobacco markets, smoking area restrictions (i.e. clean indoor air laws) have been used by policy makers. Similar to the higher taxes which increase monetary costs of smoking, smoking area restrictions also increase non-monetary costs to the smokers by creating inconvenience or additional time costs. This would affect individuals' *budget constraint* and therefore it has the potential to induce individuals to smoke less than before. However, it is also likely that the policies could have a *displacement effect* in which the bans in public places induce individuals to increase smoking in private places (i.e. cars, homes) with adverse effects on non-smokers, especially young children (Adda and Cornaglia 2010). We provide a brief review of this large body of literature below.

During the last decade, several developed countries have started to implement partial or comprehensive smoking bans in public places. In January 2005, Italy became the first

European Union country implementing a comprehensive smoking ban in public places. The anti-smoking law prohibited smoking in all public places with few exceptions for restaurants, cafes, and bars (Gallus et al. 2006). Based on surveys conducted in 2004, 2005 and 2006, Gallus et al.(2007) states that the percent of current smokers decreased from 26.2 to 24.3%, and the daily mean numbers of cigarettes smoked decreased from 15.4 to 13.9. Using Italian data, Buonanno and Ranzani (2013) also indicates that indoor smoking bans open to the public decreased smoking prevalence by 1.3% and daily cigarette consumption by 8%. This is a reduction in smoking that can be achieved by a 17% increase in price per pack.

The impact of the Italian smoking ban on sales was negligible. Although many restaurant owners and the tobacco industry were concerned with smoking restrictions` negative impact on their businesses, much research has shown that smoking restriction policies are not economically harmful (Bartosch and Pope 1999; Hyland et al. 1999; Sciacca and Ratliff 1998; Glantz and Smith 1997; Huang et al. 1995; Glantz and Smith 1994; Glantz and Charlesworth 1999; Adda et al. 2006; Pieroni et al. 2013; Bartosch and Pope 2002; Roseman 2006). Only a few studies, mostly funded by either the tobacco or restaurant industry, claim that the business will be affected under such policies (Sollars and Ingram 1998; Lilley and DeFranco 1998; Dunham and Marlow 2000). This negligible impact suggested in the literature on restaurant sales can be explained as follows: one possibility is that an increase in non-smokers demand for restaurant meals may offset the reductions in sales among smokers. Alternatively, it could be the case that smokers are not sufficiently inconvenienced by policies restricting smoking hence their demand for restaurant meals did not change substantially (Bartosch and Pope 2002).

Another body of literature studies the impact of a tobacco control program expenditures on *per capita* cigarette sales, or smoking rate. Tobacco control programs are mostly studied at the state level (Rhoads 2012) while Farrelly et al.(2003) was the first to look at tobacco control effects at the national level. Farrelly et al. find a negative correlation between tobacco control program expenditures and *per capita* cigarette sales. Later, they were followed by Rhoads (2012). Using data from the Behavioral Risk Factor Surveillance System (1991-2006), Rhoads finds that both comprehensive state tobacco control expenditures and other tobacco control policies, such as excise taxes and smoke-free air laws, were effective in reducing adult smoking prevalence.

Tauras et al. (2005) conducts a similar study for youths and used data from 1991 to 2000. Ciecierski et al. (2010) uses data for college students from 1997, 1999, and 2001, and Farrelly et al. (2008) uses data from 1985 to 2003 to test the effects of tobacco control program expenditures' impact on adult smoking prevalence. Yurekli and Zhang (2000) uses state level panel data, which cover government and private workplaces, grocery stores, restaurants, bars, shopping malls, public transportation, and health facilities. Even though the studies mentioned above use different data sets, they reach the same conclusions (inverse relationship between tobacco control program expenditures and adult smoking prevalence) with that of Farrelly et al. (2003).

In addition to results presented above, Rhoads (2012) concludes that if all states in the US had spent the CDC recommended level of funding between 1991 and 2006 on tobacco control programs, the number of smokers would have decreased somewhere between 635,000 and 3.7 million. On the other hand, based on his analysis of data from 2001 to 2005 for all 50 states, Marlow (2010) states that this negative correlation between tobacco control spending and smoking prevalence could be due to high *distaste* for smoking in the corresponding state. In other words, expenditures for tobacco control programs could be high in states where social norms against smoking could also be high which later may result in lower smoking prevalence rates in the corresponding states.

Another stream of research has focused on ban or restrictions of smoking in public places, and their impacts on smoking. Several studies suggest that smoking area restrictions are effective in controlling or reducing smoking (i.e. Chaloupka and Grossman 1996; Chaloupka and Wechsler 1997; Evans et al. 1999; Wasserman et al. 1991). For instance, Evans et al. (1999) studies workplace smoking policies using data from two large-scale national surveys in the US and concludes that workplace bans reduce smoking prevalence by 5 percentage points and daily consumption among smokers by 10%. Their findings were later supported by others (Farelly et al. 1999; Fichtenberg and Glantz 2002).

On the other hand, some of the studies which use data mostly from the US produced either little or inconclusive results (Adda and Cornaglia 2010; Chaloupka 1992; Chaloupka and Grossman 1996; Chaloupka and Saffer 1992; Jones et al. 2013; Keeler et al. 1993; Sung et al. 1994; Tauras 2006; Wasserman et al. 1991). This little effect on smoking behavior may be because individuals are substituting away from smoking in public places due to bans towards more private places (Adda and Cornaglia 2010). If this is the case, then smoking bans would have a negative impact on health (Wildman and Hollingsworth 2013).

Anger et al. (2010) reports that especially young and unmarried individuals and people in urban areas are less likely to smoke and smoke less following the introduction of smoking restrictions in public places. The degree of ban and individual smoking behavior are also negatively associated. Other studies such as Idris et al. (2007) and Han et al. (2008) also state that smoking regulations have a greater impact on the smoking habits of individuals living in urban areas, and among those who are single.

It is likely that the degree of smoking bans in public places would be an important factor in reducing smoking behavior. For instance, using panel data from OECD countries, Sari (2013) states that limited smoking bans in public places have not had significant impact on smoking while implementing a comprehensive ban (i.e. smoking ban in public places including restaurants and bars) decreases average smoking by 5.3%. However, it is also stated in the literature that comprehensive smoking bans may have *displacement effect* (i.e. induces individuals to increase smoking in private places such as in cars and homes) that may have adverse health effects for non-smokers, and especially for young children (Adda and Cornaglia 2010). On the other hand, it is also noted that comprehensive smoking bans may change smoking norms in a society over time. Smokers may become more considerate even in private places, and guests will no longer be welcomed smoking in houses. This indirect effect of comprehensive ban would not only decrease the exposure to second hand smoke, but also would create incentives for smokers to consider quitting (Sari 2013; Gallus et al. 2007).

CONCLUSION

Tobacco has been grown in 124 countries, and the industry is considered one of the biggest in the world. While it has substantial economic impacts around the world, the researchers indicate that the damage caused to society by tobacco consumption outweighs any economic benefit from its manufacturing and sale. The medical literature has also shown consistent evidence stating that smoking has adverse health effect and it reduces quality of life. In this chapter, we reviewed the larger body of literature on the economics of smoking in the context of effectiveness of anti-smoking policies in OECD countries. We summarized the smoking trend and anti-smoking policies implemented in the OECD countries, and highlighted the effectiveness of advertising bans for tobacco products and smoking bans in public places.

Consumption of tobacco products has increased more than 100 times in the last century, and 6 million people died due to tobacco consumption in 2011. Among these 6 million, 600,000 were non-smokers. By the end of the 21st century, the toll is expected to reach 1 billion people. The number of smoking-related deadly diseases has increased substantially. Over the last decades, medical literature has shown consistently that smoking shortens individuals` life expectancy, reduces their quality of life and imposes a great burden on the economy with additional negative externalities due to its impact on non-smokers. These findings raised concerns among civilian groups, health professionals and policy makers. As a result, many policy alternatives have been explored to provide a solution to this growing and damaging epidemic. Campaigns against smoking have aimed to raise awareness on negative health effects of smoking by providing scientific evidence and graphical illustrations on packages.

Additional policies such as excise taxes, and age restrictions to buy tobacco products have been implemented. These policy attempts were later followed by banning of advertisements and sponsorships of tobacco products, and smoking restrictions and/or bans in working places, and other public places.

It is shown in the literature that the banning of advertisements and sponsorships of tobacco products has limited impact on smoking. Studies based on data from various countries such as Australia, Spain, and OECD countries have reached mixed results. As some studies suggest that it has negative impact on smoking prevalence, others suggest that there is no significant impact. As we indicated earlier in the chapter, most of the literature indicates that smoking restrictions in public places generate a reduction in smoking prevalence with some possibility of *displacement effect*. The literature suggests that indoor smoking ban decreases smoking prevalence by about 1 to 5 percent. However, there are also studies indicating that these policies have had no impact on smoking prevalence.

It is important to note that the degree of smoking bans in public places would be an important factor in influencing smoking behavior among smokers. As opposed to weak ban, comprehensive smoking bans may have a persistent long term effect by changing smoking norms in a society over time. This would influence the overall smoking prevalence as well as smoking behavior among smokers. It helps to overcome displacement effects potentially generated by indoor smoking bans, hence decreases exposure to second hand smoke. The literature on economics of smoking does not provide enough evidence for long term impacts of anti-smoking policies, and their indirect effects. This area of research needs to be explored further to enhance our understanding of the ways that these policies work, and their overall long-run impacts.

REFERENCES

Adda, J. & Cornaglia, F. (2010). The effect of bans and taxes on passive smoking. *American Economic Journal: Applied Economics, 2*(1), 1-32.

Adda, J., Berlinski, S. & Machin, S. (2006). Short-run economic effects of the Scottish smoking ban. *International Journal of Epidemiology, 36*(1), 149-154.

Anger, S., Kvasnicka, M. & Siedler, T. (2010). *One Last Puff? Public smoking bans and smoking behavior.* Berlin: German Institute for Economic Research.

ANRF. (2013). American Nonsmokers` Rights Foundation.http://www.nosmoke.org/pdf/SummaryUSPopList.pdf (accessed December 26, 2013).

Bardsley, P. & Olekalns, N. (1999). Cigarette and Tobacco Consumption: Have Anti-smoking Policies made a difference? *The Economic Records, 75*, 225-240.

Bartosch, W. J. & Pope, G. C. (1999). The economic effect of smoke-free restaurant policies on restaurant business in Massachusetts. *Journal of Public Health Management Practice, 5*, 53-62.

Bartosch, W. J. & Pope, G. C. (2002). Economic effect of restaurant smoking restrictions on restaurant business in Massachusetts 1992 to 1998. *Tobacco Control, 11*, ii38-ii42.

Blecher, E. (2008). The impact of tobacco advertising bans on consumption in developing countries. *Journal of Health Economics, 27*, 930-942.

Buonanno, P. & Ranzani, M. (2013). Thank you for not smoking: Evidence from the Italian smoking ban. *Health Policy, 109*, 192– 199

CDC. (2013). *Tobacco Use and Pregnancy.* http://www.cdc.gov/ reproductivehealth/tobaccousepregnancy/ (accessed November 20, 2013).

Chaloupka, F. J. & Grossman, M. (1996). *Price, tobacco control policies and youth smoking, NBER Working Paper, No. 5740.* Cambridge, MA.: National Bureau of Economic Research

Chaloupka, F. J. & Saffer, H. (1992). Clean indoor air laws and the demand for cigarettes. *Contemporary Policy Issues, 10*, 72-83.

Chaloupka, F. J. & Warner, K. E. (2000). The Economics of Smoking. In: Culyer A, Newhouse J. (Eds), *The Handbook of Health Economics.* Elsevier: Amsterdam. 1541-1612.

Chaloupka, F. J. & Wechsler, H. (1997). Price, tobacco control policies and smoking among young adults. *Journal of Health Economics, 16*(3), 359-373.

Chaloupka, F. J. (1992). Clean indoor air laws, addiction and cigarette smoking. *Applied Economics, 24*, 193-205.

Ciecierski, C. C., Chatterji, P., Chaloupka, F. J. & Wechsler, H. (2010). Do state expenditures on tobacco control programs decrease use of tobacco products among college students? *Health Economics, 20*(3), 253-272.

Dunham, J. & Marlow, M. (2000). Smoking laws and their differential effects on restaurants, bars, and taverns. *Contemporary Economic Policy, 18*, 326-333.

Eriksen, M., Mackay, J. & Ross, H. (2012). *The Tobacco Atlas. Fourth Ed.* Atlanta, GA: American Cancer Society; New York, NY:World Lung Foundation

European Commission. (2007). Green Paper. Towards a Europe Free from Tobacco Smoke: Policy Options at the EU Level. (COM(2007) 27 final).

Evans, W. N., Farelly, M. C. & Montgomery, E. (1999) Do workplace smoking bans reduce smoking? *American Economic Review*, 89(4), 728-747.

Farrelly, M. C., Evans, W. N. & Sfekas, A. E. S. (1999). The impact of workplace smoking bans: results from a national survey. *Tobacco Control*, 8, 272-277.

Farrelly, M. C., Pechacek, T. F. & Chaloupka, F. J. (2003). The impact of tobacco control program expenditures on aggregate cigarette sales: 1981-2000. *Journal of Health Economics*, 22, 843-859.

Farrelly, M. C., Pechacek, T. F., Thomas, K. Y. & Nelson, D. (2008). The impact of tobacco control program on adult smoking. *American Journal of Public Health*, 98, 304-309.

Fichtenberg, C. M. & Glantz, S. A. (2002). Effect of smoke-free workplaces on smoking behavior: systematic review. *British Medical Journal*, 325(7357), 1-7.

Gallus, S, Zuccaro, P., Colombo, P, Apolone, G., Pacifici, R, Garattini, S, Bosetti, C. & La Vecchia, C. (2007). Smoking in Italy 2005–2006: Effects of a comprehensive National Tobacco Regulation. *Preventive Medicine*, 45, 198-201.

Gallus, S., Zuccaro, P., Colombo, P., Apolone, G., Pacifici, R. & Garattini, S. (2006). Effects of new smoking regulations in Italy. *Annals of Oncology*, 17, 346-347.

Glantz, S. A. & Charlesworth, A. (1999). Tourism and hotel revenues before and after passage of smoke-free restaurant ordinances. *Journal of American Medical Association*, 281, 1911-1918.

Glantz, S. A. & Smith, L. R. A. (1994). The effect of ordinances requiring smoke-free restaurant on restaurant sales. *American Journal of Public Health*, 84, 1081-1085.

Glantz, S. A. & Smith, L. R. A. (1997). The effect of ordinances requiring smoke-free restaurant and bars on revenues: A followup. *American Journal of Public Health*, 97, 1687-1693.

Hamilton, J. L. (1972). The demand for cigarettes: advertising, the health scare, and the cigarette advertising ban. *The Review of Economics and Statistics*, 54(4), 401-411.

Han, E. J., Rayens, M. K., Butler, K. M., Zhang, M., Durbin, E. & Steinke, D. (2008). Smoke-free laws and adult smoking prevalence. *Preventive Medicine*, 47, 206-209.

Hartocollis, A. (2013). *New York Raising Age to Buy Cigarettes to 21*. October 30, 2013. http://www.nytimes.com/2013/10/31/nyregion/new-york-approves-law-to-raise-tobacco-purchasing-age-to-21.html (accessed December 2013).

Huang, P., Tobias, S., Kohout, S., Harris, M., Satterwhite, D., Simmpson, D.M., Winn, L., Foehner, J. & Pedro, L. (1995). Assessment of the impact of a 100 percent smoke-free ordinance on restaurant sales, West Lake Hills, Texas, 1992-1994. *Morbidity and Mortality Weekly Report*, 44, 370-372.

Hyland, A. K., Cummings, M. & Nauenberg, E. (1999). Analysis of taxable sales receipts: Was New York City`s smoke-free air act bad for business. *Journal of Public Health Management Practice*, 5, 14-21.

Idris, B. I., Giskes, K., Borrell, C., Benach, J., Costa, G., Federico, B., Helakorpi, S., Helmert, U., Lahelma, E., Moussa, K. M., Ostergren, P.O., Prattala, R., Rasmussen, N. Kr., Mackenbach, J. P. & Kunst, A. E. (2007). Higher smoking prevalence in urban compared to non-urban areas: Time trends in six European countries. *Health & Place*, 13, 702-712.

Jha, P. & Chaloupka, F. J. (Eds) (2000). *Tobacco control in developing countries*. Oxford: Oxford University Press.

Jones, A. M., Laporte, A., Rice, N. & Zucchelli, E. (2013). Do public smoking bans have an impact on active smoking? Evidence from the UK. *Health Economics.* doi: 10.1002/hec.3009

Keeler, T. E., The-Wei, H., Barnett, P. G. & Manning, W. G. (1993). Taxation, regulation and addiction: a demand function for cigarettes based on time series evidence. *Journal of Health Economics, 12,* 1-18.

Laugesen, M. & Meads, C. (1991). Tobacco advertising restrictions, price, income and tobacco consumption in OECD countries, 1960–1986. *British Journal of Addiction, 86*(10), 1343-1354.

Lilley, W. & DeFranco, L. J. (1998). *The Impact of restaurant-bar smoking regulations on jobs. A study commissioned by the Massachussets Restaurant Assoc.* Washington DC: InContext Inc.

Marlow, M. L. (2010). Do expenditures on tobacco control decrease smoking prevalence? *Applied Economics, 42,* 1331-1343.

Nelson, J. P. (2003). Cigarette demand, structural change, and advertising bans: international evidence, 1970-1995. *Contributions to Economic Analysis & Policy, 2*(1), 1-27.

OECD. (2010). Healthy Choices, OECD Health Ministrerial Meeting. 2010.

OECD. (2011). *Health Data, National sources for non-OECD countries.* OECD Publishing. 2011. http://stats.oecd.org/index.aspx.

Pieroni, L., Daddi, P. & Salmasi, L. (2013). Impact of Italian smoking ban on business activity of restaurants, cafes and bars. *Economic Letters, 121,* 70-73.

Reichmann, G. & Reichmann, M. S. (2012). The Austrian Tobacco Act in practice - Analysing the effectiveness of partial smoking bans in Austria restaurants and bars. *Health Policy, 104,* 304-311.

Rhoads, J. K. (2012). The effect of comprehensive state tobacco control programs on adult cigarette smoking. *Journal of Health Economics, 31,* 393-405.

Rivero, L. R., Rivero Luis, R., Persson James, L., Romine David, C., Taylor John, T., Toole Theron, C., Trollman Christopher, J. Au. & William, W. (2006). Towards the world-wide ban of indoor cigarette smoking in public places. *International Journal of Hygiene and Environmental Health, 209,* 1-14.

Roseman, M. (2006). Consumer opinion on smoking bans and predicted impact on restaurant frequency. *International Journal of Hospitality & Tourism Administration, 6*(4), 49-69.

Saffer, H. & Chaloupka, F. (2000). The effect of tobacco advertising bans on tobacco consumption." *Journal of Health Economics, 19*(6), 1117-1137.

Sargent, J. D. (2006). Modifying exposure to smoking depicted in movies: a novel approach to preventing adolescent smoking. *Archives of Pediatrics & Adolescent Medicine, 157,* 643-648.

Sari, N. (2013). On anti-smoking regulations and tobacco consumption. *Journal of Socio-Economics, 43,* 60-67.

Sciacca, J. P. & Ratliff, R. I. (1998). Prohibiting smoking in restaurants: Effects on restaurant sales." *American Journal of Health Promotion, 12,* 176-184.

Shafey, O., Ross, H., Mackay, J. & Michael, E. (2009). *The Tobacco Atlas, 3rd edition.* Atlanta: American Cancer Society

Sollars, D. & Ingram, J. (1998). *The economic impact of the reataurant smoking ban in the city of Boston, Massachusetts. A study sponsored by the International Society of*

Restaurant Assoc. Exec. and funded by the Accom Program, Philip Morris USA Montgomery, Alabama. Montgomery: Auburn University

Stewart M. J. (1992). Tobacco Consumption and Advertising Restrictions: A Critique of Laugesen and Meads (1991). *International Journal of Advertising, 11*, 97-118.

Stewart, M. J. (1993). The effect on tobacco consumption of advertising bans in OECD countries. *International Journal of Advertising, 12*, 155-180.

Sung, H. Y., The-Wei, H. & Keeler, T. E. (1994). Cigarette taxation and demand: an empirical analysis. *Contemporary Economic Policy, 12*, 91-100.

Tauras, J. (2006). Smoke-free air laws, cigarette prices, and adult cigarette demand. *Economic Inquiry, 44*(2), 333-342.

Tauras, J. A., Chaloupka, F. J., Farrelly, M. C., Giovanni, G. A., Wakefield, M., Johnston, L. D., O`Malley, P. M., Kloska, D. D. & Pechacek, T. F. (2005). State tobacco control spending and youth smoking. *American Journal of Public Health, 95*, 338-344.

The Jeju Weekly. (2013). The smoking ban - key info. Also available at http://www.jejuweekly.com/news/articleView.html?idxno=3315 (accessed December 26, 2013)

Unites States Department of Health, Education, and Welfare. (1964). *Smoking and Health: report of the advisory committee to the Surgeon General of the Public Health Service.* Washington: US Department of Health, Education,and Welfare, Public Health Service, No.1103.

Wasserman J., Manning W. G., Newhouse J. P. & Winkler J. D. (1991). The effects of excise taxes and regulations on cigarette smoking. *Journal of Health Economics, 10*(1), 43-64.

WBJ. (2010). *Warsaw Business Journal: No Smoking in Poland.* November 10, 2010. http://www.wbj.pl/article-52021-no-smoking-in-poland.html? typ=wbj (accessed December 13, 2013).

WHO. (2012) *Global progress report on implementation of the WHO FCTC.* Geneva, Switzerland: WHO Press.

WHO. (2013a). Key messages - World No Tobacco Day 2013. http://www. who.int /campaigns/no-tobacco-day/2013/key_messages/en/index.html (accessed November 2013).

WHO. (2013b). *WHO report on the global tobacco epidemic, 2013: Enforcing bans on tobacco advertising, promotion, and sponsorship.* Luxemburg: WHO.

WHO. (2013c). *Parties to the WHO Framework Convention on Tobacco Control.* http://www.who.int/fctc/signatories_parties/en/(accessed December 13, 2013).

Wildman, J. & Hollingsworth, B. (2013). Public smoking bans and self-assessed health: Evidence from Great Britain. *Economic Letters, 118*, 209-212.

Yurekli, A. A. & Zhang, P. (2000). The impact of clean indoor-air laws and cigarette smuggling on demand for cigarettes: an empirical model. *Health Economics, 9*, 159-170.

In: Smoking Restrictions
Editor: Nazmi Sari

ISBN: 978-1-63321-148-3
© 2014 Nova Science Publishers, Inc.

Chapter 2

SMOKING BEHAVIOUR AND TOBACCO POLICY IN THE RURAL CONTEXT: THE AUSTRALIAN EXPERIENCE

Margaret Stebbing, PhD[*]

Department of Rural and Indigenous Health, School of Rural Health,
Monash University, Moe Victoria, Australia

ABSTRACT

This chapter reviews the progress in reducing the harms of tobacco use and achieving tobacco control in Australia with a particular reference to rural and remote and Indigenous Australian populations. The nature of and extent of measured inequities between metropolitan and rural Australia and the rural health deficit are summarized to highlight the relative disadvantage of rural Australians. The range of strategies included in Australia's comprehensive approach to tobacco control is described together with a review of evidence for tobacco control initiatives most likely to be effective for rural and remote populations including the particular case of Indigenous Australians living in rural and remote areas. The chapter concludes with a brief discussion of the benefits of adopting a social model of health in developing an understanding of the differences between urban and rural and remote populations and taking a social determinants approach in the development of tobacco policy.

Keywords: Rural, smoking, tobacco policy, smoking cessation, Indigenous, Australia, social determinants of health

1. INTRODUCTION

Australia is a Federation of six States and two Territories (known as the Commonwealth of Australia).Australian society is highly urbanized - about 70% of Australians live in capital

---

[*] Email: margaret.stebbing@monash.edu.

or major cities, the remainder (over 6.7 million) live in regional cities or large coastal towns, smaller country or coastal towns and a very small number in remote areas. Australia supports a diverse range of cultures across widely different geographical and climatic regions. The population in rural Australia is older than the population of Australia in general and supports a significant number of Indigenous Australians[1]. Rural Australia is also ageing at a faster rate than the cities. (Australian Institute of Health and Welfare, 2012)

Despite the fact that Australians as a whole enjoy high living standards, there are health differentials between those living in metropolitan areas and rural and remote communities. These differences can be explained in part by individual and personal characteristics and also by differences in the social, economic and environmental domains, sometimes called the social determinants of health. There is also a rural health deficit estimated to be around $2.1 billion dollars a year due to the combined effects of inequities evident in life expectancy, Medicare[2] funded services, health workforce availability, health status and health risk factors, effectiveness of health promotion, survival rates for cancer, education and educational outcomes, access to infrastructure, communications and cost of access to services (National Rural Health Alliance, 2011a, 2011b). Australians living in rural and remote areas have higher death rates and poorer health outcomes than Australians who live in metropolitan areas, and there are important differences in the availability and usage of health services (Australian Bureau of Statistics, 2011; National Rural Health Alliance, 2010). In general, the further people live away from major cities, the less healthy they are likely to be and the more difficulty they have in accessing health and community services. For example, in 2009–2010, the rate of hospitalised injury cases for residents of very remote areas (4,299 per100,000 population) was more than twice that for people in Major cities (1,728 per 100,000). There is also considerable variation within this general pattern as health status, health behavior and understanding of risks vary between arid inland areas and coastal regions and the relative prosperity of some farming groups and mining communities can be influenced by climatic conditions and the differential availability of natural resources (Australian Institute of Health and
Welfare, 2008).

Rural communities in Australia are generally understood to be less risk averse than their city counterparts. There are also many differences in the presence of and awareness of risk factors including tobacco smoking (Dobson et al., 2010; National Health Performance Authority, 2013a, 2013b) although this effect is not consistent across gender and socioeconomic groups (Migliorini et al., 2006). This may be in part because rural and remote communities reveal more clearly in their health choices the interdependence of environmental, economic, political and mental health concerns. (Anderson, 2009)

This chapter aims firstly to review the achievements of tobacco control in Australia with a particular reference to rural and remote and Indigenous Australian populations and to discuss the nature of and extent of measured inequities between metropolitan and rural Australia and the rural health deficit. Next the range of strategies included in Australia's comprehensive approach to tobacco control will be described together with a review of evidence for tobacco control initiatives most likely to be effective for rural and remote

---

[1] In Australia the term Indigenous is used to refer to Aboriginal and Torres Strait Islander people and to acknowledge that Aboriginal and Torres Strait Islander peoples are comprised of two distinct cultural groups.
[2] Medicare is the publicly funded universal health care scheme in Australia. Medicare is the primary funder of health care in Australia, funding essential primary health care for Australian citizens and permanent residents.

populations including the particular case of Indigenous Australians living in rural and remote areas. Finally the chapter discusses the benefits of adopting a social model of health in developing an understanding of the differences between urban and rural and remote populations and taking a social determinants approach in the development of tobacco policy.

2. SMOKING PREVALENCE AND ITS IMPACT IN AUSTRALIA

Tobacco smoking is the single most preventable contributor to the burden of disease in Australia contributing to cancer deaths, chronic obstructive pulmonary disease, cardiovascular disease and stroke in particular (Australian Institute of Health and Welfare, 2012). Tobacco is also sometimes combined with cannabis (Banbury et al., 2013). However recent (as yet unpublished) research found that only half of smokers can link smoking with lung cancer, one quarter can link smoking with heart attacks, and less than 10% of current smokers connect smoking with other health effects (Cancer Council Victoria, 2014).

In 2011-2012 one in six Australian adults smoked daily and this is estimated to cost government health budgets $12 million a year. The rate of decline in regular smokers is greatest for younger adults (18-29 years) and for those in lower socioeconomic groups due in part to the impact of closely targeted social marketing messages and increases in tobacco taxation and pricing. The prevalence of regular smoking remains consistently lower amongst adults with tertiary education (Australian Institute of Health and Welfare, 2012).

A number of population groups in Australia have higher smoking rates than the general population. This includes people who are unemployed, are sole parents, have a mental health issue, have a substance use problem, are in prison, are experiencing homelessness or are Aboriginal and/or a Torres Strait Islander (National Health Performance Authority, 2013b). People living in remote and very remote areas of Australia are 1.7 times more likely to smoke than those in major cities (National Rural Health Alliance, 2014b). The percentage of people who smoke daily is higher in remote areas - 14.8% of people in major cities compared with 26.5% of people in remote areas. The highest smoking rate of all (30.9%) is in the most disadvantaged rural areas (National Rural Health Alliance, 2014a). Deaths due to smoking related causes are up to 2.5 times higher in very remote areas. The rates varied across states and territories of Australia. One in ten adults smoke daily in the wealthiest inner-city areas compared with one in six in lower-income communities. In regional areas one in six smoke daily and in local rural areas one in four adults smoke daily.

2. EVIDENCE SUPPORTING THE EFFECTIVENESS OF TOBACCO POLICY IN AUSTRALIA

A number of evidence based frameworks underpin Australia's response to the harms and costs of tobacco use. Australia is a signatory to the WHO Framework Convention on Tobacco Control (FCTC) (World Health Organisation, 2003) and has an active Tobacco Control Strategy that incorporates priority driven research and policy development through the activity of the Australian National Preventive Health Agency (Australian Government National Preventative Health Taskforce, 2010; Australian National Preventive Health

Agency). The Council of Australian Governments' National Healthcare Agreement recently set two targets to be met by 2018: to reduce the proportion of Australian adults smoking daily to 10% and to halve the smoking rate among Aboriginal and Torres Strait Islanders primarily through the *Closing the Gap* program (Australian Institute of Health and Welfare, 2011, 2012). Medicare Locals plan, fund and deliver health services to meet the need of particular communities across Australia. In 2013 the National Health Performance Authority (NHPA) published adult smoking rates for Australia at Medicare Local level (National Health Performance Authority, 2013b). Medicare Locals are now funded to set targets for smoking prevalence and support local programs to augment national smoking policy.

Rates of smoking in Australia have been falling progressively since 1985 and are expected to continue to decline. This fall is generally attributed to a range of comprehensive tobacco control strategies at both the national and local level. These strategies have worked to prevent experimentation and uptake of tobacco by incrementally banning the advertisement of tobacco products on radio and television, in the print media and replaced them with health warnings and graphic anti-smoking advertisements. As commercial tobacco farming no longer occurs in Australia, the Government has increasing power to control the importation and price of tobacco products as part of its tobacco control program and has been effectively using tax policies for imported tobacco products (Federal excise and customs duty).

Smoke free environments are now the norm in Australia. Australians are much less exposed to second hand and third hand smoke. In a stepped process smoking has been banned in public spaces, cinemas, hospitals, restaurants and bars, public transport including airports and flights, schools, most workplaces, and in cars in which children are travelling. Sponsorship of sporting events by tobacco companies is banned with few exceptions. Nicotine replacement therapy has become increasingly more accessible and smoking cessation programs have been designed and implemented in a number of settings. Point of sale display and advertising is now banned. The most recent initiatives are the mandatory plain packaging of cigarettes and the replacement of brand graphics with emotive health warning messages.

There is a body of evidence to support the effectiveness of Australia's set of comprehensive tobacco policies as a whole and some of this evidence supports the differential effectiveness of different policies amongst disadvantaged communities including rural communities (see for example Scollo et al., 2012b). In the period 2005-2012 the prevalence of regular smoking declined most rapidly amongst the most disadvantaged Victorians following the use of highly emotive images in anti-smoking campaigns designed to have the most impact on low socioeconomic groups (Cancer Council Victoria, 2013). A review of the effectiveness of population wide tobacco strategies for disadvantaged groups (Scollo et al., 2012a) concluded that comprehensive tobacco policies in the State of Victoria benefited people of all ages and sex and both high and low education groups. In particular, advertising bans, bans on smoking in workplaces, removing barriers to smoking cessation programs and therapies and increasing the cost of cigarettes are policies with the most potential to reduce the socio-economic inequalities in smoking behavior.

Pricing strategies affect tobacco use across all socio-economic groups but this effect is most marked for lower socio-economic group smokers in Australia (Dunlop et al., 2011; Scollo et al., 2003; Siahpush et al., 2009). Following steady and hefty increases in fees and excise and customs duty on tobacco products since 2001 a higher percentage of people on low incomes stopped smoking in response to increases in the price of cigarettes (Scollo,

Winstanley, 2012b). During a period of high tobacco control activity (1997 – 2005), smoking prevalence decreased markedly amongst students aged 12-15 years and the effects were consistent across all SES groups (Scollo, Winstanley, 2012a).

The progressive and incremental introduction of policies designed to reduce exposure to second hand smoke in areas frequented by children and workplaces has increased quit rates in Australia with the most marked reduction in smoking in lower socio-economic groups (40% in lower socioeconomic groups compared with 24% in higher socioeconomic groups) was recorded in the State of Victoria after the introduction of smoke free policies in restaurants and pubs (McCarthy et al., 2008). Despite the fact that the nature of the workplace culture in rural and remote farming and mining communities supports a smoking norm, the combination of campaigns to create smoke-free working environments (workplaces and public spaces) and increases in cigarette prices is likely to be effective across all socio-economic groups in rural and remote areas (McCarthy, et al., 2008).

Graphic pictorial health warnings in advertisements and on cigarette packets have been shown to gain more attention among all smokers including lower education and socioeconomic groups, and these effects are likely to be greater when combined with the introduction of plain packaging policies in Australia in 2012.

A recent analysis of trends in requests for support to quit in two areas of Australia revealed a sustained increase in calls to Quit programs after the introduction of plain packaging (Young et al., 2014). A recent observational study in two Australian cities found that the rate of personal pack display in outdoor venues that allow smoking declined by 15% and the rate of active smoking declined by 23% after national plain packaging laws were introduced (Zacher et al., 2014).

Mass media campaigns can bring about change in smoking behavior both directly and indirectly across populations (Wakefield et al., 2010). Quit campaigns in Australia take care to place quit advertisements in mass media that will be attended to by people of lower socio-economic status, and to use emotional narratives and personal stories that are believed most likely to be effective in these groups (Durkin et al., 2009). Tobacco control mass media campaigns have been shown to reduce youth smoking not only by exposing young people to messages that prompt quit attempts and avoidance of smoking (Scollo,Winstanley, 2012b) but also through indirect effects that support not smoking by more generally de-normalising smoking in society (Australian National Preventive Health Agency, 2013). There is some evidence that television advertisements that graphically depict health effects and increased taxation on cigarettes can reduce smoking across all socio-economic groups, with the highest effect is in low income groups. Prominent television advertisements showing health effects of smoking and have been shown to increase knowledge of health effects of smoking amongst all levels of education.

A Cancer Council Victoria review concluded that whilst there is some evidence from the UK that programs that encourage greater use of smoking cessation treatment and counselling services, such intensive programs are unlikely to be feasible in rural and remote Australia. However, referral by health workers and General Practitioners after brief assessment and interventions to locally designed and delivered programs such as *Quit*, creating greater access to *Nicotine Replacement Therapy* by subsidizing nicotine replacement products and utilizing the comprehensive lifestyle tool SNAP (quit Smoking, better Nutrition, moderate Alcohol, more Physical activity) are effective at community level (The Royal Australian College of Practitioners, 2004).

3. Addressing Smoking Harms in Aboriginal and Torres Strait Islander Populations in Rural and Remote Australia

One in forty Australians identify themselves as being of Aboriginal or Torres Strait Islander origin. Life expectancy at birth for Indigenous Australians is much lower than for non-Indigenous Australians (Indigenous males 67.2 years compared with 79.5 years for non-Indigenous Males, and Indigenous females 72.9 years compared with 84 years for non-Indigenous females) (Australian Institute of Health and Welfare, 2012).

Since 2008, Australia's peak Indigenous and non-Indigenous health bodies, non-Government agencies and human rights organisations have worked together within a $1.6 billion National Partnership Agreement to address this health disadvantage in order to achieve health and life expectation equality for Australia's Aboriginal and Torres Strait Islander peoples. This is known as the *Close the Gap Program*. The campaign aims to address this gap through a range of initiatives and activities in six building blocks - Early childhood, schooling, economic participation, healthy homes, safe communities, and governance and leadership. The campaign's goal is to close the health and life expectancy gap between Aboriginal and Torres Strait Islander peoples and non-Indigenous Australians within a generation.

Smoking is a major contributor to the gap in life expectancy between Indigenous Australians and non- Indigenous Australians. Indigenous Australians are 2.2 times more likely to smoke tobacco than non-Indigenous Australians. In a study that aimed to quantify the extent to which the Indigenous health gap can be explained by common risk factors (Zhao et al., 2013), smoking explained 14-24% (three to four years) of the gap, and this contribution was greater for males than for females.

Higher proportions of Aboriginal and Torres Strait Islander people use cannabis (18% and 10% respectively) and Indigenous Australians are more likely to engage with smoking as part of traditional ceremony. The proportion of Indigenous women who smoke whilst pregnant is substantially higher for Indigenous women (48%) than for non-Indigenous women (13%) (Australian Institute of Health and Welfare, 2012).

The Australian experience with delivering preventive health measures across a range of health issues within Aboriginal and Torres Strait Islander populations has consistently shown the value of working in partnership with organisations that are already accessed by these groups to tailor cessation services to the different needs of disadvantaged groups and to introduce Indigenous specific elements to mainstream campaigns. This approach can assist in reducing the "implementation gap" often found when implementing tobacco policies into successful interventions in remote communities (Robertson et al., 2012). At the individual level, maintaining a long term relationship and utilizing a patient-centred approach and the adoption of flexible solutions and shared long term goals may also be important in the management of chronic disease and tobacco use in rural communities (Gould, 2014).

Anti-tobacco programs and strategies for Aboriginal and Torres Strait Islander people are more likely to be effective if they are based on appropriate evidence, acknowledge the historical context for tobacco use and socioeconomic influences on health, and involve the local community in the development, design, delivery and evaluation of the program (Ivers, 2011). The results of a study of Indigenous non-smokers by Thomas and others found that the most significant determinant of non-smoking behavior was socioeconomic position (Thomas et al., 2008), and stressful life experiences associated with poverty are not only implicated in the causal pathways between socio-economic position and smoking behavior but also hinder cessation efforts (Heath et al., 2006). This leads Bond and others to suggest that considering smoking behavior as a social practice and appreciating that the risk approach that dominates public health is insufficient to explain how risk is interpreted in making everyday life decisions (Bond et al., 2012).

The *Give Smokes the Flick* program utilised a smoking cessation strategy for Aboriginal people that directly addresses the disadvantage faced by many Aboriginal people in rural areas of Australia in a culturally appropriate way. The program addressed the issue of smoking during pregnancy directly and indirectly by developing two resources and providing training for workers who work with Aboriginal women.

The *"Give Smokes the Flick it really makes cents"* package is based on the social impact of smoking on behavior and lifestyle and targets the economic impact of smoking. The *"Happy Healthy Mums and Bubs"* resource provides information about the health impact of smoking for Aboriginal women who are pregnant.

A strength of this strategy is that it is designed to build capacity in health workers to provide cessation services that motivate smokers to reduce or quit smoking by linking quitting tobacco clearly with financial savings at the individual and household level (Hughes, 2009).

The *"Be Our Ally Beat Smoking (BOABS)"* randomized controlled trial tested the efficacy of an Aboriginal researcher delivered, locally tailored, intensive and multidimensional smoking cessation intervention conducted in a remote Aboriginal health care setting. The intervention featured face to face support over a period of 12 months in a real world setting. The intervention utilised the imagery of the resilient Boab tree – a life sustaining arid lands tree that can store water in its trunk for long periods of time. The study was underpowered and the results of the study were inconclusive and statistically insignificant due to a number of factors including the small population numbers in the trial.

However, success in smoking cessation amongst participants assigned to the intervention group was double that achieved by those assigned to usual care. In order to improve the conclusiveness of the study the results were combined in a meta-analysis of these findings with a similarly underpowered but comparable study of pregnant Indigenous Australian women. The results of the meta-analysis showed that Indigenous Australian participants assigned to intervention groups were 2.4 times (95% CI, 1.01-5.5) as likely to quit as participants assigned to usual care (Marley et al., 2014).

CONCLUSION

This chapter reviewed the progress in reducing the harms of tobacco use and achieving tobacco control in Australia with a particular reference to rural and remote and Indigenous Australian populations. Australia is a world leader in successful tobacco control, and has achieved much success through a comprehensive population and stepped approach over time. Despite this success the full range of psychological, social, economic and cultural factors that support the uptake, continuation and cessation of smoking in disadvantaged groups and rural Australians and support a smoking norm are only partly understood.

As smoking rates continue to fall and smoking behavior is confined to the most socially disadvantaged groups (including those living in rural and remote areas of Australia), even currently successful strategies may be less effective. Current surveys and monitoring tools may not adequately capture or monitor smoking rates in all populations in Australia or to separate the impacts of programs that are incremental in nature.

One valuable approach that may overcome this lack of detailed knowledge is to focus less on smoking cessation strategies and focus more on a "Supportive environments for health" approach[3] and work in comprehensive ways that view smoking and its associated risks as part of a social context rather than concentrating on influencing individual lifestyle choices.

The combined impacts of the differential in socioeconomic status and educational attainment, the higher rates of mental health problems, and the increased difficulty in engaging with health services between rural and urban populations in Australia drive differences between rural and urban smoking and quitting rates. Another way to address these factors might be to introduce strategies and policies that address social issues more directly.

The results of one Australian study suggest that there is a need to better understand the social drivers of inequality and how they are linked to both the stigmatization of smoking and smokers and other factors that might explain the inconsistent effects of area on smoking status across communities (Migliorini, Siahpush, 2006).

Overcoming the effects of these additional factors will involve developing partnerships across sectors and governments and Indigenous organisations. It may be difficult to evaluate such initiatives as they will often be implemented and assessed in part outside the health sector.

Taking a more holistic view of health[4] and taking steps to promote educational achievement, mental and connectedness, together with enlightened social and economic policy can also contribute to an environment for health that will in part support more directed tobacco policy. Adopting such a social model of health can focus attention more clearly on the networking qualities of rural life and the various definitions of wellbeing found in a culturally diverse local context to inform effective and appropriate initiatives to support tobacco control.

REFERENCES

Anderson, D. (2009). Enduring drought then coping with climate change: Lived experience and local resolve in rural mental health. *Rural Society, 19*(4), 340-352.

---

[3] The *"Supportive Environments for Health"* (sometimes called *"Supportive Settings"*) approach is a health promotion concept that challenges the notion that health is created only within the health sector. This approach recognizes that the interaction of the environment and the economy are the subject matter of sustainable development, and that we therefore need to create healthy and supportive physical and social environments, i.e. places that empower people to make healthy choices where they live, work and play (Dean et al., 1992).

[4] A "holistic" view of health embraces the broader cultural and political context of health, ill health and wellbeing and recognizes that the capacity for physical and emotional wellbeing changes over the lifespan and as a result of life challenges at a community family and individual level (Australian Government Department of Health). Elements considered in a holistic view of health include peace, shelter, education, food, income, a stable ecosystem, sustainable resources, social justice and equity.

Australian Bureau of Statistics. (2011). *Australian Social trends March 2011: Health outside major cities*. (Catalogue no. 4102.0). Retrieved from www.abs.gov.au/socialtrends.

Australian Government Department of Health. *Social and emotional wellbeing framework 2004 - 2009* Commonwealth of Australia, Retrieved from http://www.health.gov.au/internet/publications/publishing.nsf/Content/indig-sew-frame04-toc~indig-sew-frame04-1~indig-sew-frame04-1-und.

Australian Government National Preventative Health Taskforce. (2010). *Tobacco Recommendations*. Retrieved from http://www.preventativehealth.org.au/internet/preventativehealth/publishing.nsf/Content/6B7B17659424FBE5CA25772000095458/$File/tpa.pdf.

Australian Institute of Health and Welfare. (2008). *Rural, regional and remote health: indicators of health status and determinants of health*. Canberra: AIHW.

Australian Institute of Health and Welfare. (2011) 2010 National Drug Strategy Household Survey: survey report. *Series no. 5: Cat. No. PHE 145*. Canberra, Australia: AIHW.

Australian Institute of Health and Welfare. (2012). *Australia's Health 2012*. Retrieved from http://www.aihw.gov.au/WorkArea/DownloadAsset.aspx?id=10737422169.

Australian National Preventive Health Agency. *Promoting a Healthy Australia: Tobacco Control*. Retrieved from http://www.anpha.gov.au/internet/anpha/publishing.nsf/Content/tobacco-control.

Australian National Preventive Health Agency. (2013). *Tobacco control and mass media campaigns: evidence brief*. Retrieved from http://www.anpha.gov.au/internet/anpha/publishing.nsf/Content/tobacco-mass-media-campaigns-evidence-brief.

Banbury, A., Zask, A., Carter, S. M., van Beurden, E., Tokley, R., Passey, M.,Copeland, J. (2013). Smoking mull: a grounded theory model on the dynamics of combined tobacco and cannabis use among adult men. *Health Promot. J. Austr., 24*, 143-150.

Bond, C., Brough, M., Spurling, G.,Hayman, N. (2012). 'It had to be my choice' Indigenous smoking cessation and negotiations of risk, resistance and resilience. *Health Risk Soc., 14*(6), 565-581.

Cancer Council Victoria. (2013). Smoking rates in Victoria drop to record lows, new research reveals. Retrieved from http://www.cancervic.org.au/about/media-releases/2013-media-releases/august-2013/smoking-rates-victoria.html

Cancer Council Victoria. (2014). *Perceptions about the health effects of smoking and passive smoking among Victorian adults 2003 to 2011*. Cancer Council Victoria. unpublished work.

Dean, K.,Hancock, T. (1992). Major policy and research issues involved in creating health promoting environments. Geneva: WHO Regional Office for Europe. Retrieved from http://whqlibdoc.who.int/euro/-1993/EURO_HPR_1.pdf.

Dobson, A., McLaughlin, D., Vagenas, D.,Wong, K. Y. (2010). Why are death rates higher in rural areas? Evidence from the Australian Longitudinal Study on Women's Health. *Aust. N. Z. J. Public Health, 34*(6), 624-628.

Dunlop, S., Perez, D.,Cotter, T. (2011). Australian smokers' and recent quitters' responses to the increasing price of cigarettes in the context of tobacco tax increase. *Addiction, 106*(9), 1687-1695.

Durkin, S., Biener, L.,Wakefield, M. (2009). Effects of different types of antismoking ads on reducing disparities in smoking cessation among socieconomic subgroups. *Am. J. Public Health, 99*(12), 2217-2223.

Gould, G. S. (2014). Patient-centred tobacco management. *Drug Alcohol Rev., 33*, 93-98.

Heath, D. L., Panaretto, K., Manessis, V., Larkins, S., Malouf, P., Reilly, E.,Elston, J. (2006). Factors to consider in smoking interventions for Indigenous women. *Australian Journal of Primary Health, 12*(2), 131-136.

Hughes, D. (2009). *"Give Smokes the Flick" - A qualitative evaluation of two quit smoking resources for Aboriginal pregnant women*. Retrieved from http://www.heti.nsw.gov.au/Global/rural/completed-projects/denise_hughes_report.pdf.

Ivers, R. (2011). Anti-tobacco programs for Aboriginal and Torres Strait Islander people *Resource sheet no. 4 Closing the gap Clearinghouse*. Canberra: Australian Institute of Health and Welfare & Australian Institute of Family Studies.

Marley, J. V., Atkinson, D., Kitaura, T., Nelson, C., Gray, D., Metcalf, S.,Maguire, G. P. (2014). The Be Our Ally Smoking (BOABS) study, a randomised controlled trail of an intensive smoking cessation intervention in a remote aboriginal Australian health care setting. *BMC Public Health, 14*(32). Retrieved from http://www.biomedcentral.com/1471-2458/14/32

McCarthy, M., Durkin, S., Brennan, E.,Germain, D. (2008) Smokefree hospitality venues in Victoria: public approval, patronage and quitting behaviour, 2004-2007. In Cancer Council of Victoria Centre for Behavioural Research in Cancer (Series Ed.) & Q. Victoria (Vol. Ed.)*: Vol. 32. CBRC Research Paper Series*: Cancer Council Victoria.

Migliorini, C.,Siahpush, M. (2006). Smoking, not smoking: how important is where you live? *Health Promot. J. Austr., 17*(3), 226-232.

National Health Performance Authority. (2013a). *Healthy Communities: Avoidable deaths and expectations in 2009-2011*. Retrieved from www.myhealthycommunities.gov.au.

National Health Performance Authority. (2013b). *Healthy Communities: Tobacco smoking rates across Australia, 2011 - 2012*. Retrieved from www.myhealthycommunities.gov.au.

National Rural Health Alliance. (2010). *Fact Sheet No. 23: Measuring the metropolitan-rural inequity*. Retrieved from http://ruralhealth.org.au/sites/default/files/fact-sheets/Fact-Sheet-23-%20measuring%20the%20metropolitan-rural%20inequity_0.pdf.

National Rural Health Alliance. (2011a). Fact Sheet 27: The extent of the rural health deficit. Retrieved from http://ruralhealth.org.au/sites/default/files/fact-sheets/Fact-Sheet-27-%20the%20extent%20of%20the%20rural%20health%20deficit_0.pdf

National Rural Health Alliance. (2011b). *Fact Sheet 28: The determinants of health in rural and remote Australia*. Retrieved from http://ruralhealth.org.au/sites/default/files/publications/factsheet-determinants-health-rural-australia.pdf.

National Rural Health Alliance. (2014a). Daily smokers - smoking infographics reproduced from COAG Reform Council and Australian Institute of Health and Welfare, from http://ruralhealth.org.au/infographics/smoking

National Rural Health Alliance. (2014b). *Fact Sheet: Smoking and rural health*. Retrieved from http://ruralhealth.org.au/sites/default/files/publications/nrha-factsheet-smoking.pdf.

Robertson, J. A., Conigrave, K. M., Ivers, R., Usher, K.,Clough, A. R. (2012). Translation of tobacco policy into practice in disadvantaged and marginalized subpopulations: a study of challenges and opportunities in remote Australian Indigenous communities. *Health Research Policy and Systems*(10), 23.

Scollo, M.,Winstanley, M. (2012a). Chapter 9: Smoking and social disadvantage. In Cancer Council Victoria (Ed.), Tobacco in Australia: Facts and Issues (Fourth ed.). Melbourne, Victoria: Cancer Council Victoria. Retrieved from http://www.tobaccoinaustralia.org.au/chapter-9-disadvantage/9-8-are-current-strategies-to-discourage-smoking-i.

Scollo, M.,Winstanley, M. (2012b). *Tobacco in Australia: Facts and Issues* (Fourth ed.). Retrieved from http://www.tobaccoinaustralia.org.au/.

Scollo, M., Younie, S., Wakefield, M., Freeman, J.,Icasiano, F. (2003). Impact of tobacco tax reforms on tobacco prices and tobacco use in Australia. *Tob. Control, 12*(suppl. 2), ii59-66.

Siahpush, M., Wakefield, M., Spittal, M., Durkin, S.,Scollo, M. (2009). Taxation reduces social disparities in adult smoking prevalence. *Am. J. Prev. Med., 36*(4), 285-291.

The Royal Australian College of Practitioners. (2004). *SNAP: A population health guide to behavioural risk factors in General Practice*: The Royal Australian College of Practitioners,.

Thomas, D., Briggs, V., Anderson, I. P. S.,Cunningham, J. (2008). The social determinants of being an Indigenous ex-smoker. *Aust. N. Z. J. Public Health, 32*(2), 110-116.

Wakefield, M. A., Loken, B.,Hornik, R. C. (2010). Use of mass media campaigns to change behaviour. *Lancet, 376*, 1261-1271.

World Health Organisation. (2003). *WHO Framework Convention on Tobacco Control, opened for signature 16th June 2003, entered into force 27 February 2005*. Retrieved from http://www.who.int/fctc/en/.

Young, J. M., Stacey, I., Dobbins, T. A., Dunlop, S., Dessaix, A. L.,Currow, D. C. (2014). Association between tobacco plain packaging and Quitline calls: a population-based, interrupted time-series analysis. *Med. J. Aust., 200*(1). doi: 10.5694/mja13.11070

Zacher, M., Bayly, M., Brennan, E., Dono, J., Miller, C., Durkin, S., Scollo, M.,Wakefield, M. (2014). Personal tobacco pack display before and after the introduction of plain packaging with larger pictorial health warnings in Australia: an observational study of outdoor cafe strips. *Addiction, 109*, 653-662.

Zhao, Y., Wright, J., Begg, S.,Guthridge, S. (2013). Decomposing Indigenous life expectancy gap by risk factors: a life table analysis. *Population Health Metrics, 11*(1). Retrieved from http://www.pophealthmetrics.com/content/11/1/1.

PART II: SOCIO-ECONOMIC AND BEHAVIORAL DETERMINANTS

In: Smoking Restrictions
Editor: Nazmi Sari

ISBN: 978-1-63321-148-3
© 2014 Nova Science Publishers, Inc.

Chapter 3

SMOKING, SOCIOECONOMIC STATUS AND HEALTH

Lori J. Curtis, Ph.D.[*]
Department of Economics, University of Waterloo, Waterloo, Canada

ABSTRACT

This chapter, like many others, attempts to document the association between smoking and health. Unlike other studies, we do not simply control for socioeconomic status by adding income and/or education and other control variables within a multivariate framework. Using the Canadian Community Health Survey, designed to allow pooling of samples over many cross-sections to achieve large sample sizes, we examine the relationship between smoking and health within socioeconomic classes defined by 40 sex-income-education strata. We question whether income or education may be more or less moderating in the smoking-health relationship. Our results clearly indicate strong relationships between smoking and self-reported health status for males and females across the 20 income-education strata. The picture is less clear when using self-reported chronic conditions for females and even less so for males. We find that, in the Canadian context, income is more 'protective' within education strata than education is within income strata indicating that the situations afforded by increased income may be more important for smoking-health relationship than the additional knowledge and productivity associated with higher levels of education.

1. INTRODUCTION

Smoking causes ill health and death (Viscusi and Hersch, 2007); this relationship has been unquestioned for decades. "Tobacco use is the leading cause of preventable death, and is estimated to kill more than 5 million people each year worldwide" (World Health Organization, 2009, page 7). Jones, Gulbis, and Baker (2010) report that 21 and 17 percent of all deaths in Canada and the US, respectively, can be attributed to smoking. Most smoking attributable deaths are related to lung cancer and ischemic heart disease. Surprisingly, in both countries, the prevalence of smoking is highest among young adults who have grown up

---

[*] Phone: +1-519-888-4567 ext. 33162; Fax: +1-519-725-0530; E-mail: ljcurtis@uwaterloo.ca.

knowing the ills of smoking (Jones, Gulbis, and Baker, 2010). Individual and social morbidity and mortality costs of smoking are phenomenal (see for example, World Health Organization, 2009; Viscusi and Hersch, 2007). Between six and 15 percent of health care costs can be linked to smoking related diseases in high income countries (Janz, 2012). Current estimates of the private costs of smoking related mortality are estimated to be in the range of $100 to $200US per pack of cigarettes, for females and males respectively (Viscusi and Hersch, 2007). Both Canada and the US had stated policy goals of decreasing the prevalence of smoking. The US goal was an adult smoking prevalence of 13 percent by 2010, while Canada's goal was to reduce smoking prevalence to 12 percent by 2011. Smoking bans and smoking cessation programs are numerous in both countries but neither hit their goal. The latest smoking prevalence results from Canadian Tobacco Use Monitoring Survey (CTUMS) indicate that 16 percent of Canadians over the age of 15 years are smokers (Health Canada, 2013). The CDC (2013) reports that 18% of Americans, 18 years of age and older, smoke. While smoking rates have declined over the past decade or so, almost 1/6 North Americans still smoke.

The causal link between smoking and health is no longer questioned, so why do people still smoke? Economists have put forth many theories to account for the fact that rational beings continue to smoke. Models of myopic addiction state that smokers recognize their current consumption is dependent upon past consumption but ignore the fact that it has some effects on future consumption and continue to smoke (Pollack, 1975). Rational addiction models postulate that individuals know and have weighed the costs and consequences of smoking and do so because the long-term benefits outweigh the long-term costs (Becker and Murphy, 1988). Inconsistent time preferences or hyperbolic discounting may also explain smoking behaviours; if individuals change how they discount the future, choices made in one period may not be optimal choices in another period (Ainslie, 1991). Goldfarb, Leonard and Suranovic (2001) present an interesting discussion on the various theories which attempt to explain smoking behaviours and the empirical results that support and refute them. Readers may not be surprised to learn that the results are mixed.

Recently, studies have begun to examine the ties between smoking and, arguably, one of the most studied phenomena in health, the health gradient across socioeconomic status (SES) (Cutler et al., 2010). The SES gradient in health is apparent across most objective and subjective measures (Marmot et al., 1999). However, the exact causal pathways between SES and health have remained elusive (Lochner, 2011; *Stowasser* et al., 2011; Adams et al., 2004). Recently, researchers have attempted to tie the SES gradient in health behaviours such as smoking, sedentary life style, and poor nutritional status to SES gradient in health. The relationship between the two gradients seems clear, causal explanations are murkier. Endogeneity is a classic problem in this type of research. If there are unobserved characteristics that influence both health behaviour and health outcomes, the effects of one on the other cannot be estimated consistently (Jérôme and Lechene, 2004). Economists have focused much attention on investigating a causal pathway between income and/or education and health with mixed results (Brunello et al., 2011). The current hypothesis is that the education/income variation in health is a result of differences in health behaviours across income and education status. Those that find support for the health behaviours pathway find that it accounts for a small proportion of the SES variation in health (e.g., Brunello et al.,

(2011) and Tubeuf, Jusot and Bricard (2012) find that lifestyle explains about one third the variation).

Studies that fail to identify a causal link between SES and health behaviours, and consequently health find that health behaviours explain little of the health gradient, point to the explanation that unobserved characteristics within socioeconomic strata drive health differences (Lundborg, 2008; Brunello, 2011; Cutler et al, 2011; Costas, Palme and Simeonova, 2012; *Amin, Behrman, and Spector,* 2013). The unobserved differences are thought to include: access to health care (although observable, it is rarely included as a SES indicator), differential productivity in the use of health information or health care, differential vulnerability, environmental factors like pollution or chemical exposure (Seabrook and Avison, 2012; Cutler et al., 2011; Pampel, Krueger and Denny, 2010; Cutler and Lleras-Muney, 2010), and cumulative effects (e.g., individuals from lower socioeconomic situations experience more health shocks than those from higher socioeconomic situations (Currie and Hyson, 1999; Currie and Stabile, 2002; Evans and Kim, 2010; Seabrook and Avison, 2012)).

Canadian studies are limited in this literature. While Canada has excellent cross-sectional data on adult smoking (e.g., CTUMS) and health (e.g., the Canadian Community Health Survey (CCHS)), it is hindered by a lack of longitudinal health data spanning many years. The National Population Health Survey (NPHS) (Statistics Canada, 2013) was Canada's most recent longitudinal health survey of adults. The biennial survey began in 1994 with just over 17,000 respondents. The survey ended after 9 cycles with about 12,000 respondents remaining. The short time-frame, small sample and lack of siblings[5] make it difficult to use current techniques to investigate causal explanations for differences in health. Natural experiments, changes in school leaving policies or years to complete high school, have been exploited to test the causal link in health and education but a smaller population and fewer jurisdictions than the US data spanning fewer years make it more difficult to study causal relationships with Canadian data. Typically, Canadian policy makers point to evidence coming out of the US as evidence for Canadian policy. However, the very different institutional structures in health, education, and social safety systems may not make evidence from the US second best for Canadian policy makers.

Like many other Canadian studies, this chapter cannot address the causal pathways between socioeconomic status, smoking and health. Like the vast majority of studies found in the health literature, we examine the relationship between smoking and health, controlling for socioeconomic status. However, we recognize that simply controlling for socioeconomic status within regression analyses may lead to the attenuation of the relationships of some characteristics due to colinearity; socioeconomic factors such as income and education tend to be highly correlated as do health behaviours (LaVeist et al., 2007).

We use a unique approach to examine whether the relationships between health behaviours, particularly smoking status, and subjective and more objective health measures hold within socioeconomic strata measured by education and income. We pool 9 cycles of the

---

[5] Siblings' unobserved experiences are similar in that they grow up in the same family, neighbourhood, community, and attend the same schools, etc. Observing outcome differences between siblings across policy changes (e.g., one sibling attends school before a school leaving policy changes and the other after) allows researchers to 'control' for the unobserved characteristics and conclude that any observed differences are a result of the policy change not the unobserved factors. Canadian sibling studies have been completed using The National Longitudinal Survey of Children and Youth but the oldest individuals in the sample are 25 years of age in 2009, the last wave of data (Statistics Canada, 2013b).

Canadian Community Health Survey (CCHS) in order to obtain a sample large enough to examine the relationship between health behaviours and health status, controlling for age, marital status, immigrant status, province, and year of survey within sex-education-income class. Examining the relationship between health behaviours and health status within specific socioeconomic strata provides evidence on whether the relationships are similar across the socioeconomic spectrum or whether education and/or income mediate the effects of the health behaviours differently (e.g., are the relationships similar between individuals with lower levels of education and higher levels of income (a unionized construction labourer, for example) and those with higher levels of education and lower levels of income (say, a sessional lecturer?) If the literature that supposes that education provides individuals with the ability to use intermediate goods (health information, consumption goods and health behaviours) more efficiently than their counterparts is correct, the relationship between smoking and health should be weaker at higher educational levels than lower ones within income levels. However, if the fact that income allows individuals to purchase better intermediate goods (e.g., better environments, healthier food, less stress) for the production of health then the relationship between smoking and health should be mediated as incomes increase within educational levels. Our sex-education-income strata allow us to examine these trends. We hypothesize that the later explanation outweighs the first and thus, income will have a stronger mediating effect than education.

In the next section, we will describe the data and methods. Section 4 will present the results, and the final section will be devoted to the concluding remarks.

2. DATA AND METHODS

The Canadian Community Health Survey (CCHS) is an annual cross-sectional survey that collects information on health, health care utilization and the determinants of health from a large sample of Canadians over the age of 15 years (approximately 130,000). The survey ran biennially from 2001-2002 to 2007-2008. It reverted to an annual survey of about half the sample size after that. The survey is designed so that multiple years can be pooled to examine small populations or rare events. The 2001-2002, 2003-2004, 2005, 2007-2008, 2009-2010, 2010, 2011-2012 and 2012 surveys contain identical information, in most cases, on self-reported objective and subjective measures of health status, health behaviours, demographic and socioeconomic characteristics needed for this study[6].

The data include four education levels: less than high school diploma (lhs), high school graduate (hs), some post-secondary school (sps), and postsecondary graduate (psg). The levels are self explanatory except perhaps *sps* which includes anyone who undertook some education after they graduated from high school but did not obtain a college diploma or university degree. The level includes incomplete courses as well as technical and trade

---

[6] 2001-2002 and 2003-2004 contain slightly different information than later surveys. The important differences for this study are: income information is recorded in 5 income adequacy groups rather than income deciles (aggregated to quintiles for the study), and the chronic condition questions are slightly different. Any differences observed between early years these years and later years should be interpreted with care. Quantitative measures of cigarette consumption (e.g., number of years smoked or number of years reformed change over the survey as well) but the type of smoker does not (e.g., daily smoker, occasional smoker, former daily smoker, former occasional smoker and never smoker are defined similarly across the surveys).

certificates. This group is the most diverse and the most difficult to think about in terms of socioeconomic status. For example, individuals with this level of education may include estheticians earning close to minimum wage or carpenters earning substantial incomes. Psg includes college diplomas, university degrees, and advanced degrees. Income is measured by income quintiles 1 (lowest) through 5 (highest)[7].

We represent socioeconomic status by twenty education-income strata (lhs-first income quintile, lhs-second income quintile, lhs-third quintile, lhs-fourth quintile, lhs-fifth quintile, lhs-first quintile, hs-second quintile, hs-third quintile, hs-fourth quintile, and so on up to, psg-fifth income quintile). The data are further subdivided by sex. The sample is limited to those 20 years of age and older. Thus, there are forty sex-education-income subsamples. Sample sizes range from 2,309 (sps-first income quintile) to 53,972 (psg-fifth quintile) for males and 3,143 (lhs-fifth income quintile) and 50,434 (psg-fourth quintile) (sample sizes are recorded in Appendix 1).

Examining the relationship between health behaviours and health necessitates measuring both health and health behaviours as accurately as possible. Researchers have questioned whether self-reports are an accurate measure of health (Au, Crossley and Schellhorn, 2005; Baker, Stabile and Deri, 2004) or health behaviours, particularly smoking (Florescu et al., 2009). Self-reported health status is arguably the most commonly used measure of health in the empirical health literature, however we use two health measures, self-reported poor health status (the individual reports poor or very poor health status) and the presence of a chronic disease (the individual reports being diagnosed with one or more of the following 10 chronic diseases: asthma, chronic bronchitis, emphysema, chronic obstructive pulmonary disease (COPD), diabetes, heart disease, cancer, stroke, ulcers, bowel disorder).

In the current 'anti-smoking' environment, there are substantial insurance, wage and social penalties for smokers (Levine et al., 1997; van Ours, 2004; Auld, 2005; Grafova and Stafford, 2009; Cowan and Schwab, 2011) and as such, smokers may tend to underestimate their smoking behaviour. Recently, researchers have questioned whether biochemical markers would substantially improve measures of smoking behaviour. Tennekoon and Rosenman (2013) found that self-reported measures tend to be biased downwards, however, biochemical markers tend to be biased upwards by about the same margin. They concluded that biochemical markers are not necessarily a better measure than self reports and they are substantially more difficult and costly to obtain. We are constrained to using self-reported measures here.

It is likely that there is a dose response to smoking (Ostbye et al., 2002). There is also mounting evidence that reformed smokers have substantially less risk of health related consequences than current smokers (Østbye, Taylor and Jung, 2002). Measuring the quantity of cigarettes and/or the number of years smoked and/or reformed from smoking would arguably be a better measure of cigarette consumption than self-reported categories of smoking behaviour. However, the more quantitative measures of cigarette consumption contained in the data are limited and change over time and/or have large proportions of missing data. Therefore, individuals are classified as daily smokers, occasional smokers, former daily smokers, former occasional smokers, and never smokers for the multivariate analyses. We aggregate the groups to current smokers, former smokers and never smokers for the descriptive analysis for brevity.

---

[7] See footnote 2.

Smoking is highly correlated with other health behaviours such as activity status, the consumption of alcohol and nutritional status (Manuel et al., 2012). These health behaviours are also shown to have strong relationships with health (Cutler, Glaeser, and Rosen 2009; Olshansky et al. 2005; Stewart, Cutler, and Rosen 2009). The CCHS provides consistent data on physical activity and alcohol consumption but not nutritional status[8]. A physical activity index (active, moderately active, sedentary) is constructed based on the individuals' average daily energy expenditure which is calculated using an extensive list of questions on the respondent's usual leisure time physical activities in the last three months (Statistics Canada, 2013c). The relationship between alcohol consumption and health is more ambiguous (Thun et al. 1997) than other health behaviours. Moderate alcohol consumption may provide protective mechanisms but binge drinking has been more consistently linked to poor health (Naimi et al., 2003) and is included in our study. An individual is considered an occasional binge drinker if they consume more than 5 drinks in one occasion less than once per month and to binge drink often if they consume more than 5 drinks in one occasion more than once per month. Following the literature, we include controls for marital status (married including common law, previously married (divorced, separated, widow/widower) or never married), immigrant status (native born, less than 10 years in Canada, more than 10 years in Canada), age, province and a time trend.

Our methodology is straight forward. We begin by providing descriptive statistics on our key variables of interest. We then subdivide the sample into 40 sex-education-income strata. Using a probit model, we estimate the base probability of reporting poor health status or the presence of one or more chronic conditions and the change in that probability associated with each of the health behaviours, controlling for marital status, immigrant status, age, province and time trend, within each of the 40 sex-education-income strata. The complex survey sampling strategies used to select respondents for the CCHS necessitates the use of survey weigths. The weights are provided by Statistics Canada and used for all analyses.

3. RESULTS

Table 1 presents descriptive statistics for the study population. The first two columns of results provide the proportion of males and females reporting each characteristic. First note that male-female differences are significant in almost all cases. Females smoke less than males, are more likely to be in the lower income and education categories and less likely to be in the higher ones. Females report being less active and are less likely to binge drink than males. Males are more likely to be married or single while females are more likely to be previously married. The third and fourth columns report the proportion of females and males with given characteristics that report poor health (chronic conditions in the fifth and sixth columns). Once again, except for female previous smokers and previously married, the proportion reporting poor health status is significantly different than the base case (B) for each characteristic. For example, 11.4 (7.2) percent of female (male) never smokers (B) report poor health status. Just over 16 (14) percent of female (male) current smokers did the

---

[8] Some studies use obesity as a health behaviour. We believe obesity is a health outcome influenced by healthy eating and activity levels which are health behaviours. However, we performed sensitivity analysis including a measure of obesity and the main results hold.

same and that difference is significant at 0.000. Female previous smokers did not report poor health status significantly more or less than never smokers. However, male previous smokers were 5.5 percentage points more likely to report poor health status than their never smoker counterparts. There is a clear income and education gradient in reporting poor health status for both sexes and chronic conditions for females. However, only males with less than a high school diploma report chronic conditions significantly more than the other education levels. There is a health gradient across activity levels and an inverse gradient across binge drinking (those that often binge are less likely to report poor health or chronic conditions than those that occasionally binge and occasional bingers are less likely than never bingers to report negative health consequences). Mixed results have been recorded previously for alcohol consumption and health status (Thun et al. 1997)[9]. Marital and immigrant status differences are consistent with what is found in the literature.

The last six columns show the prevalence of smoking across the characteristics of interest in this study. Once again, there are fairly clear income and education gradients in smoking patterns with the prevalence of never and previous (current) smokers increasing (decreasing) as income and education increases. Smoking prevalences across health behaviours are as expected with more active individuals smoking less and higher alcohol consumers smoking more. Interestingly, many Canadians living with chronic illness do not consider themselves to be in poor health status; 25 percent of females and 18 percent of males report living with chronic health conditions while only 16 percent of females and 14 percent of males report poor health status.

Figures 1 through 4 provide an easier view of the descriptive statistics and some time trends. Figure 1 shows that females report smoking less than males. The proportion of Canadians who report smoking on a daily basis has decreased over the last decade from about one in four for males and one in five for females to about 1 in four for males and 1 in seven for females. The proportion of Canadians reporting to be occasional smokers has remained fairly constant over time and is similar across sexes. Figure 2 indicates that the proportion of Canadians reporting poor health status remained relatively constant over the decade. Unsurprisingly, smokers report poor health or chronic disease more than nonsmokers. Males (both smokers and nonsmokers) tend to report health problems less than females do.

SES gradients are explored in figures 3 and 4. Figure 3 presents the health status results by education and figure 4 by income. In each figure, the top left graph represents females reporting poor health status, top right male reports. Chronic conditions are reported similarly in the bottom panels. The most striking feature of the graphs in figure 3 is that individuals with less than high school education report poor health/chronic conditions almost twice as much as those in other education categories. Males with a postsecondary degree report poor health and chronic conditions only slightly less than those with a high school diploma or some postsecondary education; the gap is larger for females. An educational gradient is clear for the health measures when moving from the lowest educational level to the highest but is less clear for the mid-range educational categories; the gradient is clearer for females reporting chronic illness.

---

[9] We expected this had something to do with younger individuals binging substantially more than older but this was not the case. We also suspect possible reverse causality – unhealthier people may not be able to binge drink.

Table 1. Descriptive Statistics

	Sex		Poor Health		Chronic		Never Smoker		Previous Smoker		Current Smoker	
	Female	Male	Female	Male	Female	Male	Female	Male	Female	Male	Female	Male
Current Smoker	0.204	0.258	0.161	0.140	0.253	0.184						
Previous Smoker	0.381	0.449	__0.111__	0.127	0.252	0.263						
Never Smoked (B)	0.415	0.293	0.114	0.072	0.202	0.145						
Income Quantile 1	0.178	0.132	0.235	0.230	0.321	0.282	0.461	__0.296__	0.283	0.362	0.256	__0.342__
Income Quantile 2	0.182	0.155	0.148	0.156	0.268	0.259	0.441	__0.293__	0.346	0.431	0.214	__0.276__
Income Quantile 3	__0.203__	__0.199__	0.118	0.119	0.236	0.220	0.412	0.283	0.388	0.447	0.200	0.270
Income Quantile 4	0.228	0.249	0.082	0.087	0.190	0.181	0.389	0.284	0.413	0.465	__0.198__	0.251
Income Quantile 5(B)	0.209	0.265	0.055	0.055	0.166	0.160	0.384	0.307	0.453	0.489	0.163	0.204
Less than Secondary	__0.154__	__0.155__	0.273	0.247	0.383	0.346	0.407	0.171	0.338	0.476	0.255	0.352
High school grad	0.175	0.166	0.129	0.106	0.231	__0.186__	0.385	0.273	0.374	0.410	0.240	0.317
Some Post Secondary	__0.071__	__0.071__	0.121	0.110	__0.207__	__0.182__	0.370	0.286	0.359	0.416	0.271	0.298
Post Secondary Grad(B)	__0.600__	__0.607__	0.083	0.084	0.196	0.182	0.431	0.330	0.396	0.456	0.173	0.214
Active	0.217	0.271	0.054	0.058	0.181	0.161	0.392	0.321	0.424	0.461	0.184	0.217
Moderately Active	__0.256__	__0.250__	0.080	0.085	0.209	0.197	0.397	0.297	0.417	0.477	0.187	0.226
Sedentary(B)	0.527	0.479	0.163	0.149	0.258	0.230	0.425	0.271	0.351	0.428	0.224	0.301
Occasional Binge	0.180	0.261	0.064	0.076	0.160	0.153	0.270	0.278	0.445	__0.463__	0.284	0.260
Often Binges	0.099	0.261	0.072	0.083	0.149	0.135	0.204	0.188	0.414	0.414	0.421	0.397
Never Binges(B)	0.720	0.237	0.144	0.149	0.261	0.272	0.481	0.355	0.460	0.460	0.154	0.185
Previously Married	0.179	0.086	0.218	0.202	0.380	0.321	0.367	0.194	0.365	0.457	0.233	0.349
Never Married	0.181	0.221	__0.100__	0.094	0.153	0.112	0.441	0.356	__0.399__	0.292	0.277	0.352
Married (B)	0.640	0.693	0.103	0.110	0.212	0.225	0.421	0.285	0.282	0.498	0.175	0.217
Immigrant (>10 yrs)	__0.172__	__0.171__	0.164	0.142	0.243	0.239	0.622	0.343	0.404	__0.454__	0.109	0.202
Immigrant (<10 yrs)	__0.058__	__0.061__	0.085	0.047	0.093	0.085	0.767	0.480	0.269	0.298	0.076	0.222
Native Born(B)	__0.771__	__0.768__	0.117	0.114	0.239	0.211	0.341	0.266	0.158	0.460	0.236	0.274

Note: Non-bolded, non-underlined are significantly different from base at 0.000%. Underlined are significantly different at 0.05%.
Bold and underlined values are not significantly different than the *base (in italics)*. **(B)** stands for Base Case.
Source: Author's calculations using CCHS 2001-2012.

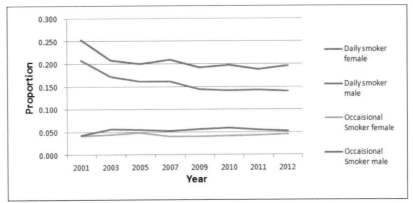

Source: Author's calculations using Canadian Community Health Survey.

Figure 1. Smokers as a Proportion of the Adult Population in Canada.

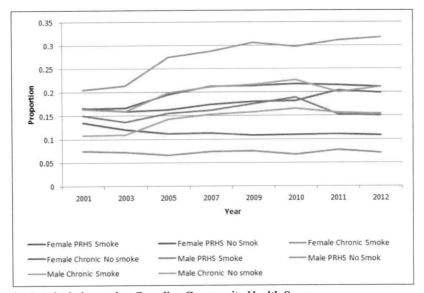

Source: Author's calculations using Canadian Community Health Survey.

Figure 2. Poor Health Status (PRHS) or Chronic Disease by Smoking Status.

The SES gradient is much more apparent when examined across income quintiles. The proportion of males and females reporting poor health status in the lowest income group is almost 20 points higher than the highest income group; the middle income groups fan out in between. The differences are not quite as large, but still worth note, for one or more chronic diseases.

As is the case elsewhere, our descriptive statistics show fairly consistent socioeconomic gradients in the prevalence of smoking and health status. In these data, income gradients are clearer than educational gradients. Smoking and activity gradients are seen in health outcomes. Demographics like marital status, immigrant status and age (not shown) are as expected. Typically, at this point, researchers argue that it is necessary to perform multivariate analyses to examine how each of these characteristics is related to health status controlling for other health behaviours and sociodemographic characteristics.

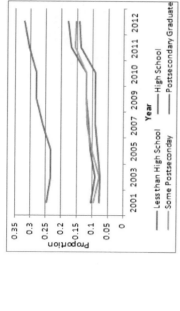
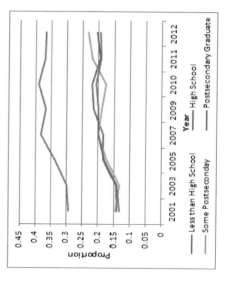
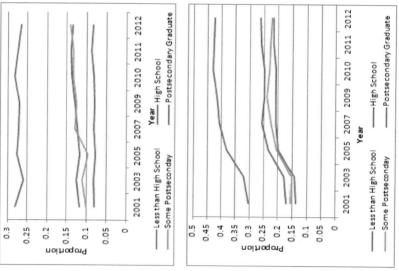

Figure 3. Poor Health Status (top) and Chronic Conditions (bottom) by Education: Female (left) and Male (right).

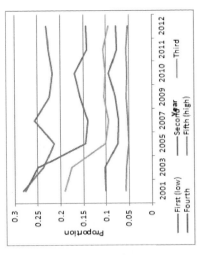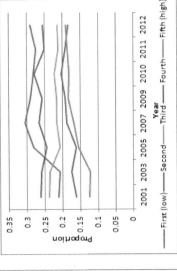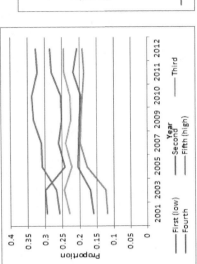

Source: Author's calculation using CCHS 2001-2012.
Figure 4. Poor Health Status (top) and Chronic Conditions (bottom) by Income Quintile: Female (left) and Male (right).

Table 2. Relationship between Poor Health Status and Health Behaviours by Education for Females

Less than High School

Poor Health Status	Quintile1	Quintile2	Quintile3	Quintile4	Quintile5
Daily Smoker	0.150***	0.111***	0.089***	0.052**	-0.022
Occasional Smoker	0.029	0.100**	0.070*	-0.016	-0.068
Former Daily	0.055***	0.062***	0.075***	0.013	-0.038
Former Occasional	0.005	-0.002	-0.024	-0.050**	-0.077**
Moderately Active	0.079**	0.025	0.031	0.040	0.027
Sedentary	0.186***	0.144***	0.120***	0.079***	0.070***
Often Binge Drink	-0.036	-0.056**	-0.031	-0.045	-0.030
Occasional Binge	-0.053**	-0.083***	-0.072***	-0.055**	-0.021
Observed Probab	0.327	0.271	0.232	0.192	0.168
Predicted Probab	0.312	0.258	0.214	0.181	0.143
# Observations	26,513	19,461	14,948	8,430	3,143

Some Post Secondary Education

Poor Health Status	Quintile1	Quintile2	Quintile3	Quintile4	Quintile5
Daily Smoker	0.201***	0.065***	0.090***	0.032**	0.021*
Occasional Smoker	0.135**	0.055	0.072**	0.014	0.007
Former Daily	0.089**	-0.006	0.037**	0.016	0.013
Former Occasional	0.066	-0.021	0.018	-0.004	-0.044***
Moderately Active	0.070*	0.016	0.043**	0.023	-0.009
Sedentary	0.107***	0.054**	0.073***	0.079***	0.053***
Often Binge Drink	-0.072**	-0.015	-0.029**	-0.055***	-0.018
Occasional Binge	-0.100**	0.026	0.001	-0.034**	-0.029**
Observed Probab	0.238	0.145	0.098	0.097	0.067
Predicted Probab	0.200	0.112	0.080	0.076	0.042
# Observations	4,486	4,245	4,699	4,950	3,456

High School Graduate

Poor Health Status	Quintile1	Quintile2	Quintile3	Quintile4	Quintile5
Daily Smoker	0.124***	0.027**	0.089***	0.022**	0.028*
Occasional Smoker	0.049	0.004	0.070*	0.002	-0.028*
Former Daily	0.036*	0.007	0.075***	0.016*	-0.007
Former Occasional	-0.015	-0.002	-0.024	-0.020**	-0.019
Moderately Active	0.086**	0.020	0.031	0.020	0.036**
Sedentary	0.152***	0.074***	0.120***	0.072***	0.093***
Often Binge Drink	-0.057**	-0.036**	-0.031	-0.040***	-0.037***
Occasional Binge	-0.107***	-0.051**	-0.072***	-0.032***	-0.020*
Observed Probab	0.233	0.271	0.127	0.089	0.078
Predicted Probab	0.213	0.258	0.119	0.071	0.058
# Observations	11,229	12,597	14,037	14,099	9,359

Post Secondary Graduate

Poor Health Status	Quintile1	Quintile2	Quintile3	Quintile4	Quintile5
Daily Smoker	0.110***	0.072***	0.058***	0.052***	0.022***
Occasional Smoker	0.056**	0.099***	0.034**	0.023**	0.100
Former Daily	0.028**	0.021**	0.020**	0.015***	0.002
Former Occasional	0.002	-0.012	0.008	0.008	-0.009**
Moderately Active	0.041**	0.024**	0.038***	0.012**	0.019***
Sedentary	0.120***	0.068***	0.081***	0.050***	0.049***
Often Binge Drink	-0.034**	-0.029**	-0.013*	-0.014***	-0.011***
Occasional Binge	-0.042	-0.011	-0.024**	-0.019***	-0.014***
Observed Probab	0.187	0.107	0.088	0.060	0.041
Predicted Probab	0.157	0.092	0.069	0.046	0.031
# Observations	23,573	29,430	40,460	51,290	50,434

Notes: *** significant at 0.000, ** significant at 0.05, and * significant at 0.10. Marginal probabilities reported – increase in the probability of reporting XX when the dummy variable changes from 0 to 1. All regressions control for marital status, immigrant status, age, and province.
Source: Author's calculation using CCHS 2001-2012.

Table 3. Relationship between Poor Health Status and Health Behaviours by Education for Males

Less than High School

Poor Health Status	Quintile1	Quintile2	Quintile3	Quintile4	Quintile5
Daily Smoker	0.162***	0.117***	0.025	0.079***	0.017
Occasional Smoker	0.179***	-0.010	-0.024	0.005	-0.055**
Former Daily	0.150***	0.072**	0.027	0.049**	-0.004
Former Occasional	0.037	-0.016	-0.059**	0.052**	-0.013
Moderately Active	-0.013	0.048**	0.028	0.041**	0.021
Sedentary	0.140***	0.107***	0.096***	0.076***	0.034**
Often Binge Drink	-0.048***	-0.079***	-0.003	-0.005	-0.037***
Occasional Binge	-0.011	-0.053**	-0.020	0.014	-0.012
Observed Probab	0.345	0.273	0.221	0.160	0.119
Predicted Probab	0.329	0.255	0.203	0.141	0.105
# Observations	13,719	12,969	14,274	11,496	6,222

Some Post Secondary Education

Poor Health Status	Quintile1	Quintile2	Quintile3	Quintile4	Quintile5
Daily Smoker	0.083*	0.065**	0.028*	0.047***	0.035**
Occasional Smoker	-0.039	-0.012	-0.010	0.030	0.028
Former Daily	-0.009	0.034*	0.006	0.034**	0.025**
Former Occasional	-0.055	-0.003	-0.006	0.049***	0.002
Moderately Active	0.133**	-0.002	0.015	0.004	0.038***
Sedentary	0.115***	0.065***	0.069***	0.035**	0.074***
Often Binge Drink	-0.090**	-0.023	-0.025**	-0.026**	-0.017**
Occasional Binge	-0.155***	-0.018	-0.008	-0.027**	-0.026***
Observed Probab	0.262	0.130	0.107	0.080	0.062
Predicted Probab	0.224	0.104	0.082	0.066	0.046
# Observations	2,472	2,700	3,779	4,815	4,074

High School Graduate

Poor Health Status	Quintile1	Quintile2	Quintile3	Quintile4	Quintile5
Daily Smoker	0.153***	0.065**	0.028*	0.047***	0.035**
Occasional Smoker	-0.015	-0.012	-0.010	0.030	0.028
Former Daily	0.142***	0.034*	0.006	0.034**	0.025**
Former Occasional	0.034	-0.003	-0.006	0.049**	0.002
Moderately Active	0.036	-0.002	0.015	0.004	0.038***
Sedentary	0.069**	0.065***	0.069***	0.035**	0.074***
Often Binge Drink	-0.100***	-0.023	-0.025***	-0.026**	-0.017**
Occasional Binge	-0.045**	-0.018	-0.008	-0.027**	-0.026***
Observed Probab	0.345	0.130	0.107	0.080	0.062
Predicted Probab	0.329	0.104	0.082	0.066	0.046
# Observations	5,300	6,802	9,961	12,974	10,766

Post Secondary Graduate

Poor Health Status	Quintile1	Quintile2	Quintile3	Quintile4	Quintile5
Daily Smoker	0.093***	0.072***	0.076***	0.035***	0.036***
Occasional Smoker	0.011	0.033	0.044***	0.004	0.004
Former Daily	0.046**	0.050***	0.055***	0.024**	0.017**
Former Occasional	0.013	0.033**	0.006	-0.015	0.002
Moderately Active	0.061***	0.008	0.030***	0.029***	0.026***
Sedentary	0.111***	0.055***	0.066***	0.056***	0.052***
Often Binge Drink	-0.015	-0.016	-0.016*	-0.017**	-0.007**
Occasional Binge	-0.030**	-0.026**	-0.019**	-0.008	-0.004
Observed Probab	0.184	0.121	0.090	0.069	0.046
Predicted Probab	0.143	0.099	0.070	0.051	0.035
# Observations	14,316	19,587	29,774	44,308	53,972

Notes: *** significant at 0.000, ** significant at 0.05, and * significant at 0.10.
Marginal probabilities reported – increase in the probability of reporting XX when the dummy variable changes from 0 to 1.
All regressions control for marital status, immigrant status, age, and province.
Source: Author's calculation using CCHS 2001-2012.

Table 4. Relationship between Chronic Health Condition and Health Behaviours by Education for Females

	Less than High School					High School Graduate				
Chronic Condition	Quintile1	Quintile2	Quintile3	Quintile4	Quintile5	Quintile1	Quintile2	Quintile3	Quintile4	Quintile5
Daily Smoker	0.138***	0.108***	0.088***	0.130***	0.002	0.107***	0.129***	0.077***	0.010***	0.032
Occasional Smoker	0.101***	0.061	0.063	0.063	-0.035	0.081	0.074	0.032	0.009	-0.032
Former Daily	0.160***	0.110***	0.010***	0.050***	-0.031	0.090***	0.085***	0.058***	0.035***	0.016
Former Occasional	0.032	0.015	0.021	0.005	-0.061	0.019	0.031	0.038***	0.000	-0.002
Moderately Active	0.019	-0.015	0.005	0.080***	0.014	0.081***	0.006	0.019	0.035**	0.084***
Sedentary	0.082***	0.075***	0.046***	0.078***	0.080***	0.063***	0.027	0.063***	0.045**	0.101***
Often Binge Drink	-0.081***	-0.023	-0.027	-0.012	0.059	-0.024	0.036	-0.037*	-0.042**	0.013
Occasional Binge	-0.129***	-0.008	-0.010	-0.052***	-0.029	-0.083***	-0.036	-0.073***	-0.029	-0.031
Observed Probab	0.457	0.121	0.347	0.291	0.277	0.301	0.265	0.249	0.199	0.194
Predicted Probab	0.442	0.099	0.334	0.273	0.262	0.270	0.237	0.227	0.179	0.175
# Observations	24,556	18,478	14,505	8,207	3,003	10,467	11,950	13,469	13,685	9,033

	Some Post Secondary Education					Post Secondary Graduate				
Chronic Condition	Quintile1	Quintile2	Quintile3	Quintile4	Quintile5	Quintile1	Quintile2	Quintile3	Quintile4	Quintile5
Daily Smoker	0.136***	0.037	0.098***	0.074**	0.096***	0.117***	0.115***	0.100***	0.076***	0.071***
Occasional Smoker	0.175***	0.057	0.106*	0.047	0.117***	0.040	0.055***	0.033***	0.013	0.020
Former Daily	0.036	0.012	0.022	0.085***	0.056***	0.039**	0.070***	0.060***	0.032***	0.033***
Former Occasional	-0.013	-0.078**	0.005	0.063**	0.008	-0.001	-0.009	0.009	0.012	0.006
Moderately Active	0.064	-0.043	-0.006	0.047*	-0.007	0.040**	0.006	0.034**	0.004	0.003
Sedentary	0.047	0.023	0.074**	0.108***	0.005	0.059***	0.041**	0.052***	0.020***	0.017**
Often Binge Drink	-0.069***	-0.047**	0.030	-0.022	0.013	-0.024	-0.022	-0.012	-0.010	-0.019**
Occasional Binge	-0.077***	-0.064**	0.011	-0.032	-0.020	-0.062**	-0.021	-0.019	-0.017	-0.018**
Observed Probab	0.322	0.211	0.232	0.2078	0.166	0.276	0.243	0.212	0.175	0.156
Predicted Probab	0.278	0.176	0.195	0.1821	0.148	0.247	0.216	0.188	0.160	0.143
# Observations	4,170	4,030	4,502	4,796	3,332	22,001	27,718	38,565	49,401	48,372

Notes: *** significant at 0.000, ** significant at 0.05, and * significant at 0.10.
Marginal probabilities reported – increase in the probability of reporting XX when the dummy variable changes from 0 to 1.
All regressions control for marital status, immigrant status, age, and province.
Source: Author's calculation using CCHS 2001-2012.

Table 5. Relationship between Chronic Health Condition and Health Behaviours by Education for Males

	Less than High School						High School Graduate				
Chronic Condition	Quintile1	Quintile2	Quintile3	Quintile4	Quintile5		Quintile1	Quintile2	Quintile3	Quintile4	Quintile5
Daily Smoker	0.055***	0.106***	0.016	0.031	0.071**		0.058**	0.013	0.022	0.002	0.065**
Occasional Smoker	0.114**	0.109*	-0.036	0.008	0.089**		-0.023	-0.033	0.042	0.093**	0.015
Former Daily	0.171***	0.101***	0.082***	0.071**	0.109***		0.103***	0.023	0.065**	0.030**	0.046**
Former Occasional	0.074**	0.013	-0.007	0.041	0.035		0.051	-0.027	-0.024	0.009	0.046**
Moderately Active	0.038	0.068**	0.014	0.026	-0.051**		0.068**	-0.023	0.022	0.009	0.039**
Sedentary	0.107***	0.070***	0.042**	0.046**	-0.032		0.066**	-0.013	0.017	0.030**	0.025*
Often Binge Drink	-0.045*	-0.069**	0.009	-0.026	-0.061**		-0.024	-0.032	-0.018	-0.014	-0.049**
Occasional Binge	-0.067***	-0.060**	-0.038*	-0.048**	-0.046**		0.021	-0.063**	-0.079***	-0.023*	-0.038**
Observed Probab	0.414	0.398	0.335	0.270	0.251		0.258	0.234	0.198	0.166	0.165
Predicted Probab	0.390	0.372	0.309	0.230	0.212		0.212	0.189	0.163	0.136	0.135
# Observations	12,679	12,160	13,731	11,107	5,946		4,994	6,429	9,486	12,560	10,351

	Some Post Secondary Education						Post Secondary Graduate				
Chronic Condition	Quintile1	Quintile2	Quintile3	Quintile4	Quintile5		Quintile1	Quintile2	Quintile3	Quintile4	Quintile5
Daily Smoker	0.153***	0.132**	0.163***	0.050*	0.146***		0.019	0.047**	0.070***	0.041***	0.059***
Occasional Smoker	0.090	-0.092**	0.157**	0.050	0.150***		0.009	0.062**	0.084**	0.039**	-0.002
Former Daily	0.070	0.158***	0.108***	0.014	0.067***		0.068***	0.072***	0.069***	0.047***	0.039***
Former Occasional	0.105*	-0.031	0.025	-0.039	0.009		-0.041*	0.052**	0.019	0.001	-0.001
Moderately Active	0.118**	0.014	-0.007	0.024	-0.015		0.060**	0.019	0.018	0.016**	0.029***
Sedentary	0.098**	0.033	0.045**	0.050**	0.019		0.066***	0.050***	0.044***	0.039***	0.037***
Often Binge Drink	-0.021	-0.076**	0.003	-0.026	-0.005		-0.039**	-0.004	-0.036**	-0.009	-0.024***
Occasional Binge	-0.092**	-0.082**	-0.046**	-0.074***	-0.067**		-0.035**	-0.030**	-0.031**	-0.011	-0.027***
Observed Probab	0.272	0.254	0.198	0.180	0.179		0.247	0.228	0.198	0.171	0.154
Predicted Probab	0.189	0.188	0.154	0.143	0.136		0.202	0.186	0.162	0.138	0.127
# Observations	2,309	2,508	3,585	4,617	3,898		13,319	18,377	28,228	42,539	51,712

Notes: *** significant at 0.000, ** significant at 0.05, and * significant at 0.10.
Marginal probabilities reported – increase in the probability of reporting XX when the dummy variable changes from 0 to 1.
All regressions control for marital status, immigrant status, age, and province.
Source: Author's calculation using CCHS 2001-2012.

All characteristics are included in the regression so that the relationships between health behaviours and sociodemographic characteristics and health can be examined, one by one (we include this analyses in Appendix Table 2). The results are consistent with the literature. As stated previously, we divide the sample into 40 sex-education-income strata instead of simply controlling for sex, education and income (results in tables 2 through 5).

This provides a better picture of the relationship between health behaviours and health status within income and education pairs[10]. Table 2 presents the results for self-reported poor health status for females. The four quadrants on the page represent education levels (less than high school graduation (top left), high school graduate (top right), some postsecondary education (bottom left), and postsecondary graduate (bottom right)). The columns contain the marginal probabilities[11] for each of the characteristics (obtained from regressions run on each sex-income-education strata – e.g., the first column of results is from the female-less than high school-first income quintile regression, the seventh column is marginal probabilities from the female-high school-second income quintile regression and so on). The bottom three rows of each quadrant present the observed and predicted probability for the base case (never smoker, active, never had 5 or more drinks at one sitting, married, 45 to 49 years of age, native born Canadian living in Ontario, in 2001) and the number of observations in each sex-education-income strata. Tables 3 through 5 are set up in an identical manner. Table 3 reports results for self-reported health status for males, Table 4 includes females reporting on chronic diseases and Table 5 is the same for males.

Some interesting information can be gleaned from the sample sizes (Appendix Table 1). First note that there are a reasonable number of observations in every cell. Some postsecondary education has the smallest sample sizes. Females with this education classification tend to be grouped into the lower income quintiles while males tend to be in the higher quintiles. Females with a postsecondary degree are about twice as likely to be in the top two quintiles than in the bottom two quintiles but males are two and a half to three times more likely to be in the higher income quintiles than in the lower. Men in the lowest educational class are about twice as likely to be in the lowest income quintile than in the top quintile. Females in this educational group are more than 8 times more likely to be in the bottom quintile than the top. For both sexes, the largest samples are in the highest educational group, a postsecondary degree. However, men in this group are most likely to be in the highest income quintile while women are most likely to be in the fourth income quintile. In sum, Table 1 and Appendix Table 1 indicate that men and women are quite similar in their educational status but are not so similar in their income status. Thus, differences in income-health relationship are also interesting from a gender perspective.

Looking across income quintiles in each female education group (Table 2), we see that the relationship between daily smoker (as compared to never smokers) and poor health status is not consistent across income groups within educational brackets. Income seems to act as a moderating force. There is a clear income gradient in the relationship between daily smoking and health for the lowest and highest educational classes with the lowest income group of daily smokers having the highest probability of reporting poor health status and the highest income group having the lowest; put simply. An income gradient is not as clear in the middle

---

[10] A multivariate framework with a complex set of interaction terms could provide the same results however, high colinearity among education, income and our explanatory variables and the large number of interactions make these types of regressions difficult to run and interpret.

[11] change in the base case probability caused by changing the value of the dummy from 0 to 1.

education groups, however if one ignores the relatively high marginal probability of reporting poor health for smokers in the third quintile, an income gradient emerges. Patterns are flatter when we move to examine the smoking-health relationship across educational levels within given income quintiles. About two percent of women smokers in income quintile 5 report poor health no matter what the educational level. Approximately 3 to 5 percent of smokers in the fourth income quintile report poor health irrespective of education. Patterns are more difficult to discern for the other smoking groups but occasional smoking is most consistently related to poor health for those with a postsecondary degree and tends to be about 2/3 of the probability of daily smokers[12]. Figure 5 and 5a present the results more succinctly. Figure 5 (6) presents the probability of reporting poor health for female (male) smokers and non-smokers by income quintile within education class and Figure 5a (6a) presents the same by education for females (males) within income quintile. There is a clear income gradient within education class indicating income is protective no matter what the education level however, the pattern is not quite as clear pattern in Figure 5a.

Females reporting a sedentary life style (as compared to an active life style) are more likely to report poor health status than are smokers for most education-income classes (surprisingly, the marginal probabilities are higher for sedentary life style than for daily smoker). Once again there seems to be a stronger income gradient within educational classes than an educational gradient within income quintiles. A woman with less than a high school education and an income in the first quintile who is a smoker has a 46 percent predicted probability of reporting poor health status.

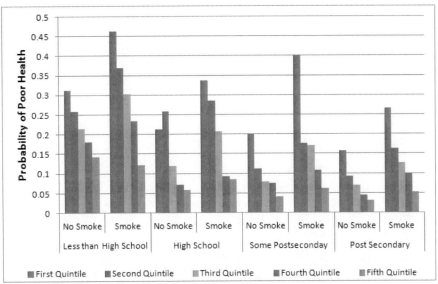

Source: Author's calculation using CCHS 2001-2012.

Figure 5. Poor Health Status by Smoking Status, Education, and Income Females.

---

[12] Ontario Ministry of Health's current "Quit the Denial" campaign claims that 'social smoking' is a ridiculous title; the commercials imply a smoker is a smoker and there is no such thing as a social smoker (occasional smoker) http://www.thestar.com/news/canada/2013/03/ 21/social_smoking_message_fart_ad_a_hit_online.html

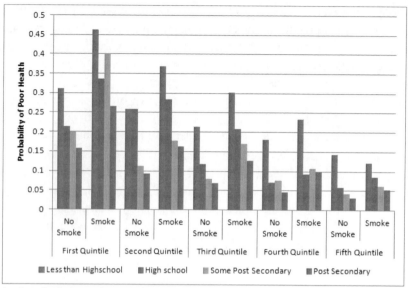

Source: Author's calculation using CCHS 2001-2012.

Figure 5a. Poor Health Status by Smoking Status, Income, and Education Females.

A non-smoking woman from the same education-income strata with a sedentary life style has a 50 percent chance. A sedentary woman with less than a high school education in the highest income quintile has a 21 percent probability of reporting poor health.

A similar female smoker has a 14 percent chance. Smoking (sedentary) women in the highest education-income strata have predicted probabilities of 5.3 (8.0). Binge drinking is either insignificantly related to poor health or is protective across education-income stratum.

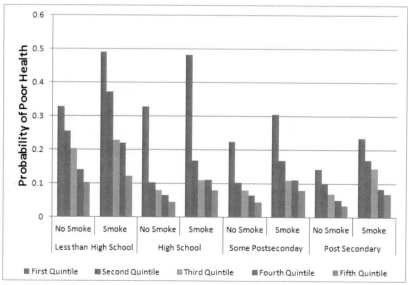

Source: Author's calculation using CCHS 2001-2012.

Figure 6. Poor Health Status by Smoking Status, Education and Income Males.

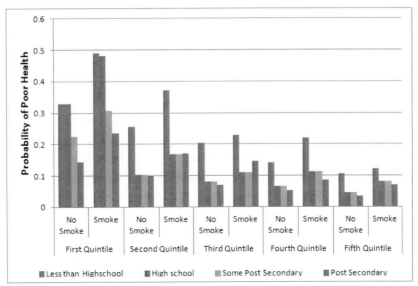

Source: Author's calculation using CCHS 2001-2012.

Figure 6a. Poor Health Status by Smoking Status, Income and Education Males.

Daily smoking is related to self-reported health status for males but there is not as consistent a gradient across income as seen with females. There are indications that within education groups, male daily smokers in higher income quintiles report poor health status less often than do smokers in lower income quintiles. Ignoring the third income quintile for a moment, there is a clear income gradient across all educational classes in the relationship between daily smoking and poor health status. However, the marginal probabilities are fairly close to one another in the higher income quintiles (e.g., except for males with less than high school education, the marginal probability of reporting poor health status for smokers is about 3 or 4 percentage points higher than nonsmokers for the third, fourth and fifth income quintiles irrespective of education and this is substantially higher in the bottom two quintiles). Probabilities that male daily smokers report poor health status are even more similar across educational levels within income quintiles (e.g., in the second (third) income quintile the daily smokers' marginal probabilities are 0.12, 0.07, 0.07, 0.07 (0.03, 0.03, 0.03, 0.08) across the educational classes). Being an occasional smoker is seldom significantly different than never smoking but being a former smoker significantly increases the likelihood of reporting poor health status for the majority of income quintiles in each education stratum. For males with a postsecondary education being a former smoker increases the probability of reporting poor health status by about 1 in 20 (first three quintiles) and about 1 in 4 (highest two quintiles). Thus, as with females, there seems to be some evidence that income is more protective than education. But, unlike females, there tends to be a dichotomy between higher and lower income levels. The graphs in Figures 6 and 6a paint the picture more clearly. Figure 6 presents the probability of reporting poor health for male smokers and non-smokers by income quintile within education class and Figure 6a by education within income quintile. As with females, there is a clear income gradient within education class indicating income is protective no matter what the education level but there is little that can be said about the pattern of education within income quintiles. Like females, males reporting a sedentary life style are consistently more likely to report poor health status. In many cases, the marginal probability is higher than that reported for current smokers. Unlike females, it is difficult to draw conclusions on income gradients within education levels or educational gradients within income quintiles. For example the probability a male with a sedentary life style and less than high school education reports poor health status is 0.14, 0.11, 0.10, 0.08, and 0.03, respectively across income quintiles one to five, more than a male with an active life style. The probability a sedentary male from the first income quintile reports poor health status is 0.14, 0.07, 0.12, and 0.11 more than an active person for less than high school, high school graduate, some postsecondary and postsecondary graduate, respectively. For a postsecondary graduate the marginal probabilities for sedentary life style are 0.11, 0.06, 0.07, 0.06, and 0.05 across income quintiles. For the highest income quintile, the marginal probabilities are 0.03, 0.07, 0.07, and 0.05 respectively across educational class. It seems income may be more protective than education for those with a sedentary life style. The predicted probability of poor health is 50 percent for a current smoker and 47 percent for a sedentary male in the lowest income-education strata. Predicted probabilities of poor health are 12 (14) percent for smoking (sedentary) males in the highest income quintile-lowest educational level stratum, 24 (25) percent in the highest education-lowest income strata and 7.1 (8.7) percent for smoking (sedentary) males in the highest education-income strata. As is the case for females, binge drinking is either insignificantly related to poor health or is protective for males across education-income stratum.

In sum, tables 2 and 3 show that daily smokers have significantly higher probabilities of reporting self-reported health status than nonsmokers. The relationship is less consistent for occasional and former smokers. Income seems to play a more protective role than education for both males and females as probabilities decline more across income strata within education levels than across educational strata for given income quintiles. Surprisingly, living a sedentary life style has almost as strong an association with poor health as being a daily smoker for both males and females and across education-income groups although this may have something to do with the downward bias of self-reported smoking measures (Tennekoon and Rosenman, 2013). The insignificant or significantly negative association between binge drinking and self-reported health status is difficult to interpret; reverse causality may be at play[13].

Tables 4 and 5 repeat the analysis for our second health outcome, self-reports of one or more chronic conditions. Although the overall conclusions are similar to those for self-reported health status, trends are more ambiguous for this 'more objective' health measure. In general, male and female daily smokers are more likely to report a chronic disease than never smokers. Female smokers in the highest income group are less likely to report a chronic condition than those in the lowest income group no matter their education level (Table 4) and, except for those with some postsecondary education, smokers in the highest income quintile are less likely to report a chronic illness than smokers in any other income quintile.

Income seems more protective in the lower educational classes than in the higher. The marginal probability of reporting a chronic disease for a daily smoker falls from 0.14 (0.11) more than a never-smoker with a less than high school (high school) education to insignificantly different from zero for the highest income group – a change of 0.14 (0.11) percentage points when moving from lowest to highest income quintile. The difference is about five percentage points for women with similar characteristics in the higher education

---

[13] see footnote 5.

levels. Moving across educational levels within the first income quintile, the probability changes from a daily smoker being 14 percentage points more likely to report a chronic illness than a never smoker to 12 percentage points if they have a postsecondary degree (a decline of only 2 percentage points). The highest income earners in the lowest educational groups are no more likely to report a chronic condition than a never smoker but they are 7 to 10 percentage points more likely if they are in the higher educational groups. The higher prevalence of chronic disease is fairly consistent across educational levels within income quintiles for the second, third and fourth income quintiles.

It is more difficult to draw conclusions when we examine males reporting chronic disease (Table 5). Surprisingly, being a daily smoker does not significantly change the probability of reporting a chronic disease for several income-education strata. When male daily smokers are significantly more likely to report a chronic illness, it is by about 6 or 7 percentage points no matter the income or educational group except for those with some postsecondary education and then it is about 15 percentage points for income quintiles one, two, three and five and about five for the fourth income quintile. There is no discernible pattern across education within income quintiles. The same holds for living a sedentary lifestyle. Where it is significantly different from living an active lifestyle, it is by about 3 to 5 percentage points across income-education strata.

Some income gradients can be seen in Figures 7 and 8 in several of the education classes for females and males, respectively. The gradients are stronger for nonsmokers than for smokers. Figures 7a and 8a show no such gradient for education within income class for either males or females.

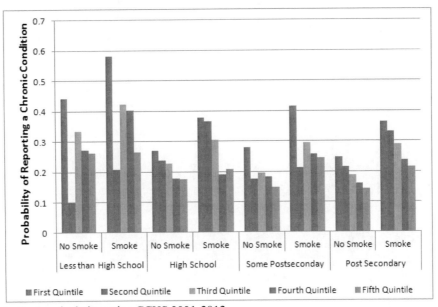

Source: Author's calculation using CCHS 2001-2012.

Figure 7. Chronic Conditions by Smoking Status, Education and Income Females.

We can glean some information on the income-education effects on chronic conditions by examining the predicted probabilities for the base case in this group. A definite income-health gradient emerges within each educational class. However, within income quintiles the probabilities of reporting a chronic disease show a shallow gradient across the three higher income levels (e.g., 0.33, 0.22, 0.20, 0.19 (0.26, 0.18, 0.17, 0.14) across educational levels in the third (fifth) income quintile. Men with base case characteristics and less than high school education report substantially higher levels of poor health than do those with other educational status.

CONCLUSION

There is no debate in the current literature on whether smoking is related to health status – it is and causal pathways have been scientifically proven.

The current debate in the empirical literature seems to focus on whether the socioeconomic gradients in smoking, and other health behaviours, can explain the socioeconomic gradient in health status; the jury is still out. Many studies have examined the question, particularly for educational gradients in health, using longitudinal data and/or natural experiments focused on changes in policies around the allowable age of school leaving or usual years of schooling for a high school diploma. The findings are mixed. Many studies find no causal link between socioeconomic status, health behaviours and health. Those that do, often find that the amount of the health variation explained by health behaviours is small to moderate at best. Studies tend to conclude that there must be unobserved individual or institutional characteristics that differ systematically within socioeconomic classes that 'cause' the differences in health status.

This chapter, like many others, focuses on attempting to document the association between smoking and health. Unlike other studies, we do not simply control for socioeconomic status by adding income and or education as control variables within a multivariate framework.

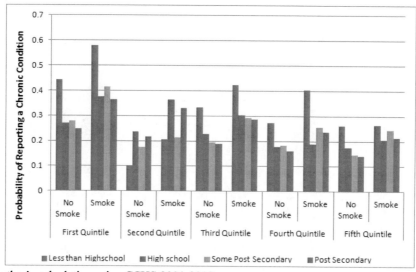

Source: Author's calculation using CCHS 2001-2012.

Figure 7a. Chronic Conditions by Smoking Status, Income and Education Females.

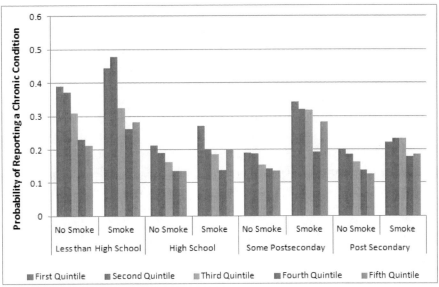

Source: Author's calculation using CCHS 2001-2012.

Figure 8. Chronic Conditions by Smoking Status, Education and Income Males.

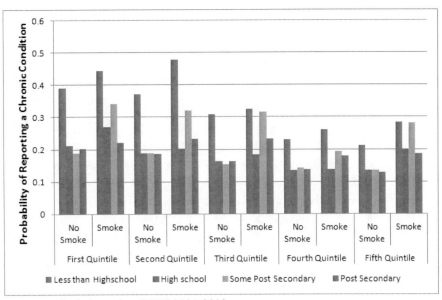

Source: Author's calculation using CCHS 2001-2012.

Figure 8a. Chronic Conditions by Smoking Status, Income, and Education Males.

Using the Canadian Community Health Survey which is specifically designed to pool samples over many cross-sections to achieve sample sizes large enough to study health questions across rare events or small populations, we examine the relationship between smoking and health within socioeconomic status defined by sex-income-education strata. We attempt to examine whether income or education may be more or less moderating in the smoking-health relationship. Our descriptive statistics show, like many before us, that men are better off when it comes to socioeconomic class but have worse health behaviours, particularly smoking. Males are less likely to report chronic health conditions than females but act similarly in reporting self-reported health status. Uniquely, we show that income gradients are clearer than educational gradients in the reporting of poor health status and one or more chronic conditions; slightly more so for females than males.

Multivariate estimation using a probit model, controlling for sex, income, education, marital status, immigrant status, province and a time trend, indicates, as many others have, that poor health behaviours such as smoking and sedentary life style, are associated with poorer health. Our results on binge drinking were unexpected but others have also found mixed results on the relationship between income and health (Thun et al. 1997).

Our main analysis used 40 sex-income-education strata to investigate whether controlling for income and education in multivariate analyses masked important information about socioeconomic class. Our results clearly indicate strong relationships between smoking and self-reported health status for males and females across income-education strata. The picture is less clear when using one or more chronic diseases as the health outcome for females and even less so for males. However, it is apparent that income is more 'protective' within educational strata than education is within income strata. There is a clear income gradient in the probability that daily smokers are more likely to report poor health than never smokers for poor self-reported health status across education levels for females and, generally, for males. Marginal probabilities are more similar across educational levels within income quintiles. The results hold much more loosely when chronic disease is used as the health measure.

We surmise, as others have, that there are unobserved characteristics within socioeconomic class that influence health (Lundborg, 2008; Brunello, 2011; Cutler et al, 2011; *Amin, Behrman,* and *Spector,* 2013). We believe our results indicate that the unobserved characteristics within income class may be more important than the unobserved characteristics within educational class when determining health.

We show that the relationship between smoking and health seems to be attenuated more by income within given levels of education than by level of education within given income quintiles. This indicates that access to health care and other consumption goods, exposure to environmental factors like pollution or chemical exposure and cumulative effects of poverty that are associated with lower income levels may be more important than the differential productivity with health information or health care that comes with increased levels of education (Currie and Hyson, 1999; Currie and Stabile, 2002; Evans and Kim, 2010; Seabrook and Avison, 2012; Cutler et al., 2011; Pampel, Krueger and Denny, 2010; Cutler and Lleras-Muney, 2010).

Essentially, we find that, in the Canadian context, income is more 'protective' within education levels than education is within income quintiles indicating that the situations afforded by increased income may be more important for smoking-health relationship than the additional knowledge/productivity associated with higher levels of education. Thus, a male construction worker (some post secondary education) is likely to have a better smoking-health relationship than a male hair stylist (same sex and education but lower income) however the results here indicate that the construction worker may also have a better smoking-health relationship than a university graduate waiter. Policy makers may need to examine more closely health relationships within income/education levels and researchers may need to be more specific about how socioeconomic gradients are measured to more thoughtfully capture possible unobserved characteristics within income and education.

Appendix Table 1. Sample Sizes

	Female					Male				
	Income1	Income2	Income3	Income4	Income5	Income1	Income2	Income3	Income4	Income5
Poor Health Status										
Less than High School	26513	19461	14948	8430	3143	13719	12969	14274	11496	6222
High School Graduate	11229	12597	14037	14099	9359	5300	6802	9961	12974	10766
Some Post Secondary	4486	4245	4699	4950	3456	2472	2700	3779	4815	4074
Post Secondary Grad	23573	29430	40460	51290	50434	14316	19587	29774	44308	53972
Chronic Condition										
Less than High School	24556	18478	14505	8207	3003	12679	12160	13731	11107	5946
High School Graduate	10467	11950	13469	13685	9033	4994	6429	9486	12560	10351
Some Post Secondary	4170	4030	4502	4796	3332	2309	2508	3585	4617	3898
Post Secondary Grad	22001	27718	38565	49401	48372	13319	18377	28228	42539	51712

Appendix Table 2. Probit Analyses

	Poor Health Status Marg Prob	p-value	Chronic Condition Marg Prob	p-value
Male	0.006	0.000	-0.013	0.000
Daily Smoker	0.062	0.000	0.080	0.000
Occasional Smoker	0.022	0.000	0.046	0.000
Former Daily Smoker	0.030	0.000	0.070	0.000
Former Occas Smoker	-0.003	0.261	0.012	0.000
Active	0.027	0.000	0.021	0.000
Moderately Active	0.073	0.000	0.042	0.000
Occasional Binge	-0.024	0.000	-0.022	0.000
Often Binges	-0.021	0.000	-0.040	0.000
Income Quantile 1	0.150	0.000	0.088	0.000
Income Quantile 2	0.079	0.000	0.046	0.000
Income Quantile 3	0.053	0.000	0.030	0.000
Income Quantile 4	0.024	0.000	0.010	0.000
Less than Secondary	0.057	0.000	0.022	0.000
High school grad	0.007	0.000	-0.009	0.001
Some Post Secondary	0.022	0.000	0.015	0.001
Previously Married	0.015	0.000	0.007	0.009
Never Married	0.025	0.000	0.007	0.015
Immigrant (>10 yrs)	-0.053	0.000	-0.106	0.000

	Poor Health Status Marg Prob	p-value	Chronic Condition Marg Prob	p-value
Immigrant (<10 yrs)	-0.050	0.000	-0.109	0.000
age 20-24*	-0.045	0.000	-0.090	0.000
age 25-29	-0.036	0.000	-0.069	0.000
age 30-34	-0.019	0.000	-0.032	0.000
age 35-39	0.021	0.000	0.045	0.000
age 40-44	0.038	0.000	0.111	0.000
age 50-54	0.043	0.000	0.169	0.000
age 55-59	0.036	0.000	0.233	0.000
age 60-64	0.048	0.000	0.286	0.000
age 65-69	0.075	0.000	0.321	0.000
age 70-74	0.083	0.000	0.343	0.000
age 75-79	-0.034	0.000	-0.080	0.000
age 80plus	0.004	0.067	-0.039	0.000
Nfld	-0.011	0.001	0.011	0.027
PEI	-0.010	0.007	0.024	0.000
NS	0.008	0.006	0.029	0.000
NB	0.017	0.000	0.009	0.025
Que	-0.023	0.000	-0.030	0.000
Man	-0.007	0.022	-0.023	0.000
Sask	-0.002	0.558	-0.011	0.004
Alb	-0.009	0.001	-0.015	0.000

Appendix Table 2. (Continued)

	Poor Health Status		Chronic Condition	
	Marg Prob	p-value	Marg Prob	p-value
BC	0.005	0.020	-0.015	0.000
year	-0.002	0.000	0.004	0.000
Observed Probabil	0.117		0.225	
Predicted Probabil	0.084		0.195	
Sample Size	635,154		604,809	

REFERENCES

Adams, Peter, Michael D. Hurd, Daniel L. McFadden, Angela Merrill, Tiago Ribeiro (2004) "Healthy, Wealthy, and Wise? Tests for Direct Causal Paths between Health and Socioeconomic Status" In Perspectives on the Economics of Aging David A. Wise, editor (p. 415 - 526) http:// www.nber.org/chapters/c10350

Adda, Jérôme and Valérie Lechene (2004) "On the Identification of the effect of smoking on mortality" Oxford University Department of Economics Working Paper series #184.

Amin, Vikesh, Jere R. Behrman, Tim D. Spector (2013) "Does more schooling improve health outcomes and health related behaviors? Evidence from U.K. twins". *Economics of Education Review*, 35:134-148.

Au, Doreen Wing Han, Thomas F. Crossley and Martin Schellhorn (2005). "The effect of health" *Health Economics,* 14(10):999-1018.

Ainslie, G. (1991). "Derivation of "rational" economic behavior from hyperbolic discount curves". *American Economic Review*, 81:134–140.

Auld M. C. 2005. Smoking, Drinking, and Income. *Journal of Human Resources,* 40: 505-518.

Baker, Michael, Mark Stabile and Catherine Deri (2004). "What Do Self-Reported, Objective, Measures of Health Measure?" *Journal of Human Resources,* 39(4):1067-1093.

Becker, G. and K. Murphy (1988). "A theory of rational addiction". *Journal of Political Economy,* 96:675-700.

Brunello, Giorgio, Margherita Fort, Nicole Schneeweis, Rudolf Winter-Ebmer (2011) "The Causal Effect of Education on Health: What is the Role of Health Behaviors?" IZA, Discussion Paper No. 5944.

CDC (2012) "Adult Cigarette Smoking in the United States: Current Estimates" Available at http://www.cdc.gov/tobacco

Cowan B. W., Schwab B. 2011. The Incidence of the Healthcare Costs of Smoking. *Journal of Health Economics*, 30(5): 1094-1102.

Currie, Janet and Rosemary Hyson (1999) "Is the Impact of Health Shocks Cushioned by Socioeconomic Status? The Case of Low Birthweight" *The American Economic Review,* Papers and Proceedings; 89(2):245-250.

Currie, Janet and Mark Stabile (2002). "Socioeconomic Status and Health: Why is the Relationship Stronger for Older Children?" *American Economic Review,* 93(5):1813-1823.

Currie, Janet and Mark Stabile (2009). "Mental health in childhood and human capital" In The problem of disadvantage The Problems of Disadvantaged Youth: An Economic Perspective, edited by Jonathan Gruber, Pp 115-148. Chicago, University of Chicago Press.

Cutler, David M., Fabian Lange, Ellen Meara, Seth Richards, Christopher J. Ruhm (2010). "Explaining the rise in educational gradients in mortality" *Journal of Health Economics,* 30:1174-1187.

Cutler, David M., Edward L. Glaeser and Allison B. Rosen. (2009). "Is the US Population Behaving Healthier?" In Social Security Policy in a Changing Environment, edited by Jeffrey Brown, R., Jeffrey Leibman and David Wise. Cambridge, MA: National Bureau of Economic Research.

Cutler, David M. and Adriana Lleras-Muney (2010) "Understanding differences in health behaviors by education". *Journal of Health Economics,* 29:1–28.

Evans, Gary W. and Pilyoung Kim (2010) "Multiple risk exposure as a potential explanatory mechanism for the socioeconomic status–health gradient" *N.Y. Acad. Sci.,* 1186:174–189.

Florescu A, Ferrence R, Einarson T, Selby P, Soldin O, Koren G. (2009). Methods for Quantification of Exposure to Cigarette Smoking and Environmental Tobacco Smoke: Focus on Developmental Toxicology. *Therapeutic Drug Monitoring,* 31:14–30.

Goldfarb, Robert S., Thomas C. Leonard and Steven M. Suranovic (2001) "Are rival theories of smoking underdetermined?" *Journal of Economic Methodology,* 8(2):229–251.

Grafova I. B. and F. P. Stafford (2009). "The Wage Effects of Personal Smoking History." *Industrial and Labor Relations Review,* 62: 381-393.

Health Canada (2013) "Tobacco use statistics" http://www.hc-sc.gc.ca/hc-ps/tobac-tabac/research-recherche/stat/_ctums-esutc_prevalence/ prevalence-eng.php#wave2_10

Janz, Teresa (2012) "Current smoking trends." Statistics Canada Catalogue no. 82-624-X.

Jones A., A. Gulbis, and E. H. Baker (2010) "Differences in tobacco use between Canada and the United States." *Int. J. Public Health,* 2010; 55(3):167-75.

Levine P. B., T. A. Gustafson, A. D. Velenchik (1997). "More Bad News for Smokers? The Effects of Cigarette Smoking on Wages." *Industrial and Labor Relations Review,* 50: 493-509.

Lundborg, Petter, Martin Nilsson, and Johan Vikström (2011). "Socioeconomic heterogeneity," Working Paper Series 2011:11, IFAU - Institute for Evaluation of Labour Market and Education Policy. http://www.ifau.se/Upload/pdf/se/2011/wp11-11-Socioeconomic-heterogeneity-in-the-effect-of-health-shocks-on-earnings.pdf

Lundborg, Petter (2008). "The Health Returns to Education: What Can We Learn from Twins?" IZA Discussion Papers 3399, Institute for the Study of Labor (IZA).

Manuel D. G., R. Perez, C. Bennett, L. Rosella, M. Taljaard, M. Roberts, R. Sanderson, M. Tuna, P. Tanuseputro, and H. Manson (2012). "Seven More Years: The impact of smoking, alcohol, diet, physical activity and stress on health and life expectancy in Ontario". ICES/PHO Report. Toronto: Institute for Clinical Evaluative Services and Public Health Ontario.

Marmot, Michael, Carold D. Ryff, Larry L. Bumpass, Martin Shipley and Nadine F. Marks (1997) Social inequalities in health: Next questions and converging evidence". *Social Sciences and Medicine*, 44(6):901-910.

Meghir, Costas, Mårten Palme and Emilia Simeonova (2012) "Education, Health and Mortality: Evidence from a Social Experiment." NBER Working Paper, 17932.

Naimi, Timothy S., Robert D. Brewer, Ali Mokdad, Clark Denny, and Mary K. Serdula (2003). "Binge Drinking Among US Adults". *JAMA.*, 289(1):70-75.

Olshansky, S. Jay, Douglas J. Passaro, Ronald C. Hershow, Jennifer Layden, et al. (2005). "A Potential Decline in Life expectancy in the United States in the 21st Century." *New England Journal of Medicine*, 352(11):1138-1145.

Østbye T., D. H. Taylor and S. H. Jung (2002) "A longitudinal study of the effects of tobacco smoking and other modifiable risk factors on ill health in middle-aged and old Americans: results from the Health and Retirement Study and Asset and Health Dynamics among the Oldest Old survey" *Preventive Medicine*, 34(3):334-45.

Pollak, R. (1975) 'The intertemporal cost of living index', *Annals of Economic and Social Measurement*, 4:179–95.

Seabrook, Jamie A. and William R. Avison (2012) "Socioeconomic status and cumulative disadvantage across the life course: Implications for health outcomes". *Canadian Review of Sociology*, 49(1):50-68.

Statistics Canada (2013a). "National Population Health Survey - Longitudinal (NPHS)" http://www23.statcan.gc.ca/imdb/ p2SV.pl?Function=getSurveyandSDDS=3225#a1

Statistics Canada (2013b). "National Longitudinal Survey of Children and Youth (NLSCY)" http://www23.statcan.gc.ca/imdb/ p2SV.pl?Function=getSurveyandSDDS=4450

Statistics Canada (2013c). "Canadian Community Health Survey - Annual Component (CCHS)" http://www23.statcan.gc.ca/imdb/p2SV.pl?Function=getSurveyandSDDS=3226

Stewart, Susan, David M. Cutler, and Allison B. Rosen (2009). "Forecasting the Effects of Obesity and Smoking on U.S. Life Expectancy," *New England Journal of Medicine*, 361(23): 2252-2260.

Stowasser, Till, Florian Heiss, Daniel McFadden, Joachim Winter (2011) "Healthy, Wealthy and Wise Revisited: An Analysis of the Causal Pathways from Socio-economic Status to Health" NBER Working Paper No. 17273.

Tennekoon, Vidhura and Robert Rosenman (2013). "Bias in measuring smoking behaviour." School of Economic Sciences Working Paper 2013-10, Washington State University.

Thun, M. J., R. Peto, A. D. Lopez, J. H. Monaco, S. J. Henley (1997). "Alcohol consumption and mortality among middle-aged and elderly U.S. adults." *New England Journal of Medicine*, 337:1705-1714.

Tubeuf, Sandy, Forence Jusot and Damien Bricard (2012) "Mediating role of education and lifestyles in the relationship between early-life conditions and health: evidence from the 1958 British Cohort". *Health Econonics*, 21(S1):129–150

van Ours J. C. (2004) "A Pint a Day Raises a Man's Pay; but Smoking Blows That Gain Away." *Journal of Health Economics*, 23:863-886.

Viscusi, W. Kip and Joni Hersch (2007) "The mortality costs to smokers" NBER Working Paper 13599 http://www.nber.org/papers/w13599

World Health Organization (2009) WHO report on the global tobacco epidemic, 2009: implementing smoke-free environments. http:// www.who.int/tobacco/mpower/2009/en/

In: Smoking Restrictions
Editor: Nazmi Sari

ISBN: 978-1-63321-148-3
© 2014 Nova Science Publishers, Inc.

Chapter 4

YOUTH SMOKING IN CANADA AND THE REVIEW OF RELATED LITERATURE

Hideki Ariizumi, Ph.D.[*]
Department of Economics, School of Business and Economics,
Wilfrid Laurier University, Canada

ABSTRACT

This article presents the recent trends of smoking behaviours among the young Canadians from 1999 to 2012, using the Canadian Tobacco Monitoring Surveys. The proportion of the daily smokers among the youth has been declining during this period, and the decline is shaper than among the older people. Then I review the youth smoking literature to help our understanding of the trends in the Canadian youth smoking behaviours.

Keywords: Youth smoking, tobacco, cigarette taxes, legal purchasing age, smoking restrictions

1. INTRODUCTION

It is a well-established fact that smoking is harmful to our health. Many toxic chemicals are identified as causing damages to our health. Given this negative relationship between smoking and health, various public policies are implemented to discourage smoking, and to help to quit smoking. Tobacco products are very addictive so that, once started, it is difficult to quit. Also the negative health problems are not necessarily immediate consequences of smoking. For example, it takes time and accumulation of smoking (that is, tar in this case) that can cause a cancer. Also smoking by someone else can harm one's health. Hence, it is important to understand the youth smoking behaviours and what policies and environments

---

[*] E-mail: hariizumi@wlu.ca.

can affect the youth smoking behaviours. In this article, I review the literature on the youth smoking in Canada, along with the recent trends of the youth smoking behaviours.

Section 2 briefly reviews the relationship between health effects and smoking. Section 3 provides the current trends in the youth smoking behaviours, using the Canadian Tobacco Monitoring Surveys. Section 4 reviews the literature on the youth smoking, focusing on the Canadian youth. Section 5 provides some conclusion.

2. Smoking and Health

Since U.S. Surgeon General Luther Terry in January 1964 released a report indicating that smoking caused illness and death, and emphasizing that the government should do something about it, medical literature has established that smoking is seriously harmful to our health. For example, Health Canada provides various health problems associated with smoking.[14] Researchers identified many toxic chemicals associated with smoking. As a report of the U.S. Surgeon General (CDC, 2010) suggests, those toxic chemicals reach our lung quickly and get into blood stream. So smoking can affect our entire body. Also the CDC report (2010) shows that about 70 chemicals in tobacco smoke can cause cancer. Smoking also alters blood chemicals and affects blood circulation. For example, carbon monoxide reduces the oxygen in our body. Hence, smoking is linked to heart attack and stroke (CDC, 2010).

Nicotine is very addictive and younger people are more sensitive to nicotine. That is, it is more likely get addicted to smoking if one starts smoking in an early age. Overall, the medical research provides strong evidence that the major causes of deaths such as cancer, coronary heart disease, and peripheral vascular disease in Canada are linked to smoking. For instance, Jones, Gublis and Baker (2010) show that 21% of all deaths over the past decade are due to smoking. The total number of deaths in Canada is just over 253,000 in 2012/13. So smoking can be responsible for about 53,000 deaths in Canada. Baliunas et al. (2007) report that 10.3 percent of all hospital diagnoses were estimated to be attributable to smoking and 7.3 percent of all acute care hospital days in 2002 in Canada. Similarly, Harrison (2003) estimated that 12 percent of hospital utilization and 7 percent of physician visits in Newfoundland in 1995 were attributable to smoking. Therefore, those studies show that smoking can cause a significant number of deaths and health problems in Canada.

3. Trend in Smoking Rates

Figure 1 shows the proportion of daily smokers in Canada from 1999 to 2012 based on Canadian Tobacco Use Monitoring Surveys (CTUMS). As in many other developed countries, the overall smoking rate is declining from over 20 percent in 1999 to less than 12 percent in 2012. The Canadian population grows from 30.5 million in 1999 to 34.88 million in 2012. Thus, the absolute number of daily smokers has declined over this period. The sales data on cigarettes in Canada (Health Canada, 2014) confirm this trend from 1999 to 2008.

---

[14] See the Health Canada web site at http://www.hc-sc.gc.ca/hc-ps/tobac-tabac/body-corps/index-eng.php.

However, since 2008, the wholesales of cigarettes are increasing: from 27.6 billion to 31 billion units between 2008 and 2011. This suggests that, despite the fact that the proportion of daily smokers are declining throughout this period, the smokers may be increasing their consumption of cigarettes in the recent years.

Table 1 shows that the average and median number of cigarettes consumed per week by the daily smokers. It appears that the average and median consumption of cigarettes were gradually declining up to 2011, and then jumped up in 2012. Although, this average and median consumption pattern does not entirely match with the whole sales pattern in terms of timing.

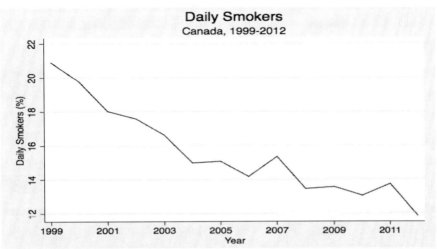

Source: Author's calculation based on Canadian Tobacco Use Monitoring Surveys, 1999 to 2012.
Figure 1.

Table 1. Weekly number of cigarettes consumed among smokers

Year	Average Consumption	Median Consumption
1999	14.87	15
2000	14.29	13
2001	13.84	12
2002	14.12	12
2003	13.28	12
2004	12.57	11
2005	13.21	12
2006	12.53	12
2007	12.87	12
2008	11.8	10
2009	11.67	10
2010	12.51	10
2011	11.8	10
2012	20.92	12

Source: Author's calculation based on Canadian Tobacco Use Monitoring Surveys, 1999 to 2012.

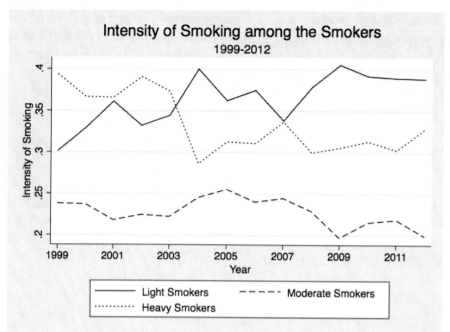

Source: Author's calculation based on Canadian Tobacco Use Monitoring Surveys, 1999 to 2012. Health Canada defines those who smoke less than 10 cigarettes per day as a light smoker, those who smoke between 10 and 19 cigarettes per day as a moderate smoker, and those who smoke more than 20 cigarettes per day as a heavy smoker.
Figure 2.

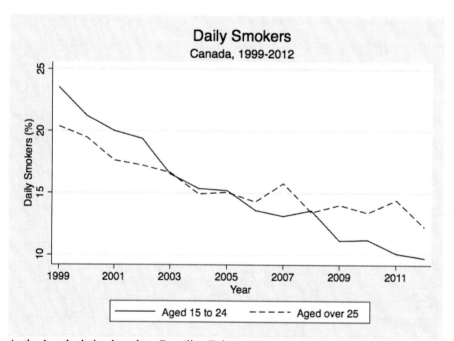

Source: Author's calculation based on Canadian Tobacco Use Monitoring Surveys, 1999 to 2012.
Figure 3.

Figure 2 shows the changes in the intensity of smoking among the smokers from 1999 to 2012.[15]

Figure 2 also seems to suggest that the consumption of cigarettes may be up again in the recent years. The proportion of heavy smokers went down sharply between 2003 and 2004, and then since 2008, it started to climb up again. Also in 2008, the proportion of light smokers went up. This change in the smoking habits was probably enough to increase the total consumption of cigarettes since 2008, even though the proportion of daily smokers keeps declining.

Figure 3 shows the same trends divided into two groups: those who are 15 to 24 years old and those who are over 25 years old. The decline in the smoking rates among the young is sharper than among the older age group between 1999 and 2012. The proportion of daily smokers among the young was 23.5 percent in 1999, and it went down to 9.8 percent in 2012.

Figure 4 shows the changes in the proportion of the daily young smokers further divided into several age groups. Similar to the overall trend, the rates of daily smokers in the all age groups among the young have been decreasing since 1999. As one expects, the proportion of daily smokers among the aged 15 to 17 is much lower than the age groups from 18 to 24 years old, and the rates are similar within this older age groups of the young. Also the age restriction for smoking is an important determinant for the youth smoking. In Canada, the legal smoking age is either 18 or 19 years old, depending on where a person lives.[16] Hence, the proportion of smokers between 15 and 17 years old is much lower than the other age groups. Unfortunately, the CTUMS public-use files grouped 18 and 19 years old together. Thus, I cannot examine the smoking rates by the different legal smoking age restrictions directly. Nonetheless, one can hypothesize that the smoking rate among the young aged from 15 to 17 years old is higher in the provinces with the legal smoking age being 18 years old than in the provinces with the legal smoking age being 19 years old. And there should not be a difference in the smoking rates among the older age groups due to the smoking age restriction. Table 2 shows the proportions of daily smokers for age 15 to 17 years old, age 18 to 19 years old and age 20 to 22 years old by the place of residence, which is divided by the legal smoking age restriction.

Table 2. The Proportion of Daily Smokers by the Place of Residence in 2012

Age Group	Legal Smoking Age is 19	Legal Smoking Age is 18	F-test statistics (P-value)
15 to 17 years old	0.0286	0.0494	3.82 (0.05)
18 to 19 years old	0.1050	0.1125	0.10 (0.76)
20 to 22 years old	0.1190	0.1508	1.96 (0.16)

Source: Author's calculation based on Canadian Tobacco Use Monitoring Survey 2012. In Alberta, Saskatchewan, Manitoba and Quebec (and the territories), the legal smoking age is 18 years old, and in the rest of Canada, the legal smoking age is 19 years old. Note that the people in the territories are excluded in the survey.

---

[15] Health Canada defines those who smoke less than 10 cigarettes per day as a light smoker, those who smoke between 11 and 19 cigarettes per day as a moderate smoker, and those who smoker more than 20 cigarettes per day as a heavy smoker.
[16] In Alberta, Saskatchewan, Manitoba and Quebec, as well as the three territories, the legal smoking age is 18 years old, and in the rest of Canada, it is 19 years old.

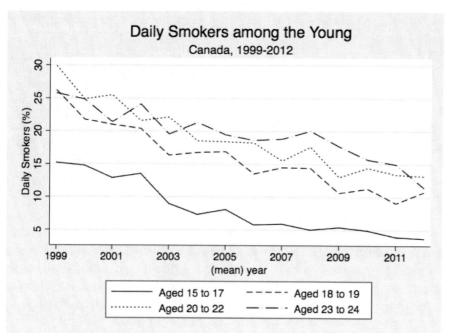

Source: Author's calculation based on Canadian Tobacco Use Monitoring Surveys, 1999 to 2012.
Figure 4.

The first row shows that the smoking rate among those who are 15 to 17 years old is 2.86% in the provinces with the legal smoking age of 19, compared with 4.94% in the provinces with the legal smoking age of 18. This difference is statistically significant at 5% level (shown in the last column).

On the other hand, the smoking rates among those who are 18 to 19 years old (in the second row) are 10.5% and 11.3%, respectively, and they are not statistically different. The proportions of daily smokers among the aged 20 to 22 are similar between the legal smoking age restrictions, as well. Hence, the legal age restriction appears to have some impact on when to start smoking. Overall, the figure suggests that some young people experiment smoking and then pick up the habit of smoking by the age of 18 to 19 years old. This can be looked at a different way.

Figure 5 shows the cohort specific profiles of the rates of daily smokers during this period for the selected cohorts. For example, the blue line refers to the changes in the daily smoking rates for those who were 15 to 17 years old in 1999, as they grew older.[17] The rate of daily smokers among 15 to 17 years old in 1999 was 15.2%, and it jumps to 20.4% when they were 18 to 19 years old in 2002, and stays around 18% when they were 20 to 22 years old in 2004 and when they were 23 to 24 years old in 2007. The cohort of 2003 (that is, those who were 15 to 17 years old in 2003) starts at a much lower smoking rate (around 9%), and then increases to 13.5% when they were 18 to 19 years old in 2006, and to 17.6% when they

---

[17] The age groups provided in CTUMS are 1) 15 to 17 years old, 2) 18 to 19 years old, 3) 20 to 22 years old, 4) 23 to 24 years old, and so on. So I am not able to follow each age group over time precisely. The graph is created to follow each cohort to match their age over time to the given age group as much as possible. For example, Cohort 1999 (in blue) plots the proportion of daily smokers who were 15 to 17 years old in 1999, its proportion when they were 18 to 19 years old in 2002, its proportion when they were 20 to 22 years old in 2004, and its proportion when they were 23 to 24 years old in 2007. The graphs for Cohort 2003 and Cohort 2007 are created similarly.

were 20 to 22 years old in 2008. In 2011 when they were 23 to 24 years old, it went down to 15%. The cohort of 2007 starts even at a lower smoking rate when they were 15 to 17 years old in 2007 than the earlier cohorts. It increases as they age, but the rates are lower than the earlier cohorts.

As briefly mentioned with respect to Figure 2, another important aspect of smoking behaviours is how much smokers smoke in a given period. The more one smokes, the more one is exposed to toxic chemicals such as tar and carbon monoxide. Hence, it increases the likelihood of one's health problems in the future.

Also more smoking means more nicotine, addictive substance, into the body, and thus it becomes harder and harder to reduce smoking and/or quit smoking.

Figure 6 and 7 show the changes of the intensity of smoking among smokers from 1999 to 2012 for the young and the old, respectively. The proportions of light smokers, moderate smokers and heavy smokers are fairly constant over this period for the young smokers. The majority of the young smokers are light smokers.

On the other hand, the trends in the intensity of smoking for smokers who are more than 25 years old are slightly different. The majority of smokers were heavy smokers before 2003 (more than 40% of the older smokers) and after that, the number of light smokers has increased towards the end of this period. The figures seem to suggest that, even though the overall number of the young smokers has been declining, the proportions of the light, moderate, and heavy young smokers did not change over time.

One important caveat is that the CTUMS is a cross-sectional survey, and thus, I am not able to follow the same individual over time. That is, I am not able to interpret that a light young smoker will always be a light smoker over time.

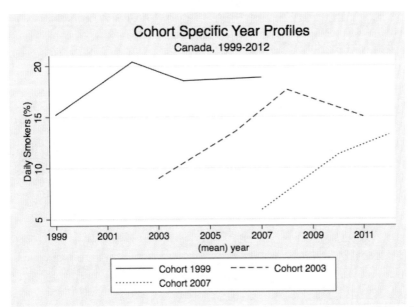

Source: Author's calculation based on Canadian Tobacco Use Monitoring Surveys, 1999 to 2012. Each line follows the changes in the proportion of daily smokers of the selected cohort. For example, Cohort 1999 refers to the proportion of daily smokers aged 15 to 17 in 1999, and then follows them when they were 18 to 19 years old in 2001, and so forth.

Figure 5.

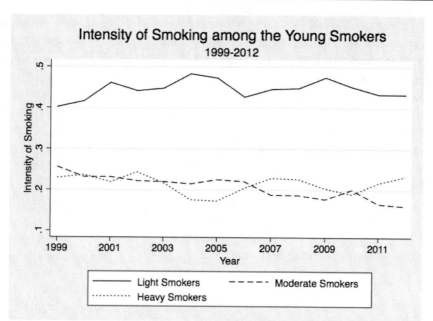

Source: Author's calculation based on Canadian Tobacco Use Monitoring Surveys, 1999 to 2012. Health Canada defines those who smoke less than 10 cigarettes per day as a light smoker, those who smoke between 10 and 19 cigarettes per day as a moderate smoker, and those who smoke more than 20 cigarettes per day as a heavy smoker.

Figure 6.

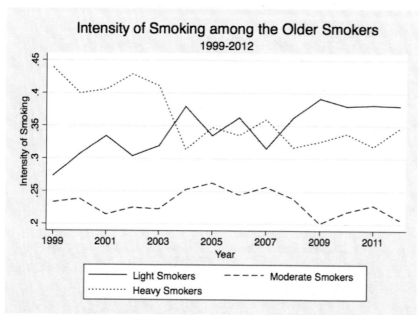

Source: Author's calculation based on Canadian Tobacco Use Monitoring Surveys, 1999 to 2012. Health Canada defines those who smoke less than 10 cigarettes per day as a light smoker, those who smoke between 10 and 19 cigarettes per day as a moderate smoker, and those who smoke more than 20 cigarettes per day as a heavy smoker.

Figure 7.

Overall, less and less young people are picking up the habit of smoking, and this is good news. For the young smokers, there seems to be a fixed proportion of light smokers, moderate smokers, and heavy smokers during this period. For the older smokers, there seems to be a declining trend of heavy smokers. Of course, there are many possible reasons for this change. Many public policies are aimed at discouraging the young people to smoke. For instance, a high tax rate on cigarettes can discourage people to smoke.

More and more smoking bans are imposed in the public spaces in Canada. It could be the case that the younger generation has a different preference on smoking compared to the older generation, which could be influenced by the public education through various channels. To evaluate each possible reason for this change and to provide a better understanding of the smoking behaviours among the young is beyond scope of this article.

Instead, I review the literature on the youth smoking to help understand this change in the next section.

4. PUBLIC POLICIES RELATED TO SMOKING

Given the negative relationship between smoking and health, understanding the effects of public policies aimed at discouraging people not to smoke, and/or to quit smoking is important.

In this section, I review the two common policies that are aimed at discouraging people to smoke, focusing especially on young people: taxes and smoking restrictions.[18]

4.1. Taxes

One of the well-researched areas related to smoking behaviours is to understand how people respond to changes in the price of cigarettes: elasticity of smoking. If we know well how people respond to the price changes, then we will be confident about how much reduction in smoking rates occurring when a further tax is imposed. Moreover, besides the health effects of tobacco products, the government in many countries are historically interested in taxing those products for the tax revenues. Partly because tobacco products are addictive, people will not decrease much of their consumption when the price increases, and hence the governments can increase the tax revenues by increasing the tax rate. Thus it is natural for the government to utilize an existing infrastructure (i.e., the tax system) in order to discourage people from smoking. To do so effectively, we need to know how smoking behaviours change in response to price/tax changes.

Many early studies from the 1980's and 1990's show the elasticity of smoking ranging from -0.3 to -0.5 (see Chaloupka and Warner (2000), and the references therein). That is, when the price of cigarettes increases by one percent, smoking will be decreased by 0.3 to 0.5 percent. With respect to the youth smoking elasticities, Lewit et al. (1981) and Lewit and Coate (1982) showed that young people are more responsive to the price/tax changes than the older people in the United States in the 1960's and 1970's. This result made sense because, for example, tobacco products are addictive and the young accumulated less of the smoking

---

[18] For broader issues related to the economics of smoking, see Chaloupka and Warner (2000).

habits than the adults, and thus the adults are less responsive to the price/tax changes than the young. There are several other possible reasons for this as well. For example, peer pressures are larger among the young than the grown-ups. Hence, with a higher price, less young people smoke, which in turn, further reduce peer smoking. Also the young have less income than the adults, which makes the young people more sensitive to the price changes of their consumption products in general.

However, in the early 1990's, upon availability of new data, Wasserman et al. (1991) indicates that the smoking behaviours with respect to the elasticity of cigarette smoking may have changed over time. They show that smoking behaviours are becoming more responsive to the price/tax. That is, the elasticity estimates are insignificant with the older portion of their data, but in 1988, they estimated the elasticity of smoking to be -0.283. Moreover, the elasticity of the youth smoking was statistically not significant. That is, their results indicate that we cannot expect the tax is effective in reducing the number of young smokers.

Since Wasserman et al. (1991), many researchers further investigated the smoking behaviours in response to the price/tax. Some studies show that the young is more responsive to the price and tax, as in the early research, while the other studies show that smoking behaviours of the young are not sensitive to the price/tax changes. For instance, Chaloupka and Wechsler (1997), Townsend (1987), Chaloupka (1991), Lewit et al. (1997), Taurus and Chaloupka (1999) showed that the young was more responsive to the price changes than the adults, similar to the earlier research. On the other hand, for example, Douglas (1998), and DeCicca, Kenkel and Mathios (2002) showed that the young did not respond to the price/tax changes.

So far the above mentioned evidence is mainly from the U.S. Now I turn to the Canadian literature on the youth smoking behaviours and taxes, although the number of studies is somewhat limited partly because of the data availability. First, Gruber, Sen and Stabile (2003) estimated the elasticity of smoking to be -0.45 to -0.47 for all ages. Hence, the general elasticity estimates are similar to the one from the other countries. Regarding to the youth smoking, Sen, Ariizumi and Driambe (2010) estimated that the elasticity of smoking participation for the aged 15 to 19 years old is -0.1 to -0.3. That is, when the tax on cigarettes increases by ten percent, the estimated elasticity suggests that the number of smokers aged 15 to 19 years old will decrease by one to three percent. Furthermore, the very young (aged 10 to 14 years old) were much more responsive to the tax changes. Sen and Wirjanto (2010) also estimated the similar elasticities with the different data set. More interestingly, Sen and Wirjanto (2010) had an access to the data that follow the same individuals over time. Using this portion of the data when people in Ontario experienced roughly 50% reduction in the provincial excise tax, they estimated the elasticity of smoking participation to be -0.2 to -0.5 among those who were non-smokers before this tax cut and became smokers after it. Hence, they conclude that the tax as a policy instrument to discourage the young people from smoking may only have a small effect.

Overall, the results in the literature suggest that the effectiveness of an increase in the tobacco taxes to reduce youth smoking may be limited given, especially the high tax rates imposed on the tobacco products.

4.2. Smoking Restrictions

Smoking bans in the public places and at work are quite common nowadays. These restrictions are aimed directly at discouraging people from smoking. It is important to understand how effective such restrictions in reducing smoking among the young people as an alternative policy instrument, along with taxes. In this section, I review the effectiveness of such restrictions on the smoking behaviours in Canada.

Lanoie and Leclair (1998) estimated that tax elasticity is -0.28, while the regulation on smoking is not statistically significant. For the subgroup of the population, tax is insignificant, but the regulation reduced smoking. Carpenter (2009) investigated the local workplace smoking laws in Ontario, and found that for the blue-colour workers, the laws reduced exposures to the environmental tobacco smoke by 28 to 33 percent. However, the results were statistically insignificant for the other types of workers. Carpenter, Postolek, and Warman (2011) showed that the restriction did not reduce smoking rates, but it did reduced the exposures of the environmental tobacco smoke in the public places, especially in bars and restaurants. Moreover, they did not find evidence that those smokers did not increase smoking at home.

The smoking restriction in the public places does not target the young people. It is targeted to the general population. There are some movements towards imposing smoking restrictions to reduce smoking exposures by children. For examples, several provinces in Canada imposed the restriction of smoking in the vehicles with children. Nguyen (2013) found that the restriction reduces smoking exposures by children in the car, and moreover, it did not increase smoking at home after the restrictions were imposed. That is, the smokers did not substitute their choice of smoking places between inside the car and at home.

Although the number of studies on the effectiveness of the anti-smoking restrictions is somewhat limited, it appears that such restrictions does not necessarily discourage smokers to quit smoking, but can reduce the exposure to smoking in the public places.

4.3. Other Related Issues on the Youth Smoking

There are many other issues related to smoking behaviours and public policies. Chaloupka and Warner (2000) provides a good detailed summary of the related issues. In this section, I review some important issues related to the youth smoking.

First, proper information regarding the negative health effects of smoking is important, and the young people tend to over- and/or under-estimate what they are getting into. Hence, providing proper information can improve the young people's decisions with regard to smoking. For example, the government can provide a health warning of smoking by making a mandatory to print the negative health effect of smoking in each cigarette package. Gospodinov and Irvine (2004) investigated the effect of such a health warning on smoking behaviours, and found that it did not reduce much smoking. Sabbane, Lowrey and Chebat (2009) studied what types of warning labels have impacts on the non-smoking adolescents' attitudes towards smoking, and found that the graphic label was most effective among the Canadian participants to their survey.

Another important issue with the youth smoking behaviours is the influence by friends, and family members. For example, even if one does not want to smoke, he/she may feel a peer pressure, and hence starts smoking despite his/her wish. It is probably easy for anyone to understand this possibility. However, it is not that easy to quantify such peer effects. Nonetheless, a few important contributions exist in the Canadian context. Krauth (2005) showed that the peer effect is an important determinant of the youth smoking behaviours. Although, taking into account of the fact that each young individual is different (that is, some are influenced by the others easily, and others are not), the peer effects are smaller than the ones found in the literature. Sen (2010) also showed that the peer effect, as well as the influence by the family member, is an important factor for the youth smoking behaviour.

Lastly, but not the least, addiction is a very important aspect of tobacco products. For example, Figure 5 can be seen as some working of the addictive nature of smoking for the Canadian youth. Note that Figure 2-4 show that the proportion of young daily smokers is declining from 1999 to 2012. However, Figure 5 shows that the proportions of light smokers, moderate smokers, and heavy smokers among the young are fairly fixed during this period.[19]

Many researchers devote their time and efforts into a better understanding of the smoking behaviours in relation to addiction (see the section in Chaloupka and Warner (2000) for the details and the references therein). However, empirical research in the Canadian context in this aspect is rather limited partly because the models are highly complex, and the available data may not be suitable for this kind of exercises. One notable exception is Auld (2005). He found that smoking is highly addictive on average for the Canadian youth.

However, if he looks at those who started smoking early (before 14 years old in his analysis), it is not as addictive as to the other group of young people. That is, his finding shows that there are selections into early initiation of smoking: those who are more immune to the addictive nature of smoking tend to start smoking early. Hence, his evidence suggests that public policies aimed at discouraging smoking can indeed reduce smoking on average for the young Canadian, but the effects may not be as large as suggested in the conventional models that do not take into account of the selection.

CONCLUSION

The proportion of daily smokers among the young has been declining since 1999, and it is less than ten percent in 2012. Less and less young generation starts picking up the habit of smoking during this period. Pinning down reasons for this change is beyond scope of this article. However, as discussed, policies aimed at discouraging smoking may be at work. For example, taxes imposed on tobacco products remain high during this period. Smoking ban in the public places is also wide-spread. Also perception that smoking is seriously harmful to our health probably becomes a norm among the young people. This article focused on cigarette smoking among the young. There are many alternatives to cigarettes: smokeless tobacco and e-cigarettes, for instance. Some of them can be used to help quitting smoking, as well. Hence, those alternatives can contribute reducing the number of smokers. However, e-cigarettes are getting the popularity. For instance, the sales of e-cigarettes will be over $1 billion in 2013, more than double of 2012.[20] Although e-cigarettes are marketed as a safer

---

[19] Since the Canadian Tobacco Monitoring Surveys are cross-sectional data, they do not follow the same individuals over time. Hence, I am not able to say definitely that the addiction is the mainly reason for this figure.

[20] Taken from http://www.cnbc.com/id/100991511, as of January 2014.

product than cigarettes, it seems that many health experts are concerned because of the chemical contents in e-cigarettes. Nonetheless, it appears too early to judge the safety concern of the e-cigarettes.

REFERENCES

Auld, C. (2005), Causal effect of early initiation on adolescent smoking patterns. *Canadian Journal of Economics*, 38(3):709-734.

Baliunas, D., Patra, J., Rehm, J., Popova, S., Taylor, B., (2007). Smoking-attributable morbidity: acute care hospital diagnoses and days of treatment in Canada, 2002. *BMC Public Health*, 7:247, doi:10.1186/1471-2458-7-247.

Carpenter, C. (2009). The Effects of Local Workplace Smoking Laws on Smoking Restrictions and Exposure to Smoke at Work. *Journal of Human Resources*, 44(4):1023-1046.

Carpenter, C., S. Postolek, C. Warman (2011). Public-place smoking laws and exposure to environmental tobacco smoke (ETS). *American Economic Journal: Economic Policy*, 3(3):35-61.

Chaloupka, F. J. (1991). Rational addictive behavior and cigarette smoking. *Journal of Political Economy*, 99(4):722-742.

Chaloupka, F. J., H. Wechsler (1997). Price, tobacco control policies and smoking among young adults. *Journal of health economics*, 16(3):359-373.

Chaloupka, J., K. E. Warner (2000). The economics of smoking. In The Handbook of Health Economics, Culyer, A. J., Newhouse, J. P., (Eds). Elsevier: Amsterdam, 1539-1627.

DeCicca, P., Kenkel, D., Mathios, A., (2002). Putting out the fires: Will higher taxes reduce the onset of youth smoking? *Journal of Political Economy*, 110(1): 144-169.

Douglas, S. (1998). The duration of the smoking habit. *Economic Inquiry*, 36(1):49-64.

Gospodinov, N., Irvine, I. (2004). Global health warnings on tobacco packaging: Evidence from the Canadian experiment. *Topics in Economic Analysis and Policy*, 4(1):1-21.

Gruber, J., Sen, A., Stabile, M., (2003). Estimating price elasticities when there is smuggling: the sensitivity of smoking price in Canada. *Journal of Health Economics*, 22(5): 821-842.

Harrison, G. (2003). Cigarette smoking and the cost of hospital and physician care. *Canadian Public Policy*, 29(1):1-20.

Health Canada (2014), http://www.hc-sc.gc.ca/hc-ps/tobac-tabac/research-recherche/indust /_sales-ventes/canada-eng.php, Retrieved January 10, 2014.

Jones, A, Gublis, A, Baker, E.,H., (2010). Differences in tobacco use between Canada and the United Staties. *Int. J. Public Health*, 55(3):167-75.

Krauth, B. (2005). Peer effects and selection effects on smoking among Canadian youth. *Canadian Journal of Economics*, 38(3):735-757.

Lanoie, P., P. Leclair, M., (1998). Taxation or regulation: looking for a good anti-smoking policy. *Economics Letters*, 58(1):85-89.

Lewit, E. M., Coate, D., Grossman, M., (1981). The effects of government regulation on teenage smoking. *Journal of Law and Economics*, 24(3):545-569.

Lewit, E. M., Coate, D., (1982). The potential for using excise taxes to reduce smoking. *Journal of Health Economics*, 1(2): 121-145.

Lewit, E. M., Hyland, A., Kerrebrock, N., Cummings, K. M., (1997). Price, public policy and smoking in young people. *Tobacco Control,* 6(S2):17-24.

Nguyen, H. (2013). Do smoke-free laws work? Evidence from a quasi-experiment. *Journal of Health Economics,* 32(1):138-148.

Sabbane, L., Lowrey, T. , Chebat, J.-C., (2009). The effectiveness of cigarette warning label threats on non-smoking adolescents. *Journal of Consumer Affairs,* 43(2): 332-345.

Sen, A. (2009). Estimating the impacts of household behavior on youth smoking: evidence from Ontario, Canada. *Review of Economics of the Household,* 7(2): 189-218.

Sen, A., Ariizumi, H., Driambe, D., (2010). Do changes in cigarette taxes impact youth smoking? Evidence from Canadian provinces. *Forum for Health Economics and Policy,* 13(2): Article 12.

Sen, A., Wirjanto, T., (2010). Estimating the impacts of cigarette taxes on youth smoking participation, initiation, and persistence: empirical evidence from Canada. *Health Economics,* 19(11):1264-1280.

Taurus, J. A., Chaloupka, F. J., (1999). Price, clean indoor air laws, and cigarette smoking: Evidence from longitudinal data for young adults. *NBER working paper,* 6937.

Townsend (1987). Cigarette tax, economic welfare, and social class patterns of smoking. *Applied Economics,* 19:355-365.

U.S. Department of Health and Human Services (2010). How Tobacco Smoke Causes Disease: What It Means to You. Atlanta: U.S. Department of Health and Human Services, Centers for Disease Control and Prevention, National Center for Chronic Disease Prevention and Health Promotion, Office on Smoking and Health.

Wasserman, J., Manning, W. G., Newhouse, J. P., Winkler, J. D., (1991). The effects of excise taxes and regulations on cigarette smoking. *Journal of Health Economics,* 10(1): 43-64.

In: Smoking Restrictions
Editor: Nazmi Sari

ISBN: 978-1-63321-148-3
© 2014 Nova Science Publishers, Inc.

Chapter 5

How Long Do Japanese Mothers Stop Smoking When They Start Raising Children? New Evidence from a Very Large National Survey[*]

Seiritsu Ogura, Ph.D.,[†] *and Sanae Nakazono*[#]
Institute on Aging, Economics Department, Hosei University,
Tokyo, Japan

Abstract

The exposure of children to secondhand smoke at home and elsewhere has been a largely overlooked problem in Japan, regardless of well spread knowledge about the health risks of secondhand smoke exposure to children. Furthermore, evidence and studies are limited and little is known about the relationship between smoking behavior and socio-economic factors in Japan. In this research, our broad perspective is to identify the important risk factors of women's smoking. We first focus on the mother, who has the greatest impact on her children's health. Thus, our main interest here is to demonstrate the mothers' behavior during the first year after the birth of a child.

We also address the association between women's smoking behavior from several different points of view including their characteristic, family or social environments. Using various years of the Comprehensive Survey of Living Conditions, and multivariate logistic regressions, we show that mothers cessation of smoking after delivery is unstable in Japan, depending on the age and the parity of a child. For a first child, more than two-thirds of women who used to smoke abstain from smoking at least for one year. For a second child, compared with a first child, only half of the mothers quit temporarily in the

---

[*] This research is funded by the Ministry of Education, Culture, Sports, Science and Technology in Japan under grant number 22000001 (principal investigator professor Noriyuki Takayama). The permission to use Survey of Living Conditions for this research is given to Seiritsu Ogura by the Ministry of Health, Labor and Welfare. All statistics in this research using the Survey are based on Ogura's own computations, and they do not necessarily coincide with official tabulation results. This chapter is based on part of the Last Lecture of Seiritsu Ogura, given on December 17, 2013.
[†] E-mail: sogura@hosei.ac.jp
[#] E-mail: sanae.miyazawa.26@stu.hosei.ac.jp

first year. In both cases, cessation efforts declined rapidly over time. By the time a mother has a third child, she barely quits smoking. Although an increasing proportion of mothers are quitting in the first year, the difference narrows considerably in subsequent years. We also found that, among Japanese women, such factors as marital status, husband's smoking status, and other smokers in the household are strongly related to smoking, while job-types, living with head of household's parents, and housing have differential impacts.

1. INTRODUCTION

The exposure of children to secondhand smoke at home and elsewhere has largely been an overlooked problem in Japan. Unlike many other external problems, this problem must be solved at home, because the most serious risk usually comes first from their mothers, second from fathers, and then from the rest of the family members. The purpose of this paper is to focus on the changes in the smoking behavior of a mother as her child grows older, at the same time identifying relevant individual and socio-economic factors that affect the prevalence of smoking in women of child-bearing age (between age 20 and 45).

For children, the health risk of mothers' smoking is the greatest during their pregnancy. It has been known for some time that smoking during pregnancy increases such risks as perinatal death, premature birth, spontaneous abortion, congenital anomaly and lower birth weight (e.g. ASH, 2011; U.S. Department of Health and Human Services, 2006). In spite of these established findings, in Japan, even the physician's response was very late in coming. After declaring its intention in 2007 to join the tobacco free movement, in 2011, Japanese Association of Obstetricians and Gynecologists finally revised its Practice Guideline. The guideline now mandates its member physicians to ask questions on the smoking status of a pregnant woman, to give a clear answer, if asked, on the harmful effects to the pre-born baby of her own and others smoking, to give her directions to stop her own and her partner's smoking, and to avoid secondhand smoke (Minakami et al., 2011).

It is fair to say that, prior to 2000, the Japanese government, most notably the powerful Ministry of Finance, in cooperation with Japan Tobacco Company, a giant partially government-owned monopoly, dragged its feet in warning the general public on the risks of tobacco smoking. Even collecting information on tobacco exposure had been a virtual taboo in national surveys, leaving pre-born children or new born children unprotected for decades. In spite of this, it turned out that, since 1990, in a little known national survey called National Growth Survey of Infants and Children, conducted only once in ten years, the Ministry of Health and Welfare (MHLW) has quietly started to ask a set of questions on the smoking of mothers and fathers/co-residents during pregnancy.

According to this survey, the proportions of smoking mothers during pregnancy almost doubled from 5.5% in 1990 to 10.0% in 2000, but fell suddenly to 5.0% in 2010. In the meantime, the proportion of unknowns, which had been 0.1% in 1990 and 0.2% in 2000, suddenly increased to 2.8% in 2010.

On average, as the survey is taken one year after the birth, and by the public health officials, however, there is some question as to the reliability of the data (Ohida et al., 2007)[21].

A prime example of the government's belittling of tobacco problems, we believe, is its smoking statistics. Using their average smoking rate of women, for example, would be very misleading in estimating the risk of secondhand smoke to children in Japan. There are a small number of solid evidences that point to a considerable downward bias in women's smoking rates in government statistics. This bias was first exposed by a survey conducted by Meiji Yasuda Life Insurance (MYLI) (Akiyama et al., 2000). The MYLI survey covered more than four million adults who purchased their life insurance policies between 1993 and 1998, getting responses from more than 96% from them.

The survey is considered to be free of unacceptability bias which we will discuss shortly, because the questions were cleverly added at the bottom of the insurance notification page, giving them an appearance of a part of the insurance notification.

The differences in smoking rates were substantial; for example, in 1997 MYLI's data, smoking rate of the women in their 20's was 27.0%, instead of 21.3% of the MHLW, and that of women in their 30's was 26.1%, instead of 15.6% of MHLW[22]. In our view, two problems, one technical and the other substantive, account for this downward bias in MHLW statistics.

The technical issue is simply a shortcoming in their sampling process. The official smoking rate statistics are computed from the samples of the National Health and Nutrition Survey (Nutrition Survey). Each year, MHLW selects only 300 survey districts in stratified random sampling for this survey. They correspond to only 0.015% of the survey districts of the National Census, and only 0.007% of Japanese households[23]. Municipal public-health officials of these districts distribute questionnaires to every household in the district, but manage to get responses from less than 70% of the households. Moreover, the response rates have huge variations across districts. If the response rates are higher in low smoking-rate districts/households, and lower in high smoking-rate districts/households, they are bound to get a sample mean much lower than the true population mean.

This bias is not corrected. Judging from the discrepancy between the results of high quality surveys like MYLI or two of Ohida's, which we will discuss shortly, this must be what has been happening.

The second problem is the unacceptability bias, a tendency to under-report socially undesirable activities in social surveys.

A number of recent studies have successfully shown that smoking is significantly under-reported among pregnant women in the U.S., in Europe, and in Japan (e.g. England et al., 2007; Ford et al., 1997; George et al., 2006; Jung-Choi et al., 2012; Kang et al., 2013; Ohashi,

---

[21] Recent studies seem to point out much higher rates than National Growth Survey's 5.0%. For example, a recent large-sample (N>5,000) study by Sasaki et al. (2011) shows that 14% of pregnant mothers were smokers in the third trimester of gestation, although their data set is limited to Hokkaido, a prefecture with one of the highest women's smoking rates. A small-sample study (N=125) by Yamashita (2012), using data from Nara prefecture, shows that 19% of women in early stages of pregnancy (10.6 ± 1.9 weeks) were smokers. According to a report by Ohashi (2009) using data from Hyogo prefecture, smoking rate was 22.6% in the early stage of pregnancy, and 15.5% in the late stage (N=460).

[22] Unfortunately, two surveys used two different definitions of smokers, making a simple comparison difficult. The MYLI's definition of smokers included those who had quit smoking within the last 12 months, while MHLW classifies them as non-smoking, ex-smokers.

[23] The number of survey districts of 2000 National Census was 939,537. Each survey district of the National Census is divided into two survey districts in Survey of Living Conditions and Nutrition Survey.

2009; Shipton et al., 2009; Yamashita)[24,25]. In Japan, however, the unacceptability bias in smoking is neither a new problem, nor limited to pregnant women. It is an old problem for the general population of women as smoking had been considered a socially unacceptable behavior for them[26]. Although the bias has been disappearing rapidly during the last decade, the older data must contain substantial under-reporting. In what follows, first, we will review the findings of the previous studies on Japanese mother's smoking, including those on smoking during pregnancy. We will pay close attention to the quality of data used, and we will argue that there is no conclusive study yet on the mother's smoking behavior after delivery. Then, we will proceed to explain the methods of our analysis, followed by the results and the discussion. Finally, we will state our conclusions and their implications next.

2. BACKGROUND AND SMOKING PREVALENCE IN JAPAN

Motivated by mounting concerns regarding the increasing prevalence of smoking among pregnant women in Japan, a large number of research papers have been published in medical journals during the last few decades. The statistical bases and findings of quality papers are summarized in the well-cited two review papers, the first one by Kurumatani et al. (1998), and the second one by Kubo and Emisu (2007). Together they reviewed 39 research papers on the topic spanning four decades, from 1965 to 2007. It is not surprising to find that the estimated prevalence rates in the reviewed papers vary substantially, as their sample sizes are typically small, usually covering narrow regions, and taken at non-uniform timing. Nevertheless, if we look at the ten papers published since 2000, they are distributed in a surprisingly narrow range. More specifically, without weighing by sample sizes, the pre-conception average smoking rate is 25.5%, and its standard deviation is 3.6%. The average smoking rate during pregnancy is 8.6%, with its standard deviation at 1.6%. Excluding Ohida's two papers to be discussed shortly changes the figure little; only the pre-conception standard error changes from 3.6% to 4.4%, but the other figures remain unchanged.

Since 2000, other than the above-mentioned National Growth Survey, we have found two nation-wide surveys that can serve as our benchmarks. Both surveys were conducted by Ohida and his associates, first in 2002 and then in 2006. Each time more than one percent of pregnant Japanese women receiving prenatal care were in their samples. They found out that, in 2002, 24.6% of would-be mothers had been smoking before they knew they were pregnant. After learning about their pregnancy, only 10% of pregnant women continued to smoke. In the 2006 survey, the pre-conception smoking rate was 25.7%, and the smoking rate during pregnancy was 7.5%. Their findings are quite informative for a number of reasons.

---

[24] As Connor Gorber et al. (2010) has noted, according to Fendrich et al. (2005), "increased public concerns about the dangers of active and passive smoking have strengthened the perception of smoking as a socially undesirable behavior, which could further undermine the validity of self-reported estimates".

[25] In Yamashita (2012), 11 out of 24 smokers claimed non-smoker status, and in Ohashi (2009), 78 out of 128 smokers claimed non-smoker status in early stages of pregnancy. Yamashita's samples were from just one hospital that gives strong messages for non-smoking to pregnant women, and Ohashi's data were collected as a part of the municipal prenatal checkups. On the other hand, in Sasaki et al. (2011), only 134 out of 709 smokers claimed non-smoker status, which is in line with a majority of literature in Europe or US.

[26] In other parts of Asia, a similar point has been made. (Barraclough 1999 for Indonesia, Chun et al., 2006 and Chung et al., 2010 for Korea).

First, their pre-conception smoking rates of 25% are much higher than the government smoking rates of women in these two years, but similar to those obtained by Akiyama et al. (2000) and the 8 other studies that appeared since 2000, surveyed by Kubo and Emisu (2007). This gave us a very good reason to suspect a downward bias in the national smoking rate statistics of MHLW. Second, their percentages of continued smokers are slightly higher than, but within one standard error of the average (8.6±1.6%) of the 8 other studies in the 2000-2007 period, mentioned above.

Third, the proportions of continued smokers are much smaller, and those of abstainers are much larger, than those reported in Europe and in the US (Cnattingius et al., 1992; Fingerhut et al., 1990; Hannover et al., 2002; Lelong et al, 2001; McLeod et al., 2003)[27]. Also Ohida found that higher education reduces the prevalence of smoking during pregnancy, as previous studies in Europe or the U.S. had found.

And finally, they found that two thirds of the pregnant women are exposed to secondhand smoke either at home or at work, but 80% of the smoke is coming from their husbands.

After giving birth, however, many Japanese mothers who quit, resumed smoking (Yasukouchi et al. 2006, Yasuda et al. 2013[28]), although not quite as quickly as in those in Western Europe or in U.S. (e.g. Colman et al., 2003; Lelong et al., 2001; Polanska et al., 2011; Solomon et al., 2007. Of course, infants and small children are vulnerable to secondhand smoke, too. The smoke increases such risks as the overall mortality, sudden infant death syndrome, respiratory infections, asthma, neurobehavioral disorders, obesity, hyper-tension, diabetes (e.g. Kabir et al., 2011; Linnet et al., 2005; Montgomery et al., 2002; Oken et al., 2005; Toschke et al., 2003; Williams et al., 1998; Yolton et al., 2005). According to a report of the Surgeon General (2006), in the U.S., almost 60% of children between 3 years old and 11 years old are exposed to secondhand smoke. We could find no comparable public information on the extent of such exposure of Japanese small children[29]. As a first step toward this goal, we will utilize the Comprehensive Survey of Living Conditions to analyze the smoking behavior of a Japanese mother starting from the delivery of her first child, until the time her third child reaches 18 years old. Using the Comprehensive Survey has several advantages over other possible alternatives.

First of all, as we have explained earlier, using MHLW statistics on smoking rates as proxies for children's exposure at home would lead to a considerable underestimation of the risk. In Figure 1, we have compared the MHLW smoking rates and JT smoking rates of women with the smoking rates of women in Comprehensive Surveys of corresponding years. The 95% confidence intervals of the latter are also shown in the figure but they are so narrow that they are hardly visible. It is clear that both nationally representative smoking statistics, particularly those of MHLW, are below those of Comprehensive Surveys.

---

[27] According to Colman and Joyce (2003), "Although the prevalence of smoking 3 months before pregnancy was stable at around 26%, quitting during pregnancy rose from 37% to 46% between 1993 and 1999". In France, Lelong et al found the smoking rate before pregnancy was 40%, but "Among the women smoking before pregnancy, about 40% quit during pregnancy (p.335)".

[28] Using a data from Fukuoka prefecture (N=191), Yasukouchi et al. (2006) found that the smoking rate was 23.1% when women learned about pregnancy, 7.9% during pregnancy, and 14.7% in four months after delivery. On the other hand, Yasuda et al. (2013) found, in their own national survey, much lower relapse rates among the quitters; the relapse rate is 22.5% in 3~4 months, 43.5% in 18 months, and 51.4% in 36 months.

[29] The only exception is the Kaneita et al. (2006) but their results are only for those born in 2001.

Another advantage is the rich socioeconomic information of the survey that we will be able to draw in our analysis. Such socioeconomic information, if available, will help us precisely identify the children at risk, and help design the efficient public intervention.

In Japan, until very recently, research on the effects of socioeconomic factors on smoking had been very difficult; in the first place, in large-scale national surveys, inclusion of questions on smoking behavior had been a virtual taboo, and in the second place, inclusion of questions on income and education, key socioeconomic indicators in health related behaviors, had been regarded as very difficult. The Comprehensive Survey of Living Conditions had been no exception. This survey was started in 1986, and has been conducted once in every three years with a sample of almost a quarter of a million households. It was not until 2001 when questions about smoking and drinking were added. It was only in 2010 that the survey included questions on education levels.

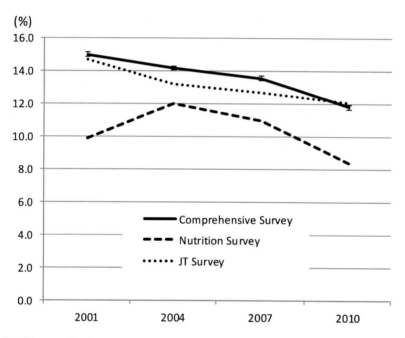

Figure 1. Smoking rate by 3 surveys.

Before we leave this survey for analysis, let us introduce some of the previous studies on the effects of socio-economic factors on the smoking behaviors of Japanese men and women. These are summarized below.

- Nakamura et al. 1994 used the forth Survey of Cardiovascular Disease conducted by MHW in 1990 (8916 samples) on general population. They analyzed regional and age group differences in the smoking prevalence of male and female populations, separately. They found significant age-group differences in the male population, but significant urban-rural differences in the female population.
- In another study, Ohida et al. (2001) utilized the Active Survey of Health and Welfare, conducted by MHW in 1996 (34,464 samples). They found out that the smoking rate of men is higher in rural communities, but the smoking rate of women

is higher in urban communities. Another interesting finding is that as household size increases, the smoking rate of women decreases.

- Ohida and his research associates conducted their own national surveys twice, first in 2002, then in 2006, on pregnant women receiving prenatal checkups. Sample sizes were 16,528 in 2002 and 19,650 in 2006, estimated to be equal to 1.4% of all pregnant women in 2002 and to 1.8% in 2006. In their 2002 survey, 500 medical institutions were randomly chosen from the list of 989 regular survey point institutions designated by the Association of Obstetricians and Gynecologists (AOG). In the 2006 survey, they asked all 940 survey point institutions to participate. The questionnaires were filled by the patients at their first prenatal checkup visits in the waiting rooms of the participating medical institutions (260 in 2002, 344 in 2006). There were no responses from one third of the contacted institutions in both surveys. The proportion of cooperating institutions went down from 56% in 2002 to 37% in 2006, probably as a result of a prominent criminal case against an obstetrician.

- Fukuda et al. (2005b) used the 2001 Comprehensive Survey to analyze the influence of individual socioeconomic factors on smoking. As they utilized income information, their sample size was limited to about 40,000 individuals. For women, they found a strong relationship between smoking and lower income, and strong effects of living with smokers and in urban areas. For younger women, having a job and being married have significantly positive effects. A second study (Fukuda et al. 2005a) examined the relationship between six "risk behaviors", including smoking and excessive drinking, and individual characteristics (age, marital status, work and household income). They found that for both men and women, divorce, employment, sales and service jobs, and lower household income are associated with a higher likelihood of risk behaviors, including smoking. They also found that higher per capita income in women was significantly associated with smoking and other risk behaviors. Another interesting finding was the marked regional differences in smoking rates that were observed in women, but not in men.

- Kaneita et al. (2006), using the very first survey of Longitudinal Survey of Newborns in the 21st Century[30], examined the effects of socio-economic factors on the mother/father's smoking behavior at 6 months after delivery. Based on 44,562 samples, they found the prevalence of smoking among the mothers and the fathers were 17.1% and 63.5%, respectively, and the percentage of mothers and fathers who smoked indoors were 12.1% and 36.2%. They pointed out that factors such as young age, smoking spouse, infants having many siblings, the mother not breastfeeding, and lower income are significantly related to parental indoor smoking. They concluded that passive smoking is common among Japanese infants and further public health measures should be taken.

---

[30] The subjects of the first survey were 53,575 babies born in 2001 and the questionnaires were mailed when babies reached 6 months old. The questionnaire covered babies' weight and height, parity, number of people who live together, parent's job, working hours and income, breastfeeding and so on. A total of 44,562 questionnaires (83.2%) were used in Kaneita et al., (2006).

3. METHODS

3.1. Data Sources

Our data set comes from four different survey years (2001, 2004, 2007, 2010) of Large Scale Comprehensive Survey of Living Conditions. This survey has been conducted by the Ministry of Health, Labour and Welfare since 1986. The Large Scale Survey is conducted once in every three years, and it consists of four different questionnaires: 1) household questionnaire, 2) health questionnaire, 3) long-term care questionnaire, and 4) income questionnaire. The questions on smoking status were added to the health questionnaire for the first time in 2001. Each time, MHLW randomly selected more than 5 thousand survey districts out of more than 930,000 survey districts of the National Census. None are repeated in consecutive surveys. Thus each large scale Comprehensive Survey provides a random cross-sectional data of about 0.6% of Japanese population, translating to 280-290 thousand households, and 750 thousand individuals, respectively. Actually, the average response rate of the Survey of these four years is 81.7%, giving us a total of 2,556,159 samples. Males account for 1,228,865, and females account for 1,327,474. The exact numbers and response rates are shown in Appendix Table A.1 and Table A.2.

Public health officials of the selected districts then distribute 1) household questionnaire and 2) health questionnaire to every household in their districts. On the other hand, the sample-sizes of 3) long-term care questionnaire and 4) income questionnaire are much smaller, because their survey districts are randomly selected from those for 1) and 2). In fact, the income questionnaire covers only 1,000 districts and hence, using the income or asset variables would have resulted in losing 13 out of every 15 possible samples in our sampling. We decided not to pay this price for income information, and to keep a much larger sample size for our empirical analysis.

3.2. Major Variables

The dependent variable in our analysis captures the smoking status of the participants. There are four categories for smoking status in the survey: 1) I do not smoke, 2) I smoke every day, 3) I smoke occasionally, and 4) I quit smoking more than one month ago. In this paper, 1) and 4) are defined as non-smokers and 2) and 3) are defined as smokers.

We also include a set of socio-economic variables in the analysis. Age, region, marital status, type of job, husband's smoking status, smokers in the same household other than the husband, living together with own or spouse's parents, health checkups, cancer checkups, age and parity of children, house-type, size of house, and household expenditure are included. We excluded self-reported health status and mental health status, subjective symptoms for possible endogeneity problem, but we included health checkups as measures for risk aversion. We excluded education level, because the question appeared for the first time in 2010 and we would have had only one-year samples.

4. SAMPLE SELECTION AND STATISTICAL ANALYSIS

As we have explained above, the survey data we have used are random samples collected in the same way, once in every three years, from the same population. In order to get the most precise estimators possible and test the statistics with the most power, we pooled all of them as an independently pooled cross section data to maximize our sample size. Compared with other studies on smoking prevalence among Japanese women, the sample size of our data is several times larger. We believe this is the strength of our study.

The purpose of our analysis is to isolate the important risk factors of women's smoking that are attributable to their own characteristics, family or social environments. In order to simplify this task, we have selected only women who are either heads of households or spouses of the head of households. If one regards a single woman as a single household, in a sense, the unit of our analysis is not an individual but rather a household.

Assuming that the maximum childbearing age is 45 years old, we have limited our samples to women born between 1938-1989. Furthermore, although the Comprehensive Survey asks questions on smoking status to anyone above 12 years old, we have chosen only those at age 20 or above. This is to minimize the possibility of misclassification of smoking status in self-reports, since the legal minimum age of smoking is age 20.

We estimated a saturated logistic regression. Our dependent variable is the binary smoking status which is equal to 0 for a nonsmoker and equal to 1 for a smoker. All our explanatory variables are indicator variables representing the individual or household characteristics, or their categories. We control women's ages by five-year age class dummy variables, and women's birth cohorts by five-year periods starting from 1936-1940 dummy variable. Besides age and birth year, the only continuous variables in our list of control variables are monthly household expenditure (in equivalent scale) and the floor size of the dwelling. Both of them are converted first to quintile categorical variables, and then to dummy variables of each category. In order to control the birth cohort effects and year effects, birth-year cohort dummy variables and survey year dummy variables are added. To analyze the time-effects, many variables interacted with survey years.

The software we used for estimating the logistic regression equations is Stata13 MP(4). Following the estimation, we computed the average marginal effects (AMEs) of the variables of our model using its *margins* command. For variables that interacted with survey year dummies, we computed their marginal effects of representative values (MERs).

Although marginal effects at means (MEMs) have been widely used, recently, the average marginal effects (AMEs) are becoming very popular, too. The MEMs measure the effects of the change in a given indicator variable, setting the other variables at their mean values. On the other hand, AMEs are obtained as the average of the marginal effects at each observation (by controlling the rest of the variables at their actual values). When substantial variability is suspected across different groups, computing marginal effects at representative values (MER) is recommended (Williams, 2012). We have followed this recommendation for variables crossed with survey years. We note here that in Stata 13, the MER option gives us confidence intervals as well.

5. RESULTS AND DISCUSSION

5.1. Main results

The descriptive statistics are shown in Appendix Table A.3. Limiting the samples to households with a woman who is either a head of household, or a spouse of household head, reduced the samples to 789,092 from 926,716. Excluding samples with missing values of explanatory variables, and outside the age and birth cohort restrictions, our sample size was reduced to 443,391[31].

In Appendix Table A.4., the results of logistic regression analysis for females are shown. In Table 1, the marginal effects of the variables are shown.

Table 1. Average marginal effects

	Delta-method dy/dx	SE	Z	P>|z|	95% CI	
Birth-cohort by 5-year (reference=1975-1979)						
1935-1939	-0.099	0.007	-14.93	0	-0.112	-0.086
1940-1944	-0.092	0.006	-15.3	0	-0.104	-0.080
1945-1949	-0.076	0.006	-13.1	0	-0.087	-0.065
1950-1954	-0.063	0.005	-11.63	0	-0.074	-0.052
1955-1959	-0.042	0.005	-8.11	0	-0.052	-0.032
1960-1964	-0.022	0.004	-4.97	0	-0.031	-0.014
1965-1969	-0.023	0.004	-5.94	0	-0.030	-0.015
1970-1974	-0.010	0.003	-3.19	0.001	-0.016	-0.004
1980-1984	-0.019	0.004	-4.74	0	-0.027	-0.011
1985-1989	-0.062	0.005	-11.37	0	-0.073	-0.051
Survey year (reference=2001)						
2004	-0.007	0.002	-4.63	0	-0.010	-0.004
2007	-0.010	0.002	-6.21	0	-0.013	-0.007
2010	-0.018	0.002	-9.37	0	-0.022	-0.014
Age group (reference=20-29)						
30-39	-0.005	0.003	-1.82	0.068	-0.011	0.000
40-49	-0.003	0.004	-0.66	0.507	-0.011	0.005
50-59	-0.013	0.005	-2.53	0.011	-0.023	-0.003
60-69	-0.027	0.006	-4.49	0	-0.039	-0.015
>70	-0.065	0.008	-7.84	0	-0.081	-0.049
Job category (reference=no work)						
Specialist	-0.007	0.002	-4.08	0	-0.010	-0.003
Management	0.041	0.005	7.82	0	0.031	0.051
Clerical	-0.012	0.002	-7.91	0	-0.015	-0.009

---

[31] One observation was dropped in the logit regression because of predicted failure.

	Delta-method				95% CI	
	dy/dx	SE	Z	P>|z|		
Sales	0.037	0.002	17.76	0	0.033	0.042
Services	0.051	0.002	29.73	0	0.048	0.055
Security	0.012	0.012	1	0.318	-0.011	0.035
AFF*	-0.032	0.003	-9.4	0	-0.039	-0.026
Production	0.019	0.002	9.81	0	0.015	0.023
Others	0.017	0.004	4.67	0	0.010	0.024
Marital status (reference=married)						
Unmarried	0.005	0.004	1.46	0.143	-0.002	0.012
Widow	0.016	0.004	3.95	0	0.008	0.023
Divorced	0.103	0.005	22.7	0	0.094	0.111
Living with parents (reference =0)						
Head of household's	-0.023	0.001	-16.22	0	-0.026	-0.020
Spouse's	-0.003	0.003	-1.14	0.256	-0.009	0.002
Number of smokers in household excluding husband (reference =0)						
1	0.045	0.002	24.94	0	0.042	0.049
2	0.076	0.004	18.22	0	0.068	0.084
3	0.091	0.014	6.69	0	0.064	0.117
4	0.140	0.048	2.92	0.003	0.046	0.234
5	(not estimable)					
Husband's smoking status (reference= no husband)						
Not smoke	-0.093	0.003	-29.42	0	-0.099	-0.086
Everyday	0.042	0.004	11.76	0	0.035	0.050
Sometimes	-0.055	0.005	-11.22	0	-0.064	-0.045
Ex-smoker	-0.090	0.004	-23.85	0	-0.098	-0.083
Health check-up	-0.024	0.001	-21.12	0	-0.026	-0.022
Cancer check-ups						
Stomach	-0.004	0.002	-2.05	0.04	-0.007	0.000
Uterus	-0.019	0.001	-13.45	0	-0.022	-0.016
Breast	-0.028	0.002	-16.06	0	-0.031	-0.024
Colon	-0.022	0.002	-11.39	0	-0.026	-0.018
House-type (reference=owner-occupied housing)						
Rented (private)	0.039	0.002	22.46	0	0.035	0.042
company-provided	-0.021	0.002	-8.56	0	-0.026	-0.016
Rented (public)	0.058	0.002	23.83	0	0.053	0.063
Others	0.036	0.003	10.82	0	0.029	0.042
Area of floor -quintile (reference=lowest)						
2	-0.007	0.001	-4.82	0	-0.010	-0.004
3	-0.012	0.002	-7.14	0	-0.016	-0.009
4	-0.020	0.002	-10.57	0	-0.023	-0.016
5	-0.030	0.002	-15.36	0	-0.034	-0.027

Table 1. (Continued)

		Delta-method					
		dy/dx	SE	Z	P>|z|	95% CI	
Household expenditure-quintile (reference=lowest)
2		-0.005	0.002	-3.19	0.001	-0.008	-0.002
3		-0.007	0.002	-4.31	0	-0.010	-0.004
4		-0.008	0.002	-5.1	0	-0.012	-0.005
5		-0.003	0.002	-1.73	0.083	-0.006	0.000
Omit region dummy
Child age	Parity						
0-2 month	1st	-0.141	0.014	-10.33	0	-0.168	-0.115
	2nd	-0.053	0.012	-4.63	0	-0.076	-0.031
	3rd	-0.008	0.014	-0.58	0.56	-0.035	0.019
3-5 month	1st	-0.115	0.010	-11.04	0	-0.135	-0.094
	2nd	-0.042	0.009	-4.48	0	-0.060	-0.024
	3rd	-0.026	0.014	-1.86	0.063	-0.054	0.001
6-8 month	1st	-0.103	0.009	-10.83	0	-0.121	-0.084
	2nd	-0.041	0.009	-4.48	0	-0.059	-0.023
	3rd	-0.020	0.013	-1.5	0.133	-0.047	0.006
9-11 month	1st	-0.069	0.008	-8.26	0	-0.086	-0.053
	2nd	-0.042	0.009	-4.51	0	-0.060	-0.024
	3rd	-0.028	0.013	-2.18	0.029	-0.053	-0.003
One	1st	-0.054	0.004	-12.61	0	-0.063	-0.046
	2nd	-0.026	0.005	-5.6	0	-0.036	-0.017
	3rd	-0.008	0.006	-1.19	0.235	-0.020	0.005
Two	1st	-0.037	0.004	-8.96	0	-0.045	-0.029
	2nd	-0.017	0.004	-3.94	0	-0.026	-0.009
	3rd	0.000	0.006	0.06	0.951	-0.012	0.013
Three	1st	-0.035	0.004	-8.31	0	-0.043	-0.027
	2nd	-0.014	0.004	-3.33	0.001	-0.023	-0.006
	3rd	0.001	0.006	0.14	0.89	-0.011	0.013
Four	1st	-0.022	0.004	-5.5	0	-0.030	-0.014
	2nd	-0.008	0.004	-2.02	0.043	-0.016	0.000
	3rd	0.000	0.006	-0.05	0.964	-0.013	0.012
Five	1st	-0.010	0.004	-2.58	0.01	-0.018	-0.002
	2nd	-0.002	0.004	-0.5	0.615	-0.010	0.006
	3rd	0.006	0.006	0.92	0.357	-0.006	0.018
6-12 year		-0.001	0.001	-0.7	0.483	-0.003	0.001
13-18 year		-0.003	0.001	-2.94	0.003	-0.005	-0.001

* Agriculture, Forestry and Fisheries

To the best of our knowledge, in Japan, so far no studies have tried to systematically analyze the effect of children's age on parent's smoking. Unfortunately, since the Survey of Living Conditions does not ask any questions about pregnancy, there is nothing to contribute on women's smoking during pregnancy. Some physicians argued that pregnancy provides a natural opportunity for smoking women to quit, particularly in the early stage of pregnancy when many suffer from nausea and vomiting (Yasukouchi and Sata 2006, 2008). Partly due to this, and partly due to medical consultations, family persuasions and social pressures, there is a consensus that at least half, and possible more than two thirds, of smoking women quit during pregnancy (Yasuda et al 2013, Ohida et al. 2007, Kaneita et al. 2007, Kurumatani et al. 1998, Kubo and Emistu, 2007). The cessation, however, may not always last throughout the pregnancy as recent studies on unacceptability bias among the Japanese pregnant women suggest (Yamashita 2012, Sasaki 2011).

Once a baby is born, however, the Survey provides information on the baby's age (by year as well as by month) and its order of birth in the family. We can evaluate the effects of the age and the parity of the baby on the mother's smoking behavior, at the same time controlling for the other socio-economic variables of the family. In order to detect the possible effects of time during the first 12 months after birth, at first we examined the effect of the baby's age in months. In spite of the fact that we have more than 16,000 zero-year-old babies in our sample, after controlling for the survey years and birth-cohorts, the resulting fluctuations in coefficients were still difficult to interpret. Hence we took a quarter of a year (three months) as our unit of measurement for baby's age in its first year. Our findings are summarized in Table 2 and Table 3.

Table 2. Average marginal effect of age (month) and parity by year

Age(month)	0-2		3-5		6-8		9-11	
			1st Child					
2001	-9.2%	***	-9.1%	***	-9.9%	***	-4.7%	***
2004	-12.3%	***	-13.0%	***	-7.5%	***	-5.7%	**
2007	-18.7%	***	-9.7%	***	-10.5%	***	-7.4%	***
2010	-16.5%	***	-14.9%	***	-12.7%	***	-10.1%	***
Average	-14.1%	***	-11.5%	***	-10.3%	***	-6.9%	***
			2nd Child					
Age(month)	0-2		3-5		6-8		9-11	
2001	-2.1%		-3.8%	*	-2.5%		-4.5%	**
2004	-6.4%	*	-2.8%		-4.0%	*	-2.8%	
2007	-6.7%	**	-4.7%	*	-3.2%		-3.3%	
2010	-6.7%	*	-5.2%	*	-7.1%	**	-6.0%	**
Average	-5.3%	***	-4.2%	***	-4.1%	***	-4.2%	***
			3rd Child					
Age(month)	0-2		3-5		6-8		9-11	
2001	-0.6%		-2.1%		-6.4%	*	-5.6%	*
2004	-1.9%		-2.2%		1.4%		0.6%	
2007	-2.1%		-6.7%	*	-2.6%		-1.6%	
2010	1.2%		0.7%		0.9%		-3.7%	
Average	-0.8%		-2.6%		-2.0%		-2.8%	*

* $p < 0.05$ ** $p<0.01$ *** $p<0.001$.

Table 3. Smoking rate of children's age (month) and parity by year

1st Child

Age(month)	0-2	3-5	6-8	9-11
2001	13.6%	13.8%	13.5%	18.6%
2004	8.1%	8.1%	12.6%	14.5%
2007	4.3%	9.5%	9.5%	11.4%
2010	3.9%	4.4%	5.7%	7.2%
Average	7.9%	9.3%	10.6%	13.2%

2nd Child

Age(month)	0-2	3-5	6-8	9-11
2001	18.2%	17.2%	18.8%	15.0%
2004	10.4%	14.4%	14.0%	15.4%
2007	9.5%	11.5%	11.8%	12.4%
2010	6.6%	9.1%	8.1%	9.0%
Average	11.8%	13.3%	13.5%	13.1%

3rd Child

Age(month)	0-2	3-5	6-8	9-11
2001	20.3%	16.5%	12.3%	13.9%
2004	15.7%	17.6%	22.2%	20.0%
2007	15.6%	12.4%	16.0%	18.8%
2010	15.5%	15.9%	17.6%	13.0%
Average	16.9%	15.5%	16.6%	16.2%

First, there are several things to note in Table 2;

- There is a clear evidence of a relapse in the mother's smoking cessation in the third and fourth quarters after the birth of her first baby. For example, in 2010, a first baby in its first or second quarters after birth would have reduced its mother's smoking rate by 16.5 and 14.9 percentage points respectively. The effect would have fallen to 12.7 percentage point in the third quarter, and to 10.1 percentage point in the fourth quarter, respectively. In other words, one out of three mothers who had quit before pregnancy, restarted six months after giving birth to first babies. Our result seems to agree with the existing Japanese literature, although it is limited to the first baby.
- Quitting rates for the first baby, particularly in the first two quarters, seem to be increasing in the last decade, subject to fluctuations. For instance, in 2001, a first baby in its first quarter would have reduced the mother's smoking rate by 9.2%, but, a similar baby in 2010 would have reduced it by 16.5%. This is probably a result of increasing public awareness on the harmful effects of second hand smoking on infants.
- As the cessation rate of the mother is smaller from the very beginning for the second baby, it does not seem to decline much in the course of the first year. For a second baby born in 2010, the corresponding negative effects are 6.7% points, 5.2% points, 7.1% points, and 6.0% points, respectively for 1st, 2nd, 3rd and 4th quarter after its

birth. Thus the mothers quitting rate does not seem to have a clear downward trend for the second baby.
- For a third baby or a baby of higher order, it seems that a smoking mother barely makes an attempt to quit. Her smoking rates in the first four quarters are almost indistinguishable from the general female smoking rate. A natural interpretation of this result is self-selection; namely, those who can quit have already quit during the two previous pregnancies and thereafter, and only the most addicted mothers are still smoking. Alternatively, by the time of a third baby, her addiction has become so entrenched that it can no longer be removed even for a limited time.

The smoking rates of mothers in the first year, at various ages (by month), and the parity of a child are shown in Table 3. Very good news is that the most recent survey (2010) suggests that a significant reduction has taken place in the mothers' smoking rate for a first child and a second.

In fact, for a first child, less than 5% of mothers were smoking in the first two quarters, compared with almost 14% of mothers during the same periods in 2001. The reduction in the smoking rates in its fourth quarter is equally impressive; in 2010, it was 7.2% compared with 18.6% in 2001. For a second child, the proportions of smoking mothers were higher than for a first child by 2% points or so, but they were still less than 10%. In contrast, for a third child, even in 2010, more than 15% of mothers were smoking in the first three quarters.

After the first year, our results are summarized in Table 4 and Table 5. For the first child aged zero, one, two, three, four and five years old, according to the latest (2010) survey, the probability of mothers to smoke **decreases** by 12.9%, 6.4%, 4.3%, 2.4%, 2.2% and 2.1%, respectively (Table 4).

Moreover, when compared with women with no children, the prevalence of smoking among women who have a first baby less than one year old is lower by almost 14% points, implying that more than two thirds of women who used to smoke abstain from smoking for at least a year. In the second year, around one half of the women who had quit (12.9% minus 6.4%, or 6.5%) resumed smoking, and in the third year, about one third of the remaining women who had quit (6.4% minus 4.3%, or 2.1%) resumed smoking, and so on. In six years after the birth, the cessation-effects have virtually disappeared.

The marginal effects of a first child are considerably different from those of a second child, or a third/higher order child. According to the latest survey (2010), the marginal effects of a second baby are -6.2%, -2.7%, -2.3%, -1.2%, -2.2% and +0.7%, at its zero, one, two, three, four and five-year-old period, respectively.

Thus compared with the first child, only half of the smoking mothers quit temporarily for the second baby in the first year. Then, in its second year, almost 60% of those that quit began to smoke again. In six years, the cessation effect disappears. Our results also indicate that by the time a mother has a third baby, she barely quit smoking.

The figures in the table also show an increasing trend for quitting immediately after delivery. For example, for a first child less than a year old, only 5.5% of mothers smoked in 2010, compared with 10.5% in 2001.

Table 4. Average marginal effect of age and parity by year

1st child

Age	Zero		One		Two		Three		Four		Five	
average	-10.1%	***	-5.4%	***	-3.7%	***	-3.5%	***	-2.2%	***	-1.0%	*
2001	-8.0%	***	-3.4%	***	-2.1%	**	-2.6%	***	-1.8%	*	-0.3%	
2004	-9.0%	***	-4.6%	***	-3.6%	***	-4.1%	***	-2.5%	**	0.3%	
2007	-10.5%	***	-7.4%	***	-5.0%	***	-5.0%	***	-2.5%	**	-1.8%	*
2010	-12.9%	***	-6.4%	***	-4.3%	***	-2.4%	**	-2.2%	**	-2.1%	*

2nd child

Age	Zero		One		Two		Three		Four		Five	
average	-4.3%	***	-2.6%	***	-1.7%	***	-1.4%	**	-0.8%	*	-0.2%	
2001	-3.3%	***	-4.1%	***	-1.3%		-2.1%	**	-0.2%		-1.9%	*
2004	-3.7%	**	-0.9%		-2.7%	**	-1.2%		-0.3%		0.1%	
2007	-4.3%	***	-2.3%	*	-0.9%		-1.0%		-0.6%		0.7%	
2010	-6.2%	***	-2.7%	**	-2.3%	*	-1.2%		-2.2%	*	0.7%	

>3rd child

Age	Zero		One		Two		Three		Four		Five	
average	-1.9%	**	-0.8%		0.0%		0.1%		0.0%		0.6%	
2001	-3.6%	**	-1.1%		-0.1%		1.5%		1.6%		0.5%	
2004	-0.3%		-0.2%		1.2%		-1.3%		1.5%		0.2%	
2007	-3.0%	*	-1.3%		1.2%		0.6%		-2.7%	*	-0.5%	
2010	-0.2%		-0.2%		-2.0%		-0.9%		-0.3%		2.1%	

* $p < 0.05$ ** $p<0.01$ *** $p<0.001$

The percentages of mothers smoking at various ages of a child (between zero and five years old) are shown in Table 5.

Table 5. Smoking rate of children's age and parity by year

			1st child			
Age	Zero	One	Two	Three	Four	Five
2001	15.0%	20.4%	20.6%	18.6%	18.9%	20.4%
2004	11.1%	16.2%	16.7%	15.3%	16.7%	20.2%
2007	9.1%	11.4%	12.9%	13.0%	15.5%	16.5%
2010	5.5%	10.1%	11.1%	12.7%	13.4%	12.9%
Average	10.5%	15.0%	15.7%	15.1%	16.3%	17.6%

			2nd child			
Age	Zero	One	Two	Three	Four	Five
2001	17.2%	16.2%	19.4%	18.9%	21.4%	18.8%
2004	13.9%	18.1%	16.2%	18.3%	19.9%	19.5%
2007	11.4%	14.1%	16.4%	17.2%	18.6%	20.1%
2010	8.3%	12.4%	13.1%	14.7%	13.7%	17.5%
Average	13.0%	15.2%	16.4%	17.3%	18.6%	19.0%

			>3rd child			
Age	Zero	One	Two	Three	Four	Five
2001	15.6%	20.1%	20.9%	21.7%	21.6%	20.1%
2004	19.1%	19.6%	19.8%	18.0%	21.5%	18.7%
2007	15.8%	18.2%	21.8%	20.4%	16.1%	18.8%
2010	15.6%	17.2%	15.8%	16.5%	17.4%	20.8%
Average	16.3%	18.8%	19.5%	19.5%	19.3%	19.7%

The difference narrows substantially for a one–year-old baby as 10.1% of mothers were smoking in 2010, compared with 15.0% of mothers in 2001. For a second child, the difference starts at around 5% in 2010, with 8.3% of mothers smoking, compared with 13.0% of mothers in 2001. For a third child, the difference is less than 1%, with 15.6% of mothers smoking, compared with 16.3% in 2001.

Thus, although in the beginning the differences are wider, the difference either narrows considerably even for a first child, or vanishes for a second and third child. As we have just shown, a number of studies in the US and in Europe have already found that a mother is more likely to quit for her first baby (Cnattingius et al., 1992; Kvalvik et al., 2008; Paterson et al., 2003). However, in Japan, this result has not yet been established (Imamura et al., 2001; Kaneko et al., 2008; Kubo et al., 2011; Suzuki et al., 2010).

There were a few studies that showed the propensity, but their data was not national and their sample sizes were relatively small (Akaike et al. 1986, Suzuki et al. 2005). Only Kaneita et al.(2006) showed, using the first wave of Survey of Babies in the 21st Century (a national panel data of 53,575 samples), that a second or third baby gives a higher ratio of adjusted odds of the mother's smoking habit compared with a first one. But their samples were taken when the babies were 6 months old, and they did not provide differential marginal effects of the parities of babies.

Thus, our study is the first to show the complete relationship between smoking behavior of women and her children's age and parity in Japan.

Moreover, our findings contradict what Fukuda et al. (2005b) had conjectured: according to them, "For women aged 25 to 39 years, marital status did not show a significant association with smoking. For men in the same age group, being married was significantly and positively associated with smoking.

Although the events of pregnancy and child bearing are related to the chance of smoking cessation (22-24), this study suggests the possibility that these events do not promote smoking cessation in the Japanese population." We have shown that pregnancy and child bearing affects the smoking habits of mothers, but behavior depends on the parity of the baby and time after the birth.

5.2. Additional Results Based on Other Control Variables

After controlling for cohort effects, age-effects, job-types, family effects, and coefficients of the year, dummies show that there are only small negative effects still unaccounted for in the four waves of Survey of Living Conditions (2001-2010).

Coefficients of birth-year dummies indicate that the peak of the female smoking prevalence had been achieved by women born between 1975 and 1980, followed by a sudden decline in subsequent cohorts.

In fact, in all the cohorts born before 1975, the smoking rates had been increasing by 2% points per each five-year cohort. In cohorts born after 1985, however, the smoking rate dropped by almost 6% points for each five-year cohort. In Japan, Marugame et al. (2006) examined the smoking trends by birth cohorts from 1900 and 1977, but they had not found the peak for women then.

Thus, our study is the first one to show that the increasing prevalence of smoking among Japanese women finally ended in the cohort born between 1975 and 1980.

After controlling for the other factors, once we control the cohort effects, the effect of age seems to be very small in female smoking behavior. In fact, our results show that the proportions of female smokers remain almost constant in their 30's and the 40's, but starts to decline a little in the 50's (-1.3% points) and modestly in the 60's (-2.7%). It is not until they reach age 70 when a substantial number of women start quitting.

With respect to marital status, the unmarried have a small, but statistically insignificant, higher risk of smoking compared with married women, but the divorced women have the highest risk of smoking, exceeding the married women by almost 9 percentage points. From the point of view of children, having mothers who experienced a divorce increases their risk of secondhand smoke exposure very substantially.

The widowed women, on the other hand, do not seem to be statistically different from married women in terms of smoking risk. Thus, if women who are divorced have children, their children have to face much greater risk of secondhand smoke. In protecting children from secondhand smoke, it is important to pay special attention to such groups as children in single mother households.

We have found almost no study that examined the effects of marital status on smoking by women in Japan, except Fukuda's article (who used the same dataset as ours). In contrast, Nystedt (2006) revealed the strong connection between marital life and smoking behavior. He stated that divorced people are more likely to smoke and getting a divorce is related to initiation of smoking, particularly for women. Moreover, the lowest cessation rates are observed for newly divorced women.

Also Lee et al. (2005) pointed out that compared with women who remained married, women who are divorced/widowed have more than a twofold greater risk of relapsing/starting smoking. In Korea, never-married, widowed and divorced women aged 25-54 showed an increased risk of smoking compared to married women (Cho et al., 2008).

As to jobs, those who work in agriculture and forestry have the lowest risk of smoking among the working female groups, followed by clerical staff, and by specialists. These three job-holders have lower risks than non-workers. In contrast, those whose jobs are characterized as "service jobs" have the highest risk of smoking, more than 5% points higher than non-workers, followed by "management" (+4.1% points), "sales" (+3.7% points), and production-line, communication and transportation workers (+1.9% point). Not surprisingly, the characteristics of these risky jobs/industries coincide with the findings of Fukuda et al. (2005a) who used part of the same data. In contrast, in Korea, according to the results of Cho et al. 2013, among the three categories of jobs (non-manual, manual and service), service workers show a higher risk of smoking than manual workers, and manual workers show a higher risk than non-manual workers.

There is a considerable amount of evidence that women's smoking behavior is strongly influenced by that of her partner's (Daly et al., 1993; Dollar et al,. 2009; Homish et al., 2005; Kahn et al., 2002; Sutton 1993,)[32]. Our results also show that smoking behaviors of husbands and wives are closely correlated.

Compared with a woman without a husband, the risk of a married woman increases substantially if her husband is a regular smoker (+4.2% points), but the risk decreases substantially if he is a non-smoker (-9.3% point), or an ex-smoker (-9.0% point). The risk also decreases significantly if he is an occasional smoker (-5.5% points). These results do not necessarily prove causal relationships, as non-smoker men are highly likely to marry non-smoker women, and smoker women who leave often marry smoker men.

We also looked into the effect of smokers other than the husband, if any, in the same household. We found that an increase in number of smokers in the household elevates the risk significantly.

One smoker in the household increases the risk by 4.5% points, two smokers by 7.6% points, three smokers by 9.1% points, and four smokers by 14.0% points[33].

One of the interesting and subtle points is the asymmetric effect of three-generation households on women's smoking: living with the parents of the heads of household reduces

---

[32] Although there is a considerable amount of literature on the smoking behaviors in married couples focusing on pregnant or postpartum women (e.g. Mcbride et al., 1998; Mullen et al., 1997; Nafstad et al., 1996; Severson et al., 1995). Similar studies also exist in Japan (e.g. Kaneko et al. 2008, Kouketsu et al. 2010, Suzuki et al. 2010, Bando et al. 2013, Imamura et al. 2011).

[33] Fukuda et al. (2005b) examined the effect of other smokers in household on smoking status by different age groups and showed significant association between other smokers and smoking status.

the smoking risk, but living with the parents of the spouses does not have a statistically significant effect.

Since an overwhelming majority of the women in our sample are not heads of household but spouses, these results imply that living with parents-in-law discourages her smoking, but living with own parents does not have a similar negative effect[34]. One of the most important factors for pregnant Japanese women to quit smoking, according to Ohida et al. (2001), is the advice given by other family members. Our results suggest that, holding the number of smokers in the family constant, while spouses cannot completely ignore the advice coming from their parents-in-law, they can ignore those coming from their own parents.

We looked at the effects of different types of residences on smoking. Compared with the owner-occupied housing, most types of rented housing tended to increase the risk of smoking. Another interesting finding of ours is that the company-provided housing decreases the risk of smoking compared with owner-occupied housing. It seems likely that wives living in company-provided housing are very conscious of their neighbor's eyes and try to avoid a socially unacceptable behavior as smoking.

With respect to health check-ups, those who have had health check-ups or cancer check-ups (except lung-cancer check-up) have lower prevalence of smoking. Although the sizes of these effects are moderate, around 2% (except 0.4% for stomach cancer) point each, they are statistically quite significant. These results are consistent with what the theory of health capital predicts; a risk-averse individual tends to invest in health-checkups and cancer-checkups and avoid risk behaviors. We note in passing that lung-cancer checkups would work in the opposite direction: in fact, the women who had check-ups have a higher risk of smoking (around 2% points).

The strong causal relationship between smoking and lung cancer has been so well-known that smokers are conscious of their own higher risk and have a lung cancer checkup as a secondary preventive measure. For this reason, we have removed this variable from the list of our regressors.

As we have explained at the outset, using income information would have reduced the size of our sample to 1/7.5 of what we are using. We traded away the luxury of income information for the sample size, believing that the household expenditure in the previous month would be sufficient for our purpose.

In so doing, just as the equivalent scale in income, we have adjusted our household expenditure by the square root of the household size[35]. Based on the equivalent scale expenditure, we have computed their quintile index and used the dummies to control for the income.

With a reference to the lowest expenditure group, all the other groups except for the highest one were less likely to smoke. According to Fukuda et al. (2005b), income was the strongest predictor of smoking and the odds ratios would become smaller as income increased on the basis of lowest income group.

Since our equivalent scale expenditure produces similar effects as their equivalent scale income, we can safely say that household expenditure could be used instead of household income.

---

[34] However, Ohida and et al. (2000) observed that more non-smoking wives tend to form three-generation households, as percentage of former smoker in three-generation households are similar to the other households.
[35] Fukuda used "OECD equivalence scale" but we used the latest "Square root scale").

CONCLUSION

This chapter employed a nationally representative survey data and examined the smoking behavior of Japanese mothers, paying close attention to their children's age and their birth orders. Thanks to the survey's large sample size, and high quality, we were able to obtain much more precise estimators with more statistical power compared to any other previous studies.

We have found that mothers smoking cessation status after delivery is quite unstable in Japan, depending on the age and the parity of a child. Based on the comparison with women with no children, we estimated that for a first child, more than two-thirds of women who used to smoke would abstain from smoking at least for one year. In the second year, around one half of the abstainers resume smoking, and in the third year, about one third of the abstainers resume smoking, and in six years after the birth, the first-child effect virtually disappears. For a second child, compared with a first child, only half of the mothers quit temporarily in their first year.

Then, in the second year, almost 60% of those who quit restart, and in six years, the second-child effect disappears. By the time a mother has a third baby, she barely quit smoking.

We have noticed, in the first decade of this century when the Japanese government started its public campaign against public smoking for the first time, there began an increasing trend for quitting among Japanese mothers immediately after delivery. The phenomenon was particularly pronounced for the first child, less so for a second child, and almost none for a third. Although in the beginning the changes are large, they seem to narrow rapidly as time goes on even for a first child, or vanishes for a second in five years. In fact, our estimation suggests that in 6 years after delivery, mothers return to the smoking habits of their cohort's.

We also found that, among Japanese women, such factors as marital status, husband's smoking status, other smokers in household are strongly related to smoking, while job-types, living with head of household's parents, and housing have differential impacts on their smoking.

There are several limitations in our analysis. First of all, as the survey data we used is not a longitudinal survey, it is inherently difficult to evaluate changes over time. We hope to have overcome much of this difficulty by controlling sample years, birth cohorts, regions, and parities, using the rich socio-economic information and the large sample-sizes of our data. But they are not perfect substitutes for a longitudinal survey.

Another limitation is that our analysis focuses only on women or mothers. From the point of view of secondhand smoke exposure of children, the husbands' smoking also affects their health significantly. A research focusing on both husbands and wives is clearly needed and we intend to carry out one shortly.

The most substantial limitation is that our statistical analyses are based on the self-reported smoking status of the survey. As we have explained at the outset, there are good reasons to suspect that a substantial proportion of Japanese women hide their true smoking status. We had no alternative but to take the self-reports at their face values.

Nevertheless, our statistical work is a considerable improvement over the official statistics as reported in Figure 1.

APPENDIX TABLES

Table A.1. Sample size of survey

(number of household)

Survey year	Number of survey objectives	Number of objects responded	Response rate	Number of objects tabulated*
2001	282,999	247,278	87.4%	247,195
2004	276,682	220,948	79.9%	220,836
2007	287,807	230,596	80.1%	229,821
2,010	289,363	229,785	79.4%	228,864
Total	1,136,851	928,607	81.7%	926,716

* excluding house which were unable to tabulate

Table A.2. Number of male and female by survey year

Survey year	Male	Female	Total
2001	338,997	364,402	703,399
2004	297,661	321,912	619,573
2007	299,936	324,232	624,168
2010	292,091	316,928	609,019
Total	1,228,685	1,327,474	2,556,159

Table A.3. Descriptive statistic

	2001 N	2001 %	2004 N	2004 %	2007 N	2007 %	2010 N	2010 %	Total N	Total %
Birth-cohort by 5-year										
1935-1939	5,905	4.99	4,640	5.14	4,710	4.01	4,069	3.47	19,324	4.36
1940-1944	17,734	14.97	13,820	15.31	15,041	12.79	13,101	11.19	59,696	13.46
1945-1949	19,558	16.51	14,739	16.33	17,735	15.09	15,989	13.65	68,021	15.34
1950-1954	18,440	15.57	13,250	14.68	16,854	14.34	15,896	13.57	64,440	14.53
1955-1959	14,787	12.48	10,654	11.8	13,868	11.8	13,681	11.68	52,990	11.95
1960-1964	13,546	11.44	9,753	10.81	12,747	10.84	12,769	10.9	48,815	11.01
1965-1969	12,532	10.58	9,015	9.99	12,346	10.5	12,554	10.72	46,447	10.48
1970-1974	10,323	8.72	8,525	9.45	12,157	10.34	12,818	10.94	43,823	9.88
1975-1979	4,747	4.01	4,290	4.75	7,930	6.75	9,092	7.76	26,059	5.88
1980-1984	874	0.74	1,573	1.74	3,326	2.83	5,023	4.29	10,796	2.43
1985-1989	0	0	0	0	842	0.72	2,138	1.83	2,980	0.67
Age group										
20-29	12,594	10.63	6,695	7.42	7,562	6.43	6,617	5.65	33,468	7.55
30-39	25,417	21.46	17,835	19.76	23,244	19.77	21,330	18.21	87,826	19.81
40-49	31,315	26.44	20,574	22.79	25,374	21.58	25,189	21.51	102,452	23.11
50-59	38,080	32.15	28,078	31.11	34,702	29.52	29,307	25.02	130,167	29.36
60-69	11,040	9.32	17,077	18.92	26,674	22.69	29,525	25.21	84,316	19.02
70-79	0	0	0	0	0	0	5,162	4.41	5,162	1.16
Total	118,446		90,259		117,556		117,130		443,391	

Table A.3. (Continued)

		2001 N	2001 %	2004 N	2004 %	2007 N	2007 %	2010 N	2010 %	Total N	Total %
Job category	No work	49,104	41.46	38,440	42.59	48,620	41.36	50,234	42.89	186,398	42.04
	Specialist	12,722	10.74	10,140	11.23	15,567	13.24	15,426	13.17	53,855	12.15
	Management	1,676	1.41	1,107	1.23	1,224	1.04	1,323	1.13	5,330	1.2
	Clerical	14,301	12.07	10,611	11.76	15,248	12.97	14,676	12.53	54,836	12.37
	Sales	10,002	8.44	7,615	8.44	6,891	5.86	6,280	5.36	30,788	6.94
	Services	13,080	11.04	9,947	11.02	15,607	13.28	15,180	12.96	53,814	12.14
	Security	484	0.41	227	0.25	112	0.1	89	0.08	912	0.21
	AFF*	3,021	2.55	2,565	2.84	2,883	2.45	2,777	2.37	11,246	2.54
	Production	12,136	10.25	8,118	8.99	8,685	7.39	8,073	6.89	37,012	8.35
	Others	1,920	1.62	1,489	1.65	2,719	2.31	3,072	2.62	9,200	2.07
Marital status	Married	100,709	85.03	77,162	85.49	98,927	84.15	97,387	83.14	374,185	84.39
	Unmarried	7,712	6.51	4,674	5.18	6,588	5.6	6,449	5.51	25,423	5.73
	Widow	4,002	3.38	3,773	4.18	5,352	4.55	6,219	5.31	19,346	4.36
	Divorced	6,023	5.09	4,650	5.15	6,689	5.69	7,075	6.04	24,437	5.51
Living with parents who are head of house	0	102,188	86.27	78,803	87.31	104,250	88.68	105,266	89.87	390,507	88.07
	1	13,008	10.98	9,326	10.33	10,958	9.32	9,869	8.43	43,161	9.73
	2	3,250	2.74	2,130	2.36	2,348	2	1,995	1.7	9,723	2.19
Total		118,446		90,259		117,556		117,130		443,391	

	2001 N	%	2004 N	%	2007 N	%	2010 N	%	Total N	%
Living with spouse's parents										
0	115,714	97.69	88,083	97.59	114,898	97.74	114,698	97.92	433,393	97.75
1	2,328	1.97	1,884	2.09	2,309	1.96	2,140	1.83	8,661	1.95
2	404	0.34	292	0.32	349	0.3	292	0.25	1,337	0.3
Number of smokers in household excluding husband										
0	99,301	83.84	76,463	84.72	101,952	86.73	104,337	89.08	382,053	86.17
1	15,944	13	11,537	13	13,382	11.38	11,110	9.49	51,973	11.72
2	2,901	2	2,053	2	2,023	1.72	1,555	1.33	8,532	1.92
3	277	0	191	0	182	0.15	113	0.1	763	0.17
4	23	0.02	14	0.02	17	0.01	15	0.01	69	0.02
5	0	0	1	0	0	0	0	0	1	0
Husband's smoking status										
Without husband	19,800	16.72	14,833	16.43	22,017	18.73	24,138	20.61	80,788	18.22
Not smoke	43,129	36.41	36,224	40	50,143	42.65	51,926	44	181,422	40.92
Smoke everyday	51,825	43.75	34,764	39	39,008	33.18	33,386	29	158,983	35.86
Smoke sometimes	1,803	1.52	1,456	2	1,862	1.58	1,708	1	6,829	1.54
Ex-smoker	1,889	1.59	2,982	3.3	4,526	3.85	5,972	5.1	15,369	3.47
Total	118,446		90,259		117,556		117,130		443,391	

Table A.3. (Continued)

		2001 N	2001 %	2004 N	2004 %	2007 N	2007 %	2010 N	2010 %	Total N	Total %
Health check-up	0	68,036	57.44	53,758	59.56	70,860	60.28	75,126	64.14	267,780	60.39
	1	50,410	42.56	36,501	40.44	46,696	39.72	42,004	35.86	175,611	39.61
Cancer check-ups											
Stomach cancer	0	93,970	79.34	71,296	78.99	88,632	75.4	86,056	73.47	339,954	76.67
	1	24,476	20.66	18,963	21.01	28,924	24.6	31,074	26.53	103,437	23.33
Lung cancer	0	102,692	86.7	78,106	86.54	91,979	78.24	90,722	77.45	363,499	81.98
	1	15,754	13.3	12,153	13.46	25,577	21.76	26,408	22.55	79,892	18
Uterus cancer	0	83,768	70.72	62,666	69.43	82,181	69.91	78,513	67.03	307,128	69.27
	1	34,678	29.28	27,593	30.57	35,375	30.09	38,617	32.97	136,263	30.73
Breast cancer	0	93,168	78.66	68,521	75.92	89,239	75.91	83,315	71.13	334,243	75.38
	1	25,278	21	21,738	24	28,317	24	33,815	28.87	109,148	24.62
Colon cancer	0	100,105	84.52	74,916	83	92,724	78.88	91,233	77.89	358,978	80.96
	1	18,341	15	15,343	17	24,832	21	25,897	22	84,413	19.04
Total		118,446		90,259		117,556		117,130		443,391	

	2001		2004		2007		2010		Total	
	N	%	N	%	N	%	N	%	N	%
House-type										
Owner-occupied housing	81,292	68.63	65,261	72.3	85,388	72.64	85,411	72.92	317,352	71.57
Rented housing (private)	22,731	19	15,149	17	20,209	17	19,679	16.8	77,768	17.54
Company-provided housing	4,861	4	3,175	4	3,636	3	3,229	2.76	14,901	3.36
Rented housing (public)	7,791	6.58	5,225	5.79	5,397	4.59	5,268	4.5	23,681	5.34
Others	1,771	2	1,449	2	2,926	2	3,543	3.02	9,689	2.19
Area of floor-quintile										
1	27,693	23.38	18,687	20.7	25,697	21.86	24,092	20.57	96,169	21.69
2	26,088	22	18,570	21	25,628	22	24,729	21.11	95,015	21.43
3	22,718	19	17,615	20	22,152	19	22,716	19.39	85,201	19.22
4	22,045	18.61	18,287	20.26	22,540	19.17	22,770	19.44	85,642	19.32
5	19,902	17	17,100	19	21,539	18	22,823	19.49	81,364	18.35
Household expenditure-quintile										
1	13,986	11.81	14,078	15.6	20,815	17.71	22,556	19.26	71,435	16.11
2	21,910	18.5	17,656	19.56	23,034	19.59	23,561	20.12	86,161	19.43
3	23,704	20.01	17,946	19.88	23,452	19.95	23,128	19.75	88,230	19.9
4	28,109	23.73	19,253	21.33	25,695	21.86	24,013	20.5	97,070	21.89
5	30,737	25.95	21,326	23.63	24,560	20.89	23,872	20.38	100,495	22.67
Total	118,446		90,259		117,556		117,130		443,391	

* Agriculture, Forestry and Fisheries

Table A.3. Descriptive statistic (continued)

Child age and Parity		2001	2004	2007	2010	Total
Zero	1st	1,810	1,221	1,476	1,388	5,895
	2nd	1,547	1,041	1,254	1,137	4,979
	3rd	602	390	513	500	2,005
One	1st	2,011	1,341	1,511	1,416	6,279
	2nd	1,605	1,131	1,265	1,199	5,200
	3rd	652	395	473	557	2,077
Two	1st	2,064	1,435	1,657	1,501	6,657
	2nd	1,569	1,158	1,458	1,303	5,488
	3rd	589	443	496	552	2,080
Three	1st	2,010	1,487	1,729	1,521	6,747
	2nd	1,601	1,098	1,447	1,347	5,493
	3rd	716	437	543	520	2,216
Four	1st	2,077	1,500	1,850	1,598	7,025
	2nd	1,638	1,161	1,363	1,274	5,436
	3rd	659	442	500	468	2,069
Five	1st	2,019	1,447	1,863	1,615	6,944
	2nd	1,654	1,164	1,465	1,427	5,710
	3rd	703	448	528	499	2,178
6-12 year		32,934	22,234	28,576	28,200	111,944
13-18 year		32,091	20,671	24,471	23,558	100,791
Total		90,551	60,644	74,438	71,580	297,213

Table A.4. Logistic regression result

	CE	SE	Z	P>|z|	95% CI	
Birth-cohort by 5-year (reference=1975-1979)						
1935-1939	-0.974	0.068	-14.34	0	-1.107	-0.840
1940-1944	-0.883	0.056	-15.87	0	-0.992	-0.774
1945-1949	-0.690	0.050	-13.87	0	-0.788	-0.593
1950-1954	-0.553	0.044	-12.43	0	-0.640	-0.466
1955-1959	-0.344	0.040	-8.52	0	-0.423	-0.265
1960-1964	-0.177	0.035	-5.13	0	-0.245	-0.109
1965-1969	-0.179	0.029	-6.17	0	-0.236	-0.122
1970-1974	-0.075	0.023	-3.24	0.001	-0.120	-0.029

	CE	SE	Z	P>|z|	95% CI	
1980-1984	-0.148	0.032	-4.58	0	-0.211	-0.085
1985-1989	-0.542	0.055	-9.83	0	-0.651	-0.434
Survey year (reference=2001)						
2004	-0.069	0.026	-2.66	0.008	-0.120	-0.018
2007	-0.084	0.025	-3.3	0.001	-0.134	-0.034
2010	-0.158	0.028	-5.59	0	-0.213	-0.102
Age group (reference=20-29)						
30-39	-0.048	0.026	-1.85	0.064	-0.098	0.003
40-49	-0.025	0.038	-0.67	0.505	-0.099	0.049
50-59	-0.122	0.047	-2.57	0.01	-0.215	-0.029
60-69	-0.265	0.059	-4.53	0	-0.380	-0.150
>70	-0.723	0.106	-6.85	0	-0.930	-0.516
Job category (reference=no work)						
Specialist	-0.067	0.031	-2.21	0.027	-0.127	-0.007
Management	0.431	0.070	6.13	0	0.293	0.569
Clerical	-0.136	0.029	-4.64	0	-0.193	-0.078
Sales	0.389	0.030	12.97	0	0.331	0.448
Services	0.464	0.027	17.34	0	0.412	0.517
Security	0.238	0.122	1.95	0.051	-0.001	0.478
AFF	-0.150	0.069	-2.17	0.03	-0.285	-0.015
Production	0.103	0.030	3.39	0.001	0.044	0.163
Others	0.056	0.067	0.83	0.406	-0.076	0.187
Marital status (reference=married)						
Unmarried	0.050	0.034	1.48	0.139	-0.016	0.116
Widow	0.146	0.036	4.07	0	0.076	0.217
Divorced	0.808	0.031	25.84	0	0.746	0.869

Note: No. of obs = 443390 Log likelihood = -154150.27 Pseudo R2 = 0.1372

Living with parents (reference =0)						
Head of household's	-0.220	0.014	-16.21	0	-0.246	-0.193
Spouse's	-0.032	0.028	-1.14	0.256	-0.087	0.023
Number of smokers in household excluding husband (reference =0)						
1	0.399	0.015	26.87	0	0.370	0.428
2	0.628	0.030	20.91	0	0.569	0.687
3	0.733	0.093	7.88	0	0.551	0.915
4	1.051	0.293	3.59	0	0.477	1.626
5	0.000	(empty)				
Husband's smoking status (reference= no husband)						
Not smoke	-1.043	0.029	-35.36	0	-1.101	-0.985
Everyday	0.315	0.028	11.12	0	0.259	0.370
Sometimes	-0.521	0.050	-10.44	0	-0.619	-0.423
Ex-smoker	-1.002	0.045	-22.25	0	-1.091	-0.914
Health check-up	-0.228	0.011	-21.31	0	-0.249	-0.207
Cancer check-ups						
Stomach	-0.035	0.017	-2.05	0.04	-0.068	-0.002
Uterus	-0.182	0.014	-13.44	0	-0.208	-0.155
Breast	-0.262	0.016	-16.05	0	-0.294	-0.230
Colon	-0.210	0.018	-11.39	0	-0.246	-0.174

Table A.4. (Continued)

House-type (reference=owner-occupied housing)							
Rented (private)		0.350	0.015	23.51	0	0.321	0.379
Company-provided		-0.228	0.028	-8.04	0	-0.283	-0.172
Rented (public)		0.505	0.019	26.25	0	0.468	0.543
Others		0.327	0.028	11.72	0	0.272	0.381
Area of floor-quintile (reference=lowest)							
2		-0.064	0.013	-4.83	0	-0.091	-0.038
3		-0.114	0.016	-7.14	0	-0.146	-0.083
4		-0.184	0.018	-10.52	0	-0.218	-0.150
5		-0.294	0.020	-15.09	0	-0.333	-0.256
Household expenditure-quintile (reference=lowest)							
2		-0.048	0.015	-3.2	0.001	-0.077	-0.019
3		-0.066	0.015	-4.32	0	-0.097	-0.036
4		-0.079	0.015	-5.12	0	-0.110	-0.049
5		-0.028	0.016	-1.73	0.083	-0.060	0.004
Omit region dummy							

Note: No. of obs = 443390 Log likelihood = -154150.27 Pseudo R2 = 0.1372

Child age	Parity						
0-2month	1st	-0.836	0.160	-5.23	0.000	-1.150	-0.523
	2nd	-0.190	0.150	-1.27	0.206	-0.484	0.104
	3rd	-0.052	0.227	-0.23	0.818	-0.497	0.392
3-5month	1st	-0.825	0.143	-5.78	0.000	-1.105	-0.545
	2nd	-0.347	0.143	-2.42	0.015	-0.628	-0.066
	3rd	-0.194	0.225	-0.87	0.387	-0.634	0.246
6-8month	1st	-0.895	0.135	-6.61	0.000	-1.160	-0.630
	2nd	-0.229	0.136	-1.68	0.092	-0.496	0.038
	3rd	-0.584	0.271	-2.16	0.031	-1.115	-0.053
9-11month	1st	-0.424	0.119	-3.56	0.000	-0.658	-0.190
	2nd	-0.403	0.142	-2.84	0.004	-0.681	-0.125
	3rd	-0.511	0.228	-2.25	0.025	-0.958	-0.065
One	1st	-0.312	0.061	-5.12	0.000	-0.432	-0.193
	2nd	-0.375	0.077	-4.85	0.000	-0.527	-0.223
	3rd	-0.101	0.105	-0.97	0.332	-0.306	0.104
Two	1st	-0.193	0.062	-3.12	0.002	-0.314	-0.072
	2nd	-0.120	0.074	-1.62	0.105	-0.264	0.025
	3rd	-0.013	0.109	-0.12	0.902	-0.227	0.200
Three	1st	-0.237	0.066	-3.58	0.000	-0.367	-0.107
	2nd	-0.190	0.072	-2.64	0.008	-0.331	-0.049
	3rd	0.134	0.098	1.37	0.171	-0.058	0.326
Four	1st	-0.165	0.066	-2.50	0.012	-0.295	-0.036
	2nd	-0.022	0.066	-0.32	0.746	-0.152	0.109
	3rd	0.143	0.102	1.40	0.160	-0.057	0.342
Five	1st	-0.025	0.066	-0.38	0.701	-0.154	0.103
	2nd	-0.173	0.069	-2.50	0.012	-0.308	-0.037

Child age	Parity						
	3rd	0.041	0.101	0.41	0.683	-0.157	0.240
6-12 year		-0.023	0.016	-1.49	0.136	-0.054	0.007
13-18 year		-0.033	0.016	-2.11	0.035	-0.064	-0.002

Note: No. of obs = 443390 Log likelihood = -154150.27 Pseudo R2 = 0.1372

* Agriculture, Forestry and Fisheries.

REFERENCES

Akiyama, N., Saitou, H., and Nagino, H. (2000). A study on smoking habits for insurance subscriber *The journal of the Association of Life Insurance Medicine of Japan,* 98, 69-75.

ASH. (2011). ASH research report: secondhand smoke ASH research reports (Vol. June).

Bando, H., Yamakawa, M., and Toshida, T. (2013). Factors related to the contribution of smoking among pregnant women: cross-sectional study in a Japanese city. *Japanese Journal of Health Education and Promotion,* 21(2), 135-141.

Barraclough, S. (1999). Women and tobacco in Indonesia. *Tob. Control,* 8(3), 327-332.

Cho, H. J., Khang, Y. H., Jun, H. J., and Kawachi, I. (2008). Marital status and smoking in Korea: the influence of gender and age. *Soc. Sci. Med.,* 66(3), 609-619. doi: 10.1016/j.socscimed.2007.10.005

Cho, Y.-S., Kim, H.-R., Myong, J.-P., and Kim, H. W. (2013). Association Between Work Conditions and Smoking in South Korea. *Safety and Health at Work,* 4(4), 197-200. doi: .http://dx.doi.org/10.1016/ j.shaw.2013.09.001

Chun, H., Doyal, L., Payne, S., Il-Cho, S., and Kim, I. H. (2006). Understanding women, health, and social change: the case of South Korea. *Int. J. Health Serv.,* 36(3), 575-592.

Chung, W., Lim, S., and Lee, S. (2010). Factors influencing gender differences in smoking and their separate contributions: evidence from South Korea. *Soc. Sci. Med.,* 70(12), 1966-1973. doi: 10.1016/j.socscimed.2010.02.025

Cnattingius, S., Lindmark, G., and Meirik, O. (1992). Who continues to smoke while pregnant? *J. Epidemiol. Community Health,* 46(3), 218-221.

Colman, G. J., and Joyce, T. (2003). Trends in smoking before, during, and after pregnancy in ten states. *Am. J. Prev. Med.,* 24(1), 29-35.

Connor Gorber, S., Schofield-Hurwitz, S., Hardt, J., Levasseur, G., and Tremblay, M. (2009). The accuracy of self-reported smoking: a systematic review of the relationship between self-reported and cotinine-assessed smoking status. *Nicotine Tob. Res.,* 11(1), 12-24. doi: 10.1093/ntr/ntn010

Daly, K. A., Lund, E. M., Harty, K. C., and Ersted, S. A. (1993). Factors associated with late smoking initiation in Minnesota women. *Am. J. Public Health,* 83(9), 1333-1335.

Dollar, K. M., Homish, G. G., Kozlowski, L. T., and Leonard, K. E. (2009). Spousal and alcohol-related predictors of smoking cessation: a longitudinal study in a community sample of married couples. *Am. J. Public Health,* 99(2), 231-233. doi: 10.2105/ajph.2008.140459

England, L. J., Grauman, A., Qian, C., Wilkins, D. G., Schisterman, E. F., Yu, K. F., and Levine, R. J. (2007). Misclassification of maternal smoking status and its effects on an epidemiologic study of pregnancy outcomes. *Nicotine Tob. Res.*, 9(10), 1005-1013. doi: 10.1080/14622200701491255

Fendrich, M., Mackesy-Amiti, M. E., Johnson, T. P., Hubbell, A., and Wislar, J. S. (2005). Tobacco-reporting validity in an epidemiological drug-use survey. *Addict. Behav.*, 30(1), 175-181. doi: 10.1016/j.addbeh.2004.04.009

Fingerhut, L. A., Kleinman, J. C., and Kendrick, J. S. (1990). Smoking before, during, and after pregnancy. *Am. J. Public Health*, 80(5), 541-544.

Ford, R. P., Tappin, D. M., Schluter, P. J., and Wild, C. J. (1997). Smoking during pregnancy: how reliable are maternal self reports in New Zealand? *J. Epidemiol. Community Health*, 51(3), 246-251.

Fukuda, Y., Nakamura, K., and Takano, T. (2005a). Accumulation of health risk behaviours is associated with lower socioeconomic status and women's urban residence: a multilevel analysis in Japan. *BMC Public Health*, 5, 53. doi: 10.1186/1471-2458-5-53

Fukuda, Y., Nakamura, K., and Takano, T. (2005b). Socioeconomic pattern of smoking in Japan: income inequality and gender and age differences. *Ann. Epidemiol.*, 15(5), 365-372. doi: 10.1016/j.annepidem.2004.09.003

George, L., Granath, F., Johansson, A. L., and Cnattingius, S. (2006). Self-reported nicotine exposure and plasma levels of cotinine in early and late pregnancy. *Acta Obstet. Gynecol. Scand.*, 85(11), 1331-1337. doi: 10.1080/00016340600935433

Hannover, W., Thyrian, J. R., Ebner, A., Roske, K., Grempler, J., Kuhl, R., John, U. (2008). Smoking during pregnancy and postpartum: smoking rates and intention to quit smoking or resume after pregnancy. *J. Womens Health (Larchmt)*, 17(4), 631-640. doi: 10.1089/jwh.2007.0419

Homish, G. G., and Leonard, K. E. (2005). Spousal influence on smoking behaviors in a US community sample of newly married couples. *Soc. Sci. Med.*, 61(12), 2557-2567. doi: 10.1016/j.socscimed.2005.05.005

Imamura, T., Washio, M., Baba, Ohsaki, Toyoshima, Y., and Ide, N. (2011). Factors related to pre-pregnancy and checkup-time smoking among the mothers who participated in the health-checkups for the four-month old and three year old children. *The Japanese Journal of Clinical and Experimental Medicine*, 88(12), 1563-1569.

Jung-Choi, K. H., Khang, Y. H., and Cho, H. J. (2012). Hidden female smokers in Asia: a comparison of self-reported with cotinine-verified smoking prevalence rates in representative national data from an Asian population. *Tob. Control*, 21(6), 536-542. doi: 10.1136/tobaccocontrol-2011-050012

Kabir, Z., Connolly, G. N., and Alpert, H. R. (2011). Secondhand smoke exposure and neurobehavioral disorders among children in the United States. *Pediatrics*, 128(2), 263-270. doi: 10.1542/peds.2011-0023

Kahn, A., Sawaguchi, T., Sawaguchi, A., Groswasser, J., Franco, P., Scaillet, S., Dan, B. (2002). Sudden infant deaths: from epidemiology to physiology. *Forensic Sci. Int.*, 130 Suppl, S8-20.

Kaneita, Y., Yokoyama, E., Miyake, T., Harano, S., Asai, T., Tsutsui, T., Ohida, T. (2006). Epidemiological study on passive smoking among Japanese infants and smoking behavior of their respective parents: a nationwide cross-sectional survey. *Prev. Med.*, 42(3), 210-217. doi: 10.1016/ j.ypmed.2005.11.017

Kaneko, A., Kaneita, Y., Yokoyama, E., Miyake, T., Harano, S., Suzuki, K., Ohida, T. (2008). Smoking trends before, during, and after pregnancy among women and their spouses. *Pediatr. Int.*, 50(3), 367-375. doi: 10.1111/j.1442-200X.2008.02582.x

Kang, H. G., Kwon, K. H., Lee, I. W., Jung, B., Park, E. C., and Jang, S. I. (2013). Biochemically-verified Smoking Rate Trends and Factors Associated with Inaccurate Self-reporting of Smoking Habits in Korean Women. *Asian Pac. J. Cancer Prev.*, 14(11), 6807-6812.

Kouketsu, T., and Matsuda, N. (2010). Postpartum smoking behavior in women and related factors. *Japanese journal of public health*, 57(2), 104-112.

Kubo, S., and Emisu, F. (2007). Trends in research on smoking among woman during pregnancy and the postpartum period in Japan: A literature review from 1995 to 2007. *The journal of Japan Academy of Health Sciences*, 10(3), 160-167.

Kubo, S., Inoue, T., Yamazaki, A., and Hata, A. (2011). Contribution of socioeconomic status to smoking behavior of parents of 4^<th> grade elementary school students in Japan. *Japanese journal of public health,* 58(5), 340-349.

Kurumatani, N., and al., e. (1998). The changes in the smoking rate of pregnant women - an examination of the Japanese literature in the last thirty years. *Perinatal medicine (Tokyo)*, 28(3), 385-389.

Kvalvik, L. G., Skjaerven, R., and Haug, K. (2008). Smoking during pregnancy from 1999 to 2004: a study from the Medical Birth Registry of Norway. *Acta Obstet. Gynecol. Scand.*, 87(3), 280-285. doi: 10.1080/ 00016340701837801

Lee, S., Cho, E., Grodstein, F., Kawachi, I., Hu, F. B., and Colditz, G. A. (2005). Effects of marital transitions on changes in dietary and other health behaviors in US women. *Int. J. Epidemiol.*, 34(1), 69-78. doi: 10.1093/ije/dyh258

Lelong, N., Blondel, B., and Kaminski, M. (2011). [Smoking during pregnancy in France between 1972 to 2003: Results from the national perinatal surveys]. *J. Gynecol. Obstet. Biol. Reprod. (Paris)*, 40(1), 42-49. doi: 10.1016/j.jgyn.2010.07.007

Lelong, N., Kaminski, M., Saurel-Cubizolles, M. J., and Bouvier-Colle, M. H. (2001). Postpartum return to smoking among usual smokers who quit during pregnancy. *Eur. J. Public Health,* 11(3), 334-339.

Linnet, K. M., Wisborg, K., Obel, C., Secher, N. J., Thomsen, P. H., Agerbo, E., and Henriksen, T. B. (2005). Smoking during pregnancy and the risk for hyperkinetic disorder in offspring. *Pediatrics*, 116(2), 462-467. doi: 10.1542/peds.2004-2054

Marugame, T., Kamo, K., Sobue, T., Akiba, S., Mizuno, S., Satoh, H., Tsugane, S. (2006). Trends in smoking by birth cohorts born between 1900 and 1977 in Japan. *Prev. Med.*, 42(2), 120-127. doi: 10.1016/ j.ypmed.2005.09.009

McBride, C. M., Curry, S. J., Grothaus, L. C., Nelson, J. C., Lando, H., and Pirie, P. L. (1998). Partner smoking status and pregnant smoker's perceptions of support for and likelihood of smoking cessation. *Health Psychol.,* 17(1), 63-69.

McLeod, D., Pullon, S., and Cookson, T. (2003). Factors that influence changes in smoking behaviour during pregnancy. *N Z Med. J.,* 116(1173), U418.

Minakami, H., Hiramatsu, Y., Koresawa, M., Fujii, T., Hamada, H., Iitsuka, Y., Yoshikawa, H. (2011). Guidelines for obstetrical practice in Japan: Japan Society of Obstetrics and Gynecology (JSOG) and Japan Association of Obstetricians and Gynecologists (JAOG) 2011 edition. *J. Obstet. Gynaecol. Res.*, 37(9), 1174-1197. doi: 10.1111/j.1447-0756.2011.01653.x

Montgomery, S. M., and Ekbom, A. (2002). Smoking during pregnancy and diabetes mellitus in a British longitudinal birth cohort. *Bmj,* 324(7328), 26-27.

Mullen, P. D., Richardson, M. A., Quinn, V. P., and Ershoff, D. H. (1997). Postpartum return to smoking: who is at risk and when. *Am. J. Health Promot.*, 11(5), 323-330.

Nafstad, P., Botten, G., and Hagen, J. (1996). Partner's smoking: a major determinant for changes in women's smoking behaviour during and after pregnancy. *Public Health,* 110(6), 379-385.

Nakamura, Y., Sakata, K., Kubo, N., Akizawa, Y., Nagai, M., and Yanagawa, H. (1994). Smoking Habits and Socioeconomic Factors in Japan. *Journal of Epidemiology,* 4(3), 157-161. doi: 10.2188/jea.4.157

Nystedt, P. (2006). Marital life course events and smoking behaviour in Sweden 1980-2000. *Soc. Sci. Med.*, 62(6), 1427-1442. doi: 10.1016/ j.socscimed.2005.08.009

Ohashi, K. (2009). An extensive survey of active and passive smoking of pregnant women and its preventive measure using the maternal and child health handbook and measurement of urine cotinine.

Ohida, T., Kamal, A. M., Takemura, S., Sone, T., Mochizuki, Y., and Kawaminami, K. (2001). Relation between smoking prevalence and various social factors in Japan. *Keio. J. Med.*, 50(4), 263-268.

Ohida, T., Sone, T., Mochizuki, Y., Kawaguchi, T., Kido, M., Harita, A., Minowa, M. (2000). Household size related to prevalence of smoking in women in Japan. *J. Epidemiol.*, 10(5), 305-309.

Ohida, T., Sone, T., Takemura, S., Ozaki, Y., Kaneita, Y., Tamaki, T., Hayashi, K. (2007). Smoking status among Japanese pregnant women. *Japanese journal of public health,* 54(2), 115-122.

Oken, E., Huh, S. Y., Taveras, E. M., Rich-Edwards, J. W., and Gillman, M. W. (2005). Associations of maternal prenatal smoking with child adiposity and blood pressure. *Obes. Res.*, 13(11), 2021-2028. doi: 10.1038/ oby.2005.248

Paterson, J. M., Neimanis, I. M., and Bain, E. (2003). Stopping smoking during pregnancy: are we on the right track? *Can. J. Public Health*, 94(4), 297-299.

Polanska, K., Hanke, W., Sobala, W., Lowe, J. B., and Jaakkola, J. J. (2011). Predictors of smoking relapse after delivery: prospective study in central Poland. *Matern. Child Health J.*, 15(5), 579-586. doi: 10.1007/s10995-010-0639-y

Sasaki, S., Braimoh, T. S., Yila, T. A., Yoshioka, E., and Kishi, R. (2011). Self-reported tobacco smoke exposure and plasma cotinine levels during pregnancy--a validation study in Northern Japan. *Sci. Total Environ.*, 412-413, 114-118. doi: 10.1016 /j.scitotenv.2011.10.019

Severson, H. H., Andrews, J. A., Lichtenstein, E., Wall, M., and Zoref, L. (1995). Predictors of smoking during and after pregnancy: a survey of mothers of newborns. *Prev. Med.*, 24(1), 23-28. doi: 10.1006/ pmed.1995.1004

Shipton, D., Tappin, D. M., Vadiveloo, T., Crossley, J. A., Aitken, D. A., and Chalmers, J. (2009). Reliability of self reported smoking status by pregnant women for estimating smoking prevalence: a retrospective, cross sectional study. *Bmj*, 339, b4347. doi: 10.1136/bmj.b4347

Solomon, L. J., Higgins, S. T., Heil, S. H., Badger, G. J., Thomas, C. S., and Bernstein, I. M. (2007). Predictors of postpartum relapse to smoking. *Drug Alcohol Depend.*, 90(2-3), 224-227. doi: 10.1016/ j.drugalcdep.2007.03.012

Sutton, G. C. (1993). Do men grow to resemble their wives, or vice versa? *J. Biosoc. Sci.*, 25(1), 25-29.

Suzuki, J., Kikuma, H., Kawaminami, K., and Shima, M. (2005). Predictors of smoking cessation during pregnancy among the women of Yamato and Ayase municipalities in Japan. *Public Health*, 119(8), 679-685. doi: 10.1016/j.puhe.2004.10.014

Suzuki, K., Sato, M., Tanaka, T., Kondo, N., and Yamagata, Z. (2010). Recent trends in the prevalence of and factors associated with maternal smoking during pregnancy in Japan. *J. Obstet. Gynaecol. Res.*, 36(4), 745-750. doi: 10.1111/j.1447-0756.2010.01206.x

Toschke, A. M., Montgomery, S. M., Pfeiffer, U., and von Kries, R. (2003). Early intrauterine exposure to tobacco-inhaled products and obesity. *Am. J. Epidemiol.*, 158(11), 1068-1074.

U.S. Department of Health and Human Services. The Health Consequences of Involuntary. Exposure to Tobacco Smoke: A Report of the Surgeon General. Atlanta, GA: U.S. Department of Health and Human Services, Centers for Disease Control and Prevention, Coordinating Center for Health Promotion, National Center for Chronic Disease Prevention and Health Promotion, Office on Smoking and Health, 2006.

Williams, G. M., O'Callaghan, M., Najman, J. M., Bor, W., Andersen, M. J., Richards, D., and U, C. (1998). Maternal cigarette smoking and child psychiatric morbidity: a longitudinal study. *Pediatrics,* 102(1), e11.

Williams, R. (2012). Using the margins command to estimate and interpret adjusted predictions and marginal effects. *Stata. Journal*, 12(2), 308-331.

Yamashita, K. (2012). A survey of smoking rates among pregnant women using self-administered questionnaires and urine cotinine measurements (Actual smoking rates among pregnant women). *Japanese journal of tobacco control*, 7(5), 134-138.

Yasuda, T., Ojima, T., Nakamura, M., Nagai, A., Tanaka, T., Kondo, N., Yamagata, Z. (2013). Postpartum smoking relapse among women who quit during pregnancy: cross-sectional study in Japan. *J. Obstet. Gynaecol. Res.*, 39(11), 1505-1512. doi: 10.1111/jog.12098

Yolton, K., Dietrich, K., Auinger, P., Lanphear, B. P., and Hornung, R. (2005). Exposure to environmental tobacco smoke and cognitive abilities among U.S. children and adolescents. *Environ. Health Perspect.*, 113(1), 98-103.

PART III: HEALTH AND ENVIRONMENTAL HAZARDS OF SMOKING

Chapter 6

POTENTIAL HEALTH HAZARDS OF IGNORING SUBMICRON PARTICLES IN LOW-TAR AND NICOTINE CIGARETTES

How classic cigarette smoke yields, as established by standardized smoking machines, are misleading.

W. D. van Dijk, M.D., Ph.D.[*]
Department of Primary and Community Care,
Radboud University Nijmegen Medical Centre, Nijmegen, Netherlands

ABSTRACT

Global smoking legislation restricts the manufacturing, presentation and sale of tobacco products. From these measures cigarette packages must display the claimed amount of tar, nicotine and carbon monoxide yields. There is ongoing discussion about categorization of cigarettes based on these mass yields. These yields are determined using smoking machines in standardised testing methods that have never been intended to predict individual exposure and disease.

A relation between tar and nicotine values of cigarettes and disease risk appears to be missing, partly due to potential smoking compensation mechanisms. Apart from insufficient evidence regarding health risks, the fundamental nature of classic smoke analyses seems questionable. Total particle mass would be an inferior predictor for toxicity compared to total particle count. Unfortunately, tar mass only represents the minority of relatively large and heavy particles and neglects the abundance of smaller (submicron) smoke particles. Indeed, analyses of size-dependent particle counts in cigarette smoke revealed that (ultra)low-tar and nicotine cigarettes have a relative increase of particle numbers when particles become smaller, exceeding the particle counts from regular-tar and nicotine cigarettes in these smaller size ranges. Altogether, current label claims underestimate true particle exposure and with that the toxicity of

---

[*] Address: Internal postal code 117, P.O. Box 9101, 6500 HB, Nijmegen, The Netherlands, e-mail: w.vandijk@aios.umcn.nl, fax:+31(0)24-3541862.

low-tar cigarettes. Present-day legislation therefore fails to meet its core objective of regulating cigarette toxicity.

In conclusion, these observations suggest that due to abundant smaller (submicron) particles, (ultra)low-tar and nicotine cigarettes are at least as hazardous to human health as regular-tar and nicotine cigarettes. It appears that this information adds to the evidence that the current categorization is misleading to smokers and should be abandoned or replaced by a more appropriate categorization.

INTRODUCTION

Smoking remains an undisputable factor in causing unnecessary disease and premature death (CDC 2013, Doll 2004, GOLD 2013). Across countries, national government policies and international agreements have been realized to develop local smoking legislation. Globally, smoking legislation aims to control and restrict the manufacturing, presentation and sale of tobacco products. Primarily these measures would affect human exposure to toxic smoke constituents in order to diminish smoking related diseases. One of these measures includes that cigarette packages must display the claimed amount of tar, nicotine and carbon monoxide mass yields from mainstream smoke per cigarette. However, there is an ongoing discussion about the usefulness of this categorization of cigarettes based on these 'classic' well-correlated yields. Some categories still refer to deceptive names such as 'light' cigarettes, despite current prohibitions for such labels (Hammond 2006).

In Europe, smoke yields for these substances are limited to 10 mg tar, 1 mg nicotine and 10 mg carbon monoxide per cigarette, as stated by a European directive (European Parliament 2001). Demanding costly and labor-intensive programs are necessary to assess if the tobacco industry obeys to the imposed legislation on cigarettes, including testing of these cigarette smoke yields as claimed on the cigarette box. The main question related to this categorization is if these measures are useful whether in serving the public by improving health or merely as a tool for the tobacco industry to mislead and avoid further tobacco restrictions.

In this chapter, a short introduction on cigarette smoke and its impact on health as well as a concise overview on the rationale of cigarette categorization is presented, followed by new insights that add to the current discussion on the usefulness of this categorization. The chapter concludes with suggestions to replace the existing categorization with an alternative method that is more appropriate to demonstrate health risk.

An Overview of Smoking and Its Characteristics

Worldwide, the percentage of smokers seems to have stabilised at 20-30% (CDC 2013, Cokkinides 2009). Over the years, large epidemiological studies identified cigarette smoking as a very important causal factor in several diseases. Cigarette smoking mainly increases the risk to develop lung cancer, cardiovascular disease and COPD (Doll 2004, GOLD 2013). The risk to develop these diseases increases both with the number of daily smoked cigarettes and with the number of cumulative smoked cigarettes (Doll 2004, Teo 2006, Willett 1987). Altogether, approximately twenty percent of total mortality can be attributed to smoking. This is illustrated in Figure 1 for selected diseases and total population (CDC 2013). In addition, passive smoking holds a significant relative risk of about 1. 3 to develop and die from smoking related diseases (Barnoya 2005, IARC 2004, McGhee 2005, Wen 2006). As indicate din subsequent studies, cessation of cigarette smoking is the best intervention to prevent the incidence and/or progression of smoking related disease (Anthonisen 1994, Cokkinides 2009, Kohansal 2009, Kuller 1991, Song 2008). However, cessation efforts are only modest. Yet fifty percent of patients with established disease continue smoking, despite intensive smoking cessation programs (Ellerbeck 2009, Schermer 2007).

Made primarily from dried tobacco leaves, over 1,000 additives, ranging from citric acid to oak moss, are available to create cigarettes with a distinctive flavour, to moisturise, to preserve and to ease manufacturing processes (PMI 2013). All ingredients finally contribute to the complex mixture of cigarette smoke constituents. Thousands of constituents have been identified yet, of which many can be hazardous (Rodgman 2006). These constituents occur in cigarette smoke as particulate matter, volatile substances or as gasses (Norman 1977, Pryor 1998). 'Tar' refers to the particulate matter which is trapped using Cambridge filters that collect 99. 9% of particles >100 nm (Pryor 1998).

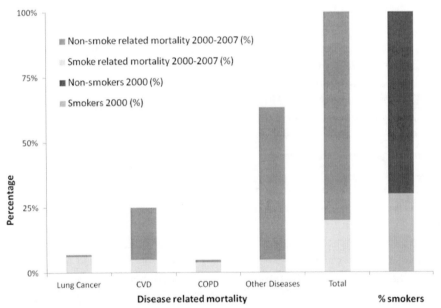

Notes: Column 1-5, percentage of mortality due to smoking and non-smoking (Y-axis) according to disease specific mortality (X-axis); Column 6, percentage of smokers amongst total population.
Abbreviations: CVD: cardiovascular disease, including coronary heart disease, stroke and heart failure; COPD: Chronic Obstructive Pulmonary Disease.
Source: Centers for Disease Control and Prevention. Smoking and Tobacco Use fact sheets. Available at http://www. cdc. gov/tobacco/data_statistics/fact_sheets/index. htm; van Gelder, B. M., Hoogenveen, R. T., van Leent-Loenen, H. M. J. A., (2005). Wat zijn de mogelijke gezondheidsgevolgen van roken?Available at www. rivm. nl/vtv/object_document/o1208n19085. html;van der Cammen, M., (2007). Documentatiemap roken. Available at http://www. oivo-crioc. org/files/nl/ 2382nl. pdf

Figure 1. Estimated relative amount of smoking-related mortality, grouped according to mortality per disease,for the period from 2000 to 2007, compared to the percentage of active smokers in 2000. Figures are based on populations of the United States, Belgium and the Netherlands.

Absolute individual smoke yields are difficult to study, since smoke characteristics are highly dynamic over time and vary across different smokers, cigarette properties and smoking conditions (Borgerding 2005, Sutton 1982). Fractional risk attributions of specific substances to develop disease are indefinite and pathogenic mechanisms of action vary across the smoke substances (Borgerding 2005, Pryor 1993). Altogether, these include local and systemic carcinogenic effects, local inflammation, and finally systemic inflammation and systemic toxic effects (Ambrose 2004, Hoffmann 1993, Jackson 2009, Pryor 1998, Smith 2000, Yanbaeva 2007). Moreover, any constructed relative risk profile to develop certain diseases from smoking certain cigarettes would be complex, crude, and incomplete, and hence would be inaccurate.

MEASUREMENT OF SMOKE YIELD MASS

The initial reasoning behind determining tar, nicotine and carbon monoxide mass yields is that they were assumed to be associated with all hazardous smoke constituents and consequently would predict total smoke exposure and subsequently the risk of smoking-related diseases (Chepiga 2000, Gregg 2004). Indeed, early reports supported such a relationship disfavoring cigarettes with more than 20 mg tar (Kaufman 1989). However, recent studies reported similar health risks for cigarettes that have even less than 20 mg tar. To begin with, blood nicotine and tar biomarkers show poor correlations with displayed yields (Harris 2004, Hecht 2005). Furthermore, while some hazardous constituents have been reported to be disproportionately high in (ultra)low-tar and nicotine cigarettes (Gendreau 2005), no fractional risk attributions have been defined that link specific constituents to the development of diseases (Borgerding 2005, Pryor 1993). Moreover, the relation between tar and nicotine values and diseases is far from absolute. Low-tar and low-nicotine cigarettes appeared to worsen outcomes in embryogenesis compared to regular-tar and nicotine cigarettes (Lin 2009), and a relation between tar values and disease was lacking or even inversed for tar values less than 21 mg per cigarette (Harris 2004, Janssen-Heijnen 2003).

These results are not surprising. Mass-based values are determined using smoking machines in standardised testing methods that have not been developed to predict individual exposure to cigarette smoke and subsequent diseases (Baker 2002, Bialous 2001, Thielen 2008). Indeed, individual exposure can be substantially modified, resulting in a final tar and nicotine exposure from low-tar and nicotine cigarettes that is almost equivalent to full blend cigarettes (Hecht 2005, Nakazawa 2004, Russell 1980, Sutton 1982). Unfortunately, the ability of tar to predict diseases clearly remains poor. Though there have been calls to change smoking standardisation, many countries still oblige manufacturers to inform consumers by displaying these claimed values on cigarette packs (Bialous 2001).

Particle Mass versus Particle Size

Apart from insufficient evidence regarding health risks, the fundamental nature of classic smoke mass analyses seems questionable. Mass is considered to be an inferior measure of toxicity compared to particle count and surface area (Schmid 2009, Stoeger 2006). Moreover, with classic smoke analyses these tar mass values are based predominantly on the weights of the larger particles (Adam 2009, Bernstein 2004, Kane 2010). However, actual particle sizes in tar range from 200 to 600 nm, with some additional particles between 100 and 1,000 nm. It would be questionable if mass values represent this whole spectrum of smoke particles, and in particular the smallest particles. In addition, these (ultra-)fine particles are particularly toxic due to deeper penetration into and transposition through the lung tissue (Schmid 2009).

Indeed, recent studies revealed that the tar weights as measured by classic smoke analyses only represent the minority of relatively large and heavy particles and neglect the smaller submicron smoke particles (van Dijk 2011, van Dijk 2012). These studies of size-dependent particle counts in mainstream cigarette smoke revealed a strong inverse correlation between particle size and the ratios of size-dependent particle counts for(ultra-)low- and regular-tar and nicotine cigarettes. The size-dependent particle counts were measured by a scanning mobility particle sizer plus faraday cup electrometer (SMPS+E) for particles less than 50 nm and by an aerosol spectrometer (1. 109) for particles higher than 250 nm, both from *Grimm Aerosol Technik*.

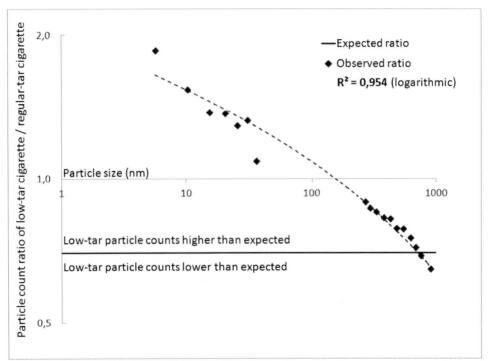

Notes: Particle counts were measured by Grimm Aerosol Technik spectrometers: 1. 109 for particles >250 nm and SMPS+E for particles <50 nm; A particle count ratio above 1 indicates higher particle counts for low-tar cigarettes compared to regular-tar cigarettes.
Source: based on results from: van Dijk, W. D. Gopal, S., Scheepers, T., (2011). Nanoparticles in cigarette smoke; real-time undiluted measurements by a scanning mobility particle sizer. Anal Bioanal Chem. 399(10), 3573-8; van Dijk, W. D., Cremers, R., Klerx, W., Schermer, T. R. J., Scheepers, P. T. J., (2012). Application of cigarette smoke characterisation based on optical aerosol spectrometry. Cur Anal Chem. 8(3), 344-50.

Figure 2. Ratios between size-dependent particle counts of low-tar (6-7 mg) versus regular-tar (10 mg) cigarettes for different particle size ranges between 5 nm and 1000 nm.

Figure 2 shows the particle count ratios between low-tar and nicotine and regular tar- and nicotine cigarettes on the Y-axis, for particle size ranges between 5 and 1000 nm (X-axis). One outlier of the particle count ratios was excluded, because the particle count exceeded the measurement capacity maximum of the spectrometer. Low-tar cigarettes contained 6-7 mg tar per cigarette whereas regular-tar cigarettes of the same brand contained 10 mg tar per cigarette. Hence, the expected particle count ratios would be 0. 7, as derived from the tar mass ratio from the two cigarette types. The expected nicotine ratio would be even lower than the expected tar ratio, i. e. 0. 5. However, most ratios observed in these studies go (far) above the expected ratio. With smaller particles, the ratio increases according to a logarithmic correlation.

For these low-tar and nicotine cigarettes, this correlation indicates a relative increase of particle counts when particles become smaller compared to regular tar- and nicotine cigarettes, with absolute particle counts of low-tar and nicotine cigarettes exceeding those of regular-tar and nicotine cigarettes for particles less than 100 nm. Similar results were observed for ultralow-tar and nicotine cigarettes. Coinciding observations from these studies also showed that puff patterns that are driven by compensation mechanisms appear to enhance the production of these smallest tar particles, thereby further increasing cigarette toxicity of (ultra-)low tar and nicotine cigarettes in particular. Moreover, exposure to smaller smoke particles in daily life would be far more than suggested by the tar mass values of (ultra)low-tar and nicotine cigarettes as claimed on cigarette boxes. Altogether, current label claims of mass based smoke yields underestimate true particle exposure and with that the toxicity of (ultra)low-tar cigarettes. Present-day legislation therefore would fail to meet its core objective of regulating smoking toxicity.

CONCLUSION

Cigarette smoking still remains an important avoidable factor in causing morbidity and mortality worldwide. The usefulness of categorizing cigarettes by mass-based tar and nicotine values is debatable. Recent observations on size-dependent particle counts in mainstream cigarette smoke suggest that due to the relative and absolute abundance of smaller (submicron) particles in cigarettes with lower tar and nicotine yields, (ultra)low-tar and nicotine cigarettes are at least as hazardous to human health as regular-tar cigarettes. These results support the evidence that the current categorization of cigarettes by tar and nicotine is misleading to smokers and should be abandoned or otherwise should be replaced by a method more appropriate to demonstrate health risk.

REFERENCES

Adam, T., McAughey, J., McGrath, C., Mocker, C., Zimmermann, R., (2009). Simultaneous on-line size and chemical analysis of gas phase and particulate phase of cigarette mainstream smoke. *Anal. Bioanal. Chem.* 394(4), 1193-1203.

Ambrose, J. A., Barua, R. S., (2004). The pathophysiology of cigarette smoking and cardiovascular disease: an update. *J. Am. Coll. Cardiol.* 43(10), 1731-7.

Anthonisen, N. R., Connett, J. E., Kiley, J. P., Altose, M. D., Bailey, W. C., Buist, A. S., Conway, W. A. Jr., Enright, P. L., Kanner, R. E., O'Hara, P., (1994). Effects of smoking intervention and the use of an inhaled anticholinergic bronchodilator on the rate of decline of FEV1. The Lung Health Study. *JAMA.* 272(19), 1497-1505.

Baker, R. R., (2002). The Development and Significance of Standards for Smoking-Machine Methodology. *Beiträge zur Tabakforschung International/ Contributions to Tobacco Research.* 20(1), 23-41.

Barnoya, J., Glantz, S. A., (2005). Cardiovascular effects of secondhand smoke: nearly as large as smoking. *Circulation.* 111(20), 2684-98.

Bernstein, D. M., (2004). A review of the influence of particle size, puff volume, and inhalation pattern on the deposition of cigarette smoke particles in the respiratory tract. *Inhal. Toxicol.* 16, 675-89.

Bialous, S. A., Yach, D., (2001). Whose standard is it, anyway? How the tobacco industry determines the International Organization for Standardization (ISO) standards for tobacco and tobacco products. *Tob. Control.* 10(2), 96-104.

Borgerding, M., Klus, H., (2005). Analysis of complex mixtures-cigarette smoke. *Exp. Toxicol. Pathol.* 57 (Suppl 1), 43-73.

CDC: Centers for Disease Control and Prevention., (2013). Smoking and Tobacco Use fact sheets. Available at http://www. cdc. gov/tobacco/data_statistics/fact_sheets/index. htm. Retrieved July 2013

Chepiga, T. A., Morton, M. J., Murphy, P. A., Avalos, J. T., Bombick, B. R., Doolittle, D. J., Borgerding, M. F., Swauger, J. E., (2000). A comparison of the mainstream smoke chemistry and mutagenicity of a representative sample of the US cigarette market with two Kentucky reference cigarettes (K1R4F and K1R5F). *Food Chem. Toxicol.* 38(10), 949-62.

Cokkinides, V., Bandi, P., McMahon, C., Jemal, A., Glynn, T., (2009). Ward, E Tobacco control in the United States-recent progress and opportunities. *CA Cancer J. Clin.* 59(6), 352-65.

Doll, R., Peto, R., Boreham, J., Sutherland, I., (2004). Mortality in relation to smoking: 50 years' observations on male British doctors. *BMJ.* 328(7455), 1519-24.

Ellerbeck, E. F., Mahnken, J. D., Cupertino, A. P., Cox, L. S., Greiner, K. A., Mussulman, L. M., Nazir, N., Shireman, T. I., Resnicow, K., Ahluwalia, J. S., (2009). Effect of varying levels of disease management on smoking cessation: a randomized trial. *Ann. Intern. Med.* 150(7), 437-46.

European parliament and council.,(2001). Directive 2001/37/EC. Available at http:// eur-lex. europa. eu/LexUriServ/LexUriServ. do?uri=OJ:L:2001:194:0026:0034:EN:PDF. RetreivedAugust 2013.

Gendreau, P. L., Vitaro, F.,(2005). The unbearable lightness of "light" cigarettes: a comparison of smoke yields in six varieties of Canadian "light" cigarettes. *Can. J. Public Health.* 96(3), 167-72.

GOLD: Global Initiative for Chronic Obstructive Lung Disease.,(2013). Global Strategy for the Diagnosis, Management and Prevention of COPD. Updated 2013. Available at www. goldcopd. org. Retrieved July 2013.

Gregg, E., Hill, C., Hollywood, M., Kearney, M., McAdam, K., McLaughlin, D., Purkis, S., Williams, M., (2004). The UK Smoke Constituents Testing Study. Summary of Results and Comparison with Other Studies. *Beiträge zur Tabakforschung International /Contributions to Tobacco Research.* 21(2), 117-38.

Hammond, D., Collishaw, N. E., Callard, C., (2006). Secret science: tobacco industry research on smoking behaviour and cigarette toxicity. *Lancet*367(9512), 781-7.

Harris, J. E., Thun, M. J., Mondul, A. M., Calle, E. E., (2004). Cigarette tar yields in relation to mortality from lung cancer in the cancer prevention study II prospective cohort, 1982-8. *BMJ.* 328(7431), 72.

Hecht, S. S., Murphy, S. E., Carmella, S. G., Li, S., Jensen, J., Le, C., Joseph, A. M., Hatsukami, D. K., (2005). Similar uptake of lung carcinogens by smokers of regular, light, and ultralight cigarettes. *Cancer Epidemiol Biomarkers Prev.* 14(3), 693-8.

Hoffmann, D., (1993). Analysis of toxic smoke constituents. In: *Toxicity testing plan vol. 5.* U. S. consumer product safety commission, D1-D38.

IARC: International Agency for Research on Cancer., (2004). *IARC Monographs on the Evaluation of Carcinogenic Risks to Humans, volume 83, Tobacco Smoke and Involuntary Smoking.* World Health Organization: Lyon.

Jackson, E., Ockene, I. S., (2009). Cardiovascular risk of smoking and benefits of smoking cessation. Available at www. uptodateonline. com. Retrieved December 2009.

Janssen-Heijnen, M. L., Coebergh, J. W., (2003). The changing epidemiology of lung cancer in Europe. *Lung Cancer* 41(3), 245-58.

Kane, D. B., Asgharian, B., Price, O. T., Rostami, A., Oldham, M. J., (2010). Effect of smoking parameters on the particle size distribution and predicted airway deposition of mainstream cigarette smoke. *Inhal. Toxicol.* 22(3), 199-209.

Kaufman, D. W., Palmer, J. R., Rosenberg, L., Stolley, P., Warshauer, E., Shapiro, S., (1989). Tar content of cigarettes in relation to lung cancer. *Am J Epidemiol.* 129(4), 703-11.

Kohansal, R., Martinez-Camblor, P., Agusti, A., Buist, A. S., Mannino, D. M., Soriano, J. B., (2009). The natural history of chronic airflow obstruction revisited: an analysis of the Framingham offspring cohort. *Am. J. Respir. Crit Care Med.* 180(1), 3-10.

Kuller, L. H., Ockene, J. K., Meilahn, E., Wentworth, D. N., Svendsen, K. H., Neaton, J. D. (1991). Cigarette smoking and mortality. MRFIT Research Group. *Prev. Med.* 20(5), 638-54.

Lin, S., Tran, V., Talbot, P., (2009). Comparison of toxicity of smoke from traditional and harm-reduction cigarettes using mouse embryonic stem cells as a novel model for preimplantation development. *Hum. Reprod.* 24(2), 386-97.

McGhee, S. M., Ho, S. Y., Schooling, M., Ho, L. M., Thomas, G. N., Hedley, A. J., Mak, K. H., Peto, R., Lam, T. H., (2005). Mortality associated with passive smoking in Hong Kong. *BMJ.* 330(7486), 287-8.

Nakazawa, A., Shigeta, M., Ozasa, K., (2004). Smoking cigarettes of low nicotine yield does not reduce nicotine intake as expected: a study of nicotine dependency in Japanese males. *BMC. Public Health.* 4, 28.

Norman, V., (1977). An overview of the vapor phase, semivolatile and novolatile components of cigarette smoke. *Rec. Advan. Tob. Sci.* 3, 28-58.

PMI: Philip Morris International Management SA., (2013). Available at www. philipmorrisinternational. com. Retrieved August 2013.

Pryor, W. A., Stone, K.,(1993). Oxidants in cigarette smoke. Radicals, hydrogen peroxide, peroxynitrate, and peroxynitrite. *Ann. N. Y. Acad. Sci.* 686, 12-27.

Pryor, W. A., Stone, K., Zang, L. Y., Bermudez, E., (1998). Fractionation of aqueous cigarette tar extracts: fractions that contain the tar radical cause DNA damage. *Chem. Res. Toxicol.* 11(5), 441-8.

Rodgman, A., Perfetti, T. A., (2006). The Composition of Cigarette Smoke: A Catalogue of the Polycyclic Aromatic Hydrocarbons. *Beiträge zur Tabakforschung International /Contributions to Tobacco Research.* 22(3), 13-69.

Russell, M. A., Jarvis, M., Iyer, R., Feyerabend, C., (1980). Relation of nicotine yield of cigarettes to blood nicotine concentrations in smokers. *BMJ.* 280(6219), 972-6.

Schermer, T., Heijdra, Y., Zadel, S., van den Bemt, L., Boonman-de Winter, L., Dekhuijzen, R., Smeele, I., (2007). Flow and volume responses after routine salbutamol reversibility testing in mild to very severe COPD. *Respir. Med.* 101(6), 1355-62.

Schmid, O., Möller, W., Semmler-Behnke, M., Ferron, G. A., Karg, E., Lipka, J., Schulz, H., Kreyling, W. G., Stoeger, T., (2009). Dosimetry and toxicology of inhaled ultrafine particles. *Biomarkers.* 14(suppl 1), 67-73.

Smith, L. E., Denissenko, M. F., Bennett, W. P., Li, H., Amin, S., Tang, M., Pfeifer, G. P., (2000). Targeting of lung cancer mutational hotspots by polycyclic aromatic hydrocarbons. *J. Natl. Cancer Inst.* 92(10), 803-11.

Song, Y. M., Sung, J., Cho, H. J., (2008). Reduction and cessation of cigarette smoking and risk of cancer: a cohort study of Korean men. *J Clin. Oncol.* 26(31), 5101-6.

Stoeger, T., Reinhard, C., Takenaka, S., Schroeppel, A., Karg, E., Ritter, B., Heyder, J., Schulz, H., (2006). Instillation of six different ultrafine carbon particles indicates a surface area threshold dose for acute lung inflammation in mice. *Environ. Health Perspect.* 114(3), 328-33.

Sutton, S. R., Russell, M. A., Iyer, R., Feyerabend, C., Saloojee, Y., (1982). Relationship between cigarette yields, puffing patterns, and smoke intake: evidence for tar compensation? *BMJ (Clin. Res. Ed).* 285(6342), 600-3.

Teo, K. K., Ounpuu, S., Hawken, S., Pandey, M. R., Valentin, V., Hunt, D.,Diaz, R., Rashed, W., Freeman, R., Jiang, L., Zhang, X., Yusuf, S., (2006). Tobacco use and risk of myocardial infarction in 52 countries in the INTERHEART study: a case-control study. *Lancet.* 368(9536), 647-58.

Thielen, A., Klus, H., Muller, L., (2008). Tobacco smoke: unraveling a controversial subject. *Exp. Toxicol. Pathol.* 60(2-3)., 141-56.

van Dijk, W. D., Gopal, S., Scheepers, T., (2011). Nanoparticles in cigarette smoke; real-time undiluted measurements by a scanning mobility particle sizer. *Anal Bioanal Chem.* 399(10), 3573-8.

van Dijk, W. D., Cremers, R., Klerx, W., Schermer, T. R. J., Scheepers, P. T. J., (2012). Application of cigarette smoke characterisation based on optical aerosol spectrometry. *Cur Anal Chem.* 8(3), 344-50.

Wen, W., Shu, X. O., Gao, Y. T., Yang, G., Li, Q., Li, H., Zheng, W., (2006). Environmental tobacco smoke and mortality in Chinese women who have never smoked: prospective cohort study. *BMJ.* 333(7564), 376.

Willett, W. C., Green, A., Stampfer, M. J., Speizer, F. E., Colditz, G. A., Rosner, B., Monson, R. R., Stason, W., Hennekens, C. H., (1987). Relative and absolute excess risks of coronary heart disease among women who smoke cigarettes. *N Engl J Med.* 317(21), 1303-9.

Yanbaeva, D. G., Dentener, M. A., Creutzberg, E. C., Wesseling, G., Wouters, E. F., (2007). Systemic effects of smoking. *Chest.* 131(5), 1557-66.

In: Smoking Restrictions
Editor: Nazmi Sari
ISBN: 978-1-63321-148-3
© 2014 Nova Science Publishers, Inc.

Chapter 7

PSYCHOPATHOLOGICAL DISORDERS, TOBACCO SMOKING, SMOKING CESSATION AND REDUCTION

P. Caponnetto[1,3], G. Minutolo[2,3,•], R. Auditore[3],
M. Maglia[1,3], A. Alamo[1], F. Benfatto[1], M. D'Alessandro[4],
G. Nasca[4], V. Palumbo[4], C. Russo[1,3] and R. Polosa[1]

[1]Centro per la prevenzione e la cura del tabagismo(CPCT),
AOU Policlinico-Vittorio Emanuele of Catania,
University of Catania, Italy
[2]Department of Psychiatry, AOU Policlinico-Vittorio Emanuele of Catania,
University of Catania, Italy
[3]CTA Villa Chiara, Psychiatric Rehabilitation Center and Research, Italy
[4]Mental Health Department, ASP 3 Paternò-Gravina (CT), Italy

ABSTRACT

Tobacco smoking among patients with psychiatric disorders is more common than in the general population. The neurobiological and psychosocial links to smoking appear stronger in certain comorbidities, notably anxiety, affective disorders (specifically depression and bipolar disorder), schizophrenia, substance abuse disorders and personality disorders. Tobacco smoking may have certain beneficial effects across a range of mental health domains in these patients, including improved concentration and cognition, relief of stress and depressive affect, and feeling pleasurable sensations. This chapter describes the relationship between tobacco smoking and the more common psychopathological disorders and their mutual influence.

Keywords: Schizophrenia, Tobacco, Smoking Cessation and Reduction, Psychiatric disorders, Psychopathology

---

[•] E-mail: giuseppeminutolo@hotmail.com.

INTRODUCTION

Tobacco smoking among patients with psychopathological disorders is more common than in the general population. The neurobiological and psychosocial links to smoking appear stronger in certain comorbidities, notably anxiety, affective disorders (specifically depression and bipolar disorder), schizophrenia, substance abuse disorders and personality disorders. (Aubin et al., 2012; Dierker et al., 2005; Zvolensky et al., 2011).

Tobacco smoking may have certain beneficial effects across a range of mental health domains in these patients, including improved concentration and cognition, relief of stress and depressive affect, and feeling pleasurable sensations (Aubin et al., 2012).

This chapter describes the relationship between tobacco smoking and the more common psychopathological disorders (schizophrenia, depression, anxiety, and alcoholism), and their mutual influence. In the following sections, we will discuss relationship between smoking and each of these disorders. In the last section of the chapter, we will present the summary and conclusion.

SCHIZOPHRENIA

Schizophrenia is a mental disorder characterized by a breakdown of thought processes and by poor emotional responsiveness. It is well established in studies across several countries that tobacco smoking is more prevalent among schizophrenic patients than the general population (Zvolensky et al., 2011). For example, in the US, 80% or more of schizophrenics smoke, compared to approximately 20% of the general population (De Leon.; Diaz, 2005). Many social, psychologic and biologic explanations have been proposed, but today research focuses on neurobiological action of nicotine and its pharmacodynamic interactions. For example, it was hypothesized that schizophrenic patients smoke to reduce symptoms and/or to mitigate the negative effects of neuroleptic therapy (Keltner, Grant, 2006), that smoking may contribute to development of the disorder by altering neurochemical systems in the brain, (Glassman, 1993) and that both conditions could arise from a common genetic vulnerability (Zvolensky et al. 2001). Smoking is often accepted as a customary social activity in many psychiatric treatment facilities, sometimes despite smoking bans and schizophrenic patients are seldom encouraged to quit smoking (Kelly, McCreadie 1999). As a consequence, smoking related morbidity and mortality are particularly high in patients with schizophrenia (Addington, 1998).

As the risk of serious disease diminishes rapidly after quitting and life-long abstinence is known to reduce the risk of lung cancer, heart disease, strokes, chronic lung disease and other cancers (Brown, et al., 2000; United States Public Health Service,1990) , smoking cessation in these patients is mandatory.

Although there is little doubt that currently-marketed smoking cessation products increase the chance of committed smokers to stop smoking (Brown, et al., 2000), they are not particularly effective in schizophrenic patients who smoke (Addington, 1998; Lightwood, Glantz, 1997; United States Public Health Service 1990). This scenario is further complicated by the belief that quitting smoking will worsen psychiatric symptoms, or that these patients have little or no interest in quitting. Moreover, the prescribing information for bupropion and varenicline, two important first-line medications for nicotine dependence, carry a "black-box" warning highlighting an increased risk of psychiatric symptoms and suicidal ideation in patients reporting any history of psychiatric illness (Casella, Caponnetto, Polosa, 2010).

DEPRESSION

The association between nicotine dependence and affective disorders, particularly major depressive disorder, is well known, with high prevalence rates being reported for smokers (Breslau et al., 1993; Anda et al., 1990) . The reason for this association is not clear, but it has been argued that smoking may help individuals to cope with stress (Revell, Warburton, Wesnes, 1985) or medicate depressed mood (Covey, Glassman, Stetner, 1997). In support of this hypothesis, it has been shown that smokers with a history of depression who abstain from smoking are at a significantly increased risk of developing a new episode of major depression and this risk remains high for at least 6 months (Kinnunen et al.,1990; Glassman et al., 2001). Until recent years, the belief that a history of depression greatly decreases the likelihood of quitting smoking has been widely promoted (Fergusson, Lynskey, Horwood, 1996). Although it is generally assumed that a history of depression may be a barrier to quitting smoking, contradictory evidence also exists (Murphy et al., 2003; Glassman 1993). It must be noted that the process of cessation itself produces withdrawal symptoms, which include a variety of mood disturbances and affective symptoms (e.g., depressed mood, anxiety, nervousness, restlessness, irritability, fatigue and drowsiness); these are more pronounced in the days immediately following cessation and generally return to baseline levels within a month of continued abstinence. These differences in mood disturbance appear to be related to successful cessation as well.

Predictably, smokers reporting higher levels of negative mood and depressive symptoms were less likely to quit than were smokers with less mood disturbance (Covey, Glassman, Stetner , 1997). The meta-analysis by Hitsman et al. (2003) shows that lifetime history of major depression does not appear to be an independent risk factor for cessation failure in smoking-cessation treatment. Likewise, a recent article showed that the presence of depressive symptoms did not have a significant impact on smoking cessation (Kinnunen et al., 2006). During consultation, it is advised to ascertain systematically whether a history of depression is present by using simple validated questionnaires, such as the Beck Depression Inventory II (Beck, Steer, Brown, 1996). Smokers in this category are likely to experience intense withdrawal symptoms and will benefit from intensive pharmacological treatment for smoking cessation during the first 2–3 weeks of abstinence. Moreover, a judicious use of antidepressants should be considered and a referral to a specialist for the most challenging cases is advised (Blondal et al., 1999; Hughes 2007).

ANXIETY

Smoking is highly prevalent across most anxiety disorders and varies widely, depending on the specific diagnosis and the sample selected (Morissette et al., 2007). Smokers with anxiety disorders have more severe withdrawal symptoms during smoking cessation than smokers without anxiety disorders (Breslau, Kilbey, Andreski, 1992).

Moreover, smokers commonly implicate anxiety as a risk factor for relapse to smoking (Morissette et al., 2007; Brandon 1990). In these cases, psychological treatments that incorporate cognitive restructuring of automatic thoughts may also have considerable utility (Morissette et al., 2007). Understanding the functional relationship between smoking behavior and anxiety is important to improve assistance to those who are trying to quit, but additional research is also needed to understand factors contributing to the development, maintenance and relapse of smoking that are important to smokers with anxiety disorders.

During consultation, it is advised to ascertain the level of anxiety by using simple validated questionnaires such as the Hamilton Anxiety Scale (Hamilton, 1959). Be aware that anxiety is one of the nicotine withdrawal symptoms and smokers should be advised that their level of anxiety may increase within the first couple of weeks after smoking cessation. Smokers in this category will benefit from pharmacological treatment for smoking cessation during the first 2–3 weeks of abstinence. Moreover, a judicious use of anxiolytic drugs may be considered in individual cases (Hughes, Stead, Lancaster, 2000).

ALCOHOLISM

Current alcoholism is a negative prognostic factor for successful smoking cessation, and discontinuation of alcoholism is likely to increase the potential for successful smoking cessation. After correcting for sex, age and race, population studies have shown that smokers with active alcoholism in the preceding year were 60% less likely to quit than were smokers with no history of alcoholism. It was also interesting to observe that smokers whose alcoholism had remitted were at least as likely to quit as smokers reporting no alcohol use, with a greater than threefold increase in the likelihood of subsequent smoking cessation compared with smokers with current alcohol use. The notion that current alcoholism may interfere with the success of smoking cessation was confirmed in subsequent studies of smokers attending smoking cessation clinics, which predicted smoking relapse not only for smokers with current alcoholism at baseline but also for any alcohol use during cessation treatment (Hughes, Stead, Lancaster, 2000). Conversely, it appears that smoking cessation did not precipitate an alcoholic relapse (Martin et al., 1997) and, in actual fact, smoking cessation programs appear to improve quit rates in abusers undergoing alcohol treatment (Humfleet et al, 1999; Hurt et al. 1996).

Although the reasons for the detrimental effect of alcoholism on smoking cessation are unclear, controlled studies have shown that alcohol has the ability of producing a generalized increase in reported urge to smoke (Joseph 1993; Joseph et al.,1990). There is currently increasing support for addressing smoking cessation in alcohol-dependent persons, but the most efficacious strategies for smoking cessation in this population are not clear (Burton, Tiffany, 1997) . Behavioral therapy strategies are clearly important in smoking cessation programs for the general population, but it appears that low intensity programs are not effective in patients in alcohol treatment (Sayette et al., 2005).

Behavioral therapy for smoking cessation that is similar to standard counseling approaches for alcohol dependence has been shown to be very effective in recovering alcoholics, with quit rates at 1 year that are comparable with persons without an alcohol addiction history, at approximately 25% (Hurt Patten 2003).

All smokers should be advised to quit by their physician, but if a history of current alcoholism is present, a referral to a specialist center may be recommended because smokers in this category have been shown to perform poorly in smoking-cessation programs (Bobo 1998; Martin 1997). However, a smoker with a mild alcohol problem probably would not need to be referred to a specialist. In addition, the notion that even low-to-moderate levels of alcohol consumption during smoking cessation may decrease treatment success calls for a sensible plan against alcohol use during smoking-cessation efforts.

CONCLUSION

Tobacco smoking among patients with psychopathological disorders is more common than in the general population. The reason for this association is not clear, but it has been argued that smoking may help individuals to cope with stress (smokers reporting higher levels of negative mood and depressive symptoms are less likely to quit than those without these problems). Many social, psychologic and biologic explanations have been proposed, but today research focuses on neurobiological action of nicotine and its pharmacodynamic interactions. Further research are needed in order to provide a more detailed explanation of the relationship between tobacco smoking and more common psychopathological disorders, specifically for psychiatric chronic disorders such as schizophrenia and related disorders.

REFERENCES

Addington, J. (1998) Group treatment for smoking cessation among persons with schizophrenia. *Psychiatr. Services,* 1998, 49, 925–928.

Anda R. F., Williamson D. F., Escobedo L. G., Mast E. E., Giovino G. A., Remington P. L. (1990). Depression and the dynamics of smoking. *JAMA,* 264(12), 1541–1545.

Aubin H. J., H. Rollema H, T. H. Svensson, T. H., G. Winterer G. (2012) Smoking, quitting, and psychiatric disease: A review. *Neuroscience and Biobehavioral Reviews,* 36 271–284.

Beck A. T., Steer R. A., Brown G. K. (1996). Manual for the Beck Depression Inventory-II. The Psychological Corporation, TX, USA.

Blondal T., Gudmundsson L. J., Tomasson K. et al. (1999). The effects of fluoxetine combined with nicotine inhalers in smoking cessation a randomized trial. *Addiction,* 94(7), 1007–1015.

Bobo J. K., McIlvain H. E., Lando H. A., Walker R. D., Leed- Kelly A. (1998). Effect of smoking cessation counseling on recovery from alcoholism: findings from a randomized community intervention trial. *Addiction,* 93(6), 877–887.

Brandon T. H., Tiffany S. T., Obremski K. M., Baker T. B. (1990). Postcessation cigarette use: the process of relapse. *Addict. Behav.,* 15(2), 10514.

Breslau N., Kilbey M., Andreski P. (1993). Nicotine dependence and major depression. *Arch. Gen. Psychiat.,* 50, 31–35.

Breslau N., Kilbey M. M., Andreski P. (1992). Nicotine withdrawal symptoms and psychiatric disorders: findings from an epidemiologic study of young adults. *Am. J. Psychiat.*, 149(4), 464–469.

Breslau N., Peterson E., Schultz L., Andreski P., Chilcoat H. (1996). Are smokers with alcohol disorders less likely to quit? *Am. J. Public Health*, 86(7), 985–990.

Brown, S.; Inskip, H.; Barraclough, B. (2000) Causes of the excess mortality of schizophrenia. *Brit. J. Psychiat.*, 177, 212–217.

Burton S. M., Tiffany S. T. (1997).The effect of alcohol consumption on craving to smoke. *Addiction*, 92(1), 15–26.

Casella, G.; Caponnetto, P.; Polosa, R. (2010) Therapeutic advances in the treatment of nicotine addiction: Present and future. *Ther. Adv. Chronic Dis.*, 1, 95–106.

Covey L. S., Glassman A. H., Stetner F. (1997). Major depression following smoking cessation. *Am. J.Psychiat.*, 209–224 (1985).

Covey L. S., Glassman A. H., Stetner F., Becker J. (1993).Effect of history of alcoholism or major depression on smoking cessation. *Am. J. Psychiat.*, 150(10), 1546–1547.

De Leon, J.; Diaz, F. J. (2005), A meta-analysis of worldwide studies demonstrates an association between schizophrenia and tobacco smoking behaviors. *Schizophr. Res.*, 76, 1351–1357.

Dierker L. C. et al. (2005) Association between psychiatric disorders and smoking stages among Latino adolescents. *Drug and Alcohol Dependence*, 80 361–368.

Fergusson D. M., Lynskey M. T., Horwood L. J. (1996). Comorbidity between depressive disorders and nicotine dependence in a cohort of 16 years olds. *Arch. Gen. Psychiat.*, 53(11), 1043–1047.

Glassman, A. H. (1993)Cigarette smoking: Implications for psychiatric illness. *Am. J. Psychiatry*, 1993,150, 546–553.

Glassman A. H., Covey L. S., Stetner F., Rivelli S. (2001). Smoking cessation and the course of major depression: a follow-up study. *Lancet*, 357(9272), 1929–1932.

Hamilton M. (1959).The assessment of anxiety states by rating. *Br. J. Med. Psychol.*, 32, 50–55.

Hitsman B., Borrelli B., McChargue D. E., Spring B., Niaura R. (2003).History of depression and smoking cessation outcome: a meta-analysis. *J. Consult. Clin. Psychol.*, 71(4), 657–663.

Hughes J. R., Stead L. F., Lancaster T. (2000). Anxiolytics for smoking cessation. *Cochrane Database Syst. Rev.*, 4, CD000031.

Hughes J. R., Stead L. F., Lancaster T. (2007).Antidepressants for smoking cessation. *Cochrane Database Syst. Rev.*, 24(1), CD000031 .35.

Humfleet G., Munoz R., Sees K., Reus V., Hall S. (1999). History of alcohol or drug problems, current use of alcohol or marijuana, and success in quitting smoking. *Addict. Behav.*, 24(1), 149–154.

Hurt R. D., Eberman K. M., Croghan I. T. et al. *(1994)*. Nicotine dependence treatment during inpatient treatment for other addictions: a prospective intervention trial. *Alcohol Clin. Exp. Res.*, 18(4), 867–872.

Hurt R. D., Patten C. A. (2003). Treatment of tobacco dependence in alcoholics. *Rec. Dev. Alcohol*, 16, 335–359.

Joseph A. M. (1993).Nicotine treatment at the drug dependency program of the Minneapolis VA Medical Center. A researcher's perspective. *J. Subst. Abuse Treat.*, 10(2), 147–152.

Joseph A. M., Nichol K. L., Willenbring M. L., Korn J. E., Lysaght L. S. (1990). Beneficial effects of treatment of nicotine dependence during an inpatient substance abuse treatment program. *JAMA*, 263(22), 3043–3046.

Kelly, C.; McCreadie, R. G. (1999) Smoking habits, current symptoms, and premorbid characteristics of schizophrenic patients in Nithsdale, Scotland. *Am. J. Psychiatry*, 156, 1751–1757.

Keltner. N. L.; Grant, J. S.(2006) Smoke, smoke, smoke that cigarette. *Perspect. Psychiatr. Care*, 42, 256–261.

Kinnunen T., Henning L., Nordstrom B. L. (1999). Smoking cessation in individuals with depression: recommendations for treatment. *CNS Drugs*, 11, 93–103.

Kinnunen T., Haukkala A., Korhonen T., Quiles Z. N., Spiro A., Garvey A. J. (2006).Depression and smoking across 25 years of the Normative Aging Study. *Int. J. Psychiat. Med.*, 36(4), 413–426.

Lightwood, J. M.; Glantz, S. A. (1997) Short-term economic and health benefits of smoking cessation:Myocardial infarction and stroke. *Circulation*, 96, 1089–1096.

Martin J. E., Calfas K. J., Patten C. A. *et al. (1997).* Prospective evaluation of three smoking interventions in 205 recovering alcoholics: one-year results of Project SCRAP-Tobacco. *J. Consult. Clin. Psychol.*, 65(1), 190–194.

Medical Center. A researcher's perspective. (1993) *J. Subst. Abuse Treat.*, 10(2), 147–152.

Morissette S. B., Tull M. T., Gulliver S. B., Kamholz B. W., Zimering R. T. (2007).Anxiety, anxiety disorders, tobacco use, and nicotine: a critical review of interrelationships. *Psychol. Bull.*, 133(2), 245–272.

Murphy J. M., Horton N. J., Monson R. R. (2003). Cigarette smoking in relation to depression: historical trends from the Stirling County Study. *Am. J. Psychiat.*, 160(9), 1663–1669.

Revell A. D., Warburton D. M., Wesnes K. (1985)Smoking as a coping strategy. *Addict. Behav.* 10(3), smoking across 25 years of the Normative Aging Study. *Int. J. Psychiat. Med.*, 36(4), 413–426.

Sayette M. A., Martin C. S., Wertz J. M., Perrott M. A., Peters A. R. (2005). The effects of alcohol on cigarette craving in heavy smokers and tobacco chippers. *Psychol. Addict. Behav.*, 19(3), 263–270.

United States Public Health Service. The Health Benefits of Smoking Cessation; United States Public Health Service. Office on Smoking and Health: Atlanta, GA, USA, 1990. historical trends from the Stirling County Study. *Am. J. Psychiat.*, 160(9), 1663–1669.

Wilhelm K., Arnold K., Niven H., Richmond R. (2004). Grey lungs and blue moods: smoking cessation in the context of lifetime depression history. *Aust. NZ J. Psychiat.*, 38(11E12), 896–905.

Zvolensky M. J. et al. (2011) Personality disorders and cigarette smoking among adults in the United States. *Journal of Psychiatric Research*, 45 835e841.

In: Smoking Restrictions
Editor: Nazmi Sari

ISBN: 978-1-63321-148-3
© 2014 Nova Science Publishers, Inc.

Chapter 8

IMPACTS OF SMOKING ON PERIODONTAL AND PERI-IMPLANT HEALTH

Mirella Lindoso Gomes Campos[1*], *Mônica Grazieli Corrêa*[2] *and Antonio Wilson Sallum*[3]

[1]University of Sacred Heart – USC, Jardim Brasil. Bauru, São Paulo, Brasil
[2]Paulista University – UNIP, Aquarela Tower. São Paulo, São Paulo, Brazil
[3]Piracicaba Dental School, State University of Campinas - UNICAMP
Limeira Avenue, Areião. Piracicaba, São Paulo, Brazil

ABSTRACT

Smoking is considered a risk factor for several leading causes of death in the world and has been considered a public health problem worldwide. Tobacco smoke contains numerous components which are harmful not only to the systemic health of the individual, but also to periodontal health. The smoking habit, therefore, is also recognized as a risk factor in Periodontics having relation of cause and effect proven in longitudinal clinical studies and provides increasing incidence and severity of periodontal diseases. Smoker patients with periodontal disease when compared to non-smoker and former-smoker patients have more extensive and severe alveolar bone loss, deeper periodontal pockets, greater number of teeth with furcation involvement, more periodontal clinical attachment loss, and several postoperative complications and implant failure in oral peri-implant sites such as less of osseo-integration and more peri-implantitis. Therefore, this chapter aims to critically review the literature, contextualizing the impact of smoking within periodontics and the specific action of chemical compounds on periodontal cells proliferation, emphasizing the damage in the periodontal insertion and protection and the importance of motivation in the dentist to advise smoking cessation.

Keywords: Smoking; adverse effects; Periodontitis; Peri-implantitis; Osseointegration

---

[*] Corresponding author: Email: mirellalindoso@gmail.com, Phone: 55 14 21077340.

1. Introduction

Tobacco is a plant with a scientific classification of *Nicotina tabacum*. It is legally marketed worldwide in the form of cigars, cigarettes, pipes and several chewable forms. Nicotine is the main component of tobacco and it is responsible for causing addiction in users as well as physiologic and psychological dependence. Indiscriminate selling and the easy access to purchase the final product cause the numbers of smokers to increase every year.

Smoking is considered a risk factor for several of the leading causes of death in the world and has been considered a public health problem not only in developing countries but also in developed countries. Tobacco smoke contains numerous components besides nicotine such as acrolein and acetaldehyde, which are harmful not only to the systemic health of the individual, but also to periodontal health. Its relation to periodontal disease has been extensively studied and is well elucidated in the scientific literature. The smoking habit is related to increasing progression and the severity of periodontal diseases; the harmful habit of smoking also worsens the biological response of the periodontium to the periodontal pathogens. Smoker patients with periodontal disease, when compared to non-smoker and former-smoker patients, have more extensive and severe alveolar bone loss, deeper periodontal pockets, a greater number of teeth with furcation involvement and more periodontal clinical attachment loss, which is considered the gold standard parameter for identifying the progression of periodontitis.

Nowadays, with the advent and popularization of rehabilitation with oral implants, this interrelation needs to be scientifically assessed again. Several postoperative complications and implant failure in oral peri-implant sites, such as less of osseo-integration and more peri-implantitis, have been described in literature but a true interaction is still controversial. In this way, the interaction of tobacco with oral implants should be better explored to consider whether the smoking habit acts as a risk factor for peri-implant disease and thus interferes with the rehabilitation prognosis.

The clinician should be familiar with these interactions to clarify the disease process to the patient and the interaction of the smoking habit in the development of periodontal and peri-implant diseases and its relationship with the periodontal prognosis. Therefore, this chapter aims to critically review the literature by contextualizing the impact of smoking within Periodontics and the specific action of chemical compounds on periodontal cell proliferation, emphasizing the damage in the periodontal and peri-implant insertion and protection. We will also focus on the importance of the role of dentists in successful smoking cessation programs.

2. Impact of Tobacco Consumption on General Health and Characteristics of Cigarette Smoke

Smoking is a risk factor for six of the eight leading causes of death worldwide (WHO, 2008) and has been considered a public health problem not only in developed countries but also in developing ones. Smokers have a 70% higher risk of death from cancer, cardiovascular or pulmonary disease compared to non-smokers (WHO, 2008).

Nicotine, one of the toxic substances present in tobacco, is responsible for causing similar effects such as drug addiction to heroin or cocaine. According to the World Health Organization, there are about 1.1 billion smokers in the world and this population is increasing, especially in developing countries (WHO, 2003). The prevalence of current tobacco smoking is an important predictor of the future burden of tobacco-related diseases. Active or direct tobacco smoking is responsible for the death of 5 million people. According to the 2004 WHO estimate, among the global deaths attributed to all causes observed in individuals aged 30-44 years, 7% were related to tobacco and, in the USA, the proportion found in individuals of the same age group was about 14% (WHO, 2012).

Cigarette smoke is a complex mixture of gases and particles from burning tobacco, which contains over 4000 potentially toxic substances including 43 carcinogens (Haverstoch & Mandracchia, 1998). The gas phase consists of carbon monoxide, carbon dioxide, nitrogen, oxygen, hydrogen cyanide, acrolein, acetaldehyde, and formaldehyde (Silverstein, 1992). In the particulate phase water, nitrates, nitrosamines, and aromatic hydrocarbons are found (Hanes et al., 1991). Nicotine is found both in the particulate phase and in the gas phase. Free nicotine that is found mainly in the gas phase is the most active type that is rapidly absorbed and it intensifies the degree of dependence (Robertson & Richard, 1998). More than 600 additives are used by the tobacco industry to make it more palatable and several have the function of releasing more nicotine, ammonia being the most important one.

Nicotine is the primary reason for smoking. This substance can be absorbed through the skin, mucous membranes (stomach and intestine), the lungs, and is transported through the bloodstream. Nicotine reaches the central nervous system (CNS), through the blood-brain barrier and exerts its effects in approximately 7 seconds (Brunton, Chabner, Knollmann, 2011). About 70% of the inhaled nicotine is metabolized in the liver and, to a lesser extent in the lungs and kidneys (Furtado, 2002). Nicotine distribution in tissue is fast and provides a cumulative effect in the body (Focchi, 2003).

Chronic intake of nicotine has a complex effect on the human body leading to psychological and physical dependence due to its neurobiological and psycho-stimulant characteristics (Robbers, Speedie, Tyler, 1997). This toxic component acts especially on dopaminergic mesolimbic centers and cholinergic nucleus accumbens, causing increased production of norepinephrine, dopamine and other psychoactive hormones, leading to addiction due to its euphoric anxiolytic properties (Rosenberg, 2004; Furtado, 2002). In the International Classification of Disease 10 (ICD-10), the World Health Organization classifies the addiction to tobacco as F-12 category "Mental and behavioral disorders due to use of tobacco" (WHO, 1992). In The Diagnostic and Statistical Manual of Mental Disorders IV (DSM-IV), the American Psychiatric Association classifies the nicotine-addiction (not the influence of tobacco use) as a "substance-related disorder" in a subgroup of "substance dependence and substance abuse" (American Psychiatric Association, 2000).

Benowitz & Hennigfield (1994) found that the average concentration of nicotine in the blood of dependent smokers is 300ng per milliliter. One cigarette produces blood concentrations of about 14ng/ml, reaching 70ng/ml in five cigarettes smoked per day. Thus, it could be estimated that the levels of 50 to 70ng/ml would be the minimum concentration to create addiction. These levels correspond to 4mg to 6mg of daily nicotine inhalation.

Nicotine is a tertiary amine and is constituted by pyridine and pyrolidine rings and has a short half-life (Rosenberg, 2004). In *Nicotiana tabacum* stereoisomers the most important pharmacological compounds are found including anabasine, anabatine, nornicotine, myosin,

N- metilanabasina nicotirine and nornicotirine (Rosenberg, 2004). The activity of nornicotine and anabasine is similar to that of nicotine (Rosenberg, 2004). The type of tobacco, and the mode and frequency of puffs influence the quantification of these alkaloids. Quantitatively and qualitatively, the most important metabolites are cotinine and nicotine-N-oxide (Benowitz, 1998).

Both nicotine and cotinine can be detected in urine, blood and saliva. The detection of nicotine is more limited since its half-life in the plasma after inhalation is 30 to 60 minutes (Furtado, 2002), which could extend to 2 hours (Focchi, 2003). On the other hand, the plasma half-life of cotinine extends, on average, to 36 to 40 hours and sometimes even longer, and can be detected several hours after smoking cessation (Benowitz, 1998). In active or passive smokers, the levels of cotinine concentration are linear with the amount of tobacco consumed and the degree of exposure to environmental tobacco smoke by passive smokers (Benowitz, 1998).

The carbon monoxide (CM) is 4% of cigarette smoke (Haverstoch & Mandracchia, 1998). It is a toxic, odorless, colorless, tasteless and non-irritating gas that interferes with oxygen transported in blood and its use. The CM affinity to hemoglobin (Hb) is 220 times greater than for oxygen (Brunton, Chabner, Knollmann, 2011). Even at low concentrations of alveolar CM, smokers have significant levels of carboxyhemoglobin (COHb) (5-15% in smokers; 0.5 to 3% in nonsmokers), due to the metabolism of Hb and air pollution (Beckers & Camu, 1991). CM is only eliminated by breathing and its binding with Hb is a very stable connection, which can be detected even after the patient's death (Klaassen, 1996). This set of phenomena, by reducing the availability of oxygen to the damaged tissues, may interfere directly with tissue repair.

Hydrogen cyanide is a colorless and highly toxic compound present in cigarette smoke. It was used in World War II as a genocidal agent (Martin, 2008) and is also used as an insecticide. When absorbed by human cells it reacts with trivalent iron cytochrome oxidase in mitochondria. Cellular respiration is then inhibited, resulting in cytotoxic hypoxia and lactic acidosis (Brunton, Chabner, Knollmann, 2011). These enzymatic changes in cellular respiration can affect the process of tissue repair.

Aldehydes, volatile components present in the composition of cigarette smoke, are hydrocarbons formed from the incomplete combustion of tobacco and by oxidation by sunlight (Brunton, Chabner, Knollmann, 2011). Acetaldehyde, the initial product of the oxidation of ethanol, and acrolein, are potent toxic compounds even in small quantities. Such aldehydes have cytotoxic and genotoxic effects in cultured human bronchial cells and fibroblasts (Grafström et al., 1994).

Smoke not only affects those who actively use tobacco manufactured derivates, but also others who are exposed to tobacco smoke. The environmental tobacco smoke (ETS) is a major contributor to the increase in concentration and exposure to particles indoors. It is composed of a mixture of smoke produced by the combustion of tobacco and that exhaled by smokers. Arguably, many of its compounds are toxic or carcinogenic chemicals and inhaling them can cause various health hazards (WHO, 2000). The air polluted by tobacco smoke contains, on average, three times more nicotine, three times more carbon monoxide, and up to fifty times more carcinogens than the smoke that enters the mouth of the smoker after going through the filter of the cigarette (WHO, 2007).

The subjects exposed to ETS are known as passive smokers or second hand smokers. Second hand smoking (SHS) is seen as a cause of 600,000 deaths per year (Oberg et al.,

2011). In 2007, the World Health Organization (WHO) and the Centers of Disease Control and Prevention (CDC) supported the implementation of the Global Adult Tobacco Survey (GATS) in 14 countries: Bangladesh; Brazil; China; Egypt; Russia; Philippines; India; Mexico; Poland; Thailand; Turkey; Ukraine; Uruguay and Vietnam. Results from GATS help countries in formulation, tracking and implementation of effective tobacco control interventions. For example, 22 million people in Brazil were exposed to SHS in at least one of the environments studied in the survey. The survey showed that 9 million people were exposed to tobacco smoke in the workplace, 5 million in health facilities, 12 million in restaurants, 5.5 million in public transport and 4.3 million in buildings or government offices (Brasil, 2010). It is estimated that there are about 2 billion passive smokers worldwide; 700 million of them are children (Organización Panamericana de Salud, 2000). It is proven that there are no safe levels of ETS exposure and even short period of exposure can trigger cardiovascular lesions and significant contamination by carcinogens among non-smokers.

SHS can cause heart disease by increasing inflammation and acute changes in the endothelium, vasoconstriction and increased platelet aggregation capacity. This can trigger acute manifestations of cardiovascular diseases such as myocardial infarction and stroke, especially for people who already suffer from acute coronary syndromes (Raupach et al., 2006). The effects of SHS on the cardiovascular system generate proportionately higher risk for a low exposure and they are comparable to chronic smoking, which is equivalent to the risk of smoking one to nine cigarettes per day (Barnoya et al., 2005). Likewise, it is responsible for lung disease in adults and worsening the risk of middle ear and acute respiratory infections, asthma problems with lung development in children (especially among asthmatics). It is also associated with an increased risk of sudden infant death, nasal cancer and morbidity/mortality from lung cancer and cardiovascular diseases. Also, in pregnant women the exposure is associated with decreased weight of the newborn (WHO, 2007). Carcinogens such as NNK (4- (methylnitrosamin) -1 - (3-pyridyl)-1-butanone), tobacco-specific lung carcinogens found in the urine of smokers, are also detected in the urine of non-smokers immediately after contact with SHS and its concentration increases by 6% for every hour of exposure (Stark et al., 2007).

3. THE INFLUENCE OF CIGARETTE SMOKE IN PERIODONTOLOGY

The etiology of Periodontitis is multifactorial, resulting from the interaction of the biofilm with the host immune-inflammatory response, which can be modulated by environmental and systemic factors, such as smoking (Armitage, 1999) as seen in Figure 1.

Cigarette smoking is a known risk factor for the development of periodontal disease (Tonetti, 1998; Genco, 1996). There is a clear relationship reported in literature between the severity and extent of periodontal disease and the direct influence of smoking in worsening periodontal conditions. Authors have shown in clinical studies that smokers and patients with periodontal disease have more extensive and severe alveolar bone loss (Baljoon et al., 2004; Rosa et al., 2008), deeper periodontal pockets and greater number of teeth with furcation involvement (van der Weijden et al., 2001; Calsina et al., 2002; Axselsson et al., 1998; Kerdvongbundit & Wikesjö, 2000).

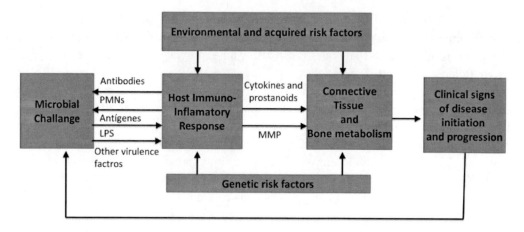

Figure 1. Etiopathogenesis of Periodontal disease adapted from Page & Kornman, 1997.

Smokers also have greater clinical attachment loss compared to non-smokers and patients who were former smokers, suggesting a local action of cigarettes (Haffajee & Sockransky, 2001a). However, more studies elucidating the action mechanism of cigarette smoke on the periodontal structures, the interference with the cell metabolism, and the interference with the metabolism of the periodontal tissues and the periodontal immune response are needed. Therefore, *in vitro* and *in vivo* studies are still needed to better answer how cigarette smoke and isolating cigarette compounds could lead to tissue destruction due to its direct toxic effects or acting indirectly and being responsible for initiating the inflammatory response.

3.1. In Vitro Studies

In vitro studies are the first step to unravel cell physiology and their behavior in the face of certain conditions and drugs. They have great importance in science because the researchers can artificially control the temperature, pressure, concentration, amount of substance, time and the choice of samples and thus better study the phenomenon with greater focus. Several studies have been conducted to evaluate the impact of nicotine, cotinine and other toxic smoke compounds on periodontal cells. Differentiation, proliferation, cell adhesion and cytotoxicity are some of the issues studied.

Ramp et al. (1991) studied the effect of nicotine on cultured osteoblast type cells. The results showed that nicotine inhibited alkaline phosphatase activity and collagen synthesis in a dose-dependent pattern. There were no effects of nicotine on non-collagenous proteins and the authors observed a stimulation of DNA synthesis. Fang et al. (1991) examined the effects of nicotine on the proliferation of osteoblasts and the alkaline phosphatase activity. The results suggest that nicotine might have critical effects on bone metabolism to inhibit osteoblast-like cell proliferation and stimulate, in a dose-dependent manner, the formation of tartrate-resistant acid phosphatase (TRAP) positive cells (osteoclasts).

In another study, Liu et al. (2001) isolated osteoprogenitor cells from the bone marrow of the iliac crest donated by three healthy donors. These cells were cultured and exposed to cigarette smoke extract (CSE). The authors noted that CSE inhibited the proliferation of osteoprogenitor cells incubated in control conditions and on those incubated in the presence of osteogenic supplements in a dose-concentration dependent manner. The effects were reversible, indicating that the inhibition was not triggered by cellular toxicity or non-specific cell death. Gullihorn et al. (2005) studied the effect of different doses of nicotine and CSE condensate in osteoblast-like cells. Nicotine stimulated in a dose-dependent manner the bone cell metabolism on all samples and its negative effect could be observed in low concentrations of nicotine (12.5ng/ml of nicotine, half the concentration observed on smokers). The preparations with CSE condensate with similar concentrations of nicotine reduced the metabolic activity showing inhibitory effect at all levels. The authors speculate on its conclusion that the delay observed in clinical healing of skeletal injuries on patients who smoke may be in part a consequence of the absorption of other toxic components of the cigarette besides nicotine.

Tanaka et al. (2006) found that expression of macrophage colony stimulated factor (M-CSF) and prostaglandin E_2 (PGE_2), inflammatory markers related to bone resorption, increased in cells cultured with lipopolysaccharides (LPS) and nicotine compared to those which were grown only on nicotine. The expression of osteoprotegerin (OPG), a protein that in humans inhibits osteoclastogenesis, increased in the early stage of culture with nicotine and LPS, but decreased in the final stage. The medium containing M-CSF and PGE_2 produced by human osteoblasts treated with nicotine and soluble receptor activators of nuclear factor kappa-B ligand (RANKL) increased marking osteoclasts-like cells compared with that produced by nicotine treatment alone. The results suggest that nicotine and LPS stimulate osteoclast formation by increased production of M-CSF and PGE_2 and this association produces a greater stimulation compared to the effect of nicotine alone.

Some studies have been conducted to investigate the effects of cigarette smoke and its components on fibroblasts, whose function is critical in the metabolism of connective tissue and in tissue repair. Several researchers have been investigating the effect of tobacco components on gingival fibroblast and periodontal ligament fibroblast cultures. Tipton & Dabbous (1995) studied the effect of nicotine on the proliferation of gingival fibroblasts cultivated from healthy individuals without gingival inflammation, the production of fibronectin and type I collagen turnover. The authors found that nicotine causes cell death at concentrations greater than 0.075%. At concentrations from 0.001 to 0.075%, nicotine significantly inhibited the proliferation of fibroblasts. The production of fibronectin and type I collagen were significantly inhibited at nicotine concentrations $\geq$ 0.05% and $\geq$ 0.025% and concentrations $\geq$ 0.025% of nicotine were able to significantly increase the activity of colagenase. These results suggest that even in low amounts, nicotine can increase the destruction of the gingival fibroblasts for smoker patients and worsen gingivitis.

Cattaneo et al. (2000), Rota et al. (2001) and Poggi et al. (2002) evaluated the effect of components of the volatile phase of cigarette smoke, acrolein and acetaldehyde on the cytoskeleton of human gingival fibroblasts (HGFs). In these three studies the authors obtained HGFs from healthy subjects with non-inflamed gingiva and the cells were incubated in different concentrations of acrolein and acetaldehyde. Two of these studies found that both substances produced similar effects, resulting in inhibition of adhesion and proliferation of HGFs in a dose-dependent manner showing the cytotoxic effect of these volatile components. Cattaneo et al. (2000) also observed that the cytotoxic effect on HGFs could be reversed in 3 days after removal of these substances. The final consequences of these volatile compounds could be impairment of the maintenance, integrity and remodeling of the oral connective tissue (Poggi et al., 2002). In a recent research, Anand et al. (2011) also confirmed the cytotoxic effect of acrolein in a dose-dependent manner on HGFs leading to a complete inhibition of attachment and proliferation at higher concentrations.

In other research, Zhang et al. (2009) evaluated the influence of cigarette smoke condensation (CSC) on the collagen-degrading ability of HGFs cultured from a healthy subject and its mechanism. The authors observed that cell proliferation decreased and cytotoxicity increased in HGFs with increasing concentrations of CSC implying an increase in the collagen-degrading ability of HGFs by altering the production and localization of matrix metalloproteinases (MMPs) and tissue inhibitors of metalloproteinases (TIMPs).

Giannopoulou et al. (1999) showed adverse effects of nicotine on various functions of the periodontal ligament fibroblasts (PLF). The authors observed a dose-dependent inhibition of cell proliferation and cell proliferation at concentrations $\geq$ 100ng/ml. The alkaline phosphatase activity and chemotaxis decreased significantly in a concentration-dependent manner. The authors concluded that these results partially explain the increased incidence and severity of chronic periodontitis in smokers. In another study, James et al. (1999) investigated the action of nicotine and its primary metabolite, cotinine, on cultures of human PLF. The results showed that nicotine inhibits the adhesion and growth of PFL in all concentrations tested. On the other hand, cotinine appears to inhibit the growth and adhesion of PFL at the highest concentration studied but this result was not statistically significant.

Gamal & Bayomy (2002) cultured PLF from smoker patients with periodontal disease. The authors cultured cells on root segments of extracted teeth, and found that the samples of the fibroblasts of the groups who smoked up to 19 cigarettes/day and 20 cigarettes or more cigarettes/day were less adherent to the root surface compared with the positive control groups and PLF cultured from non-smokers. In 2010, Yanagita et al. evaluated by real time protein chain reaction (RT-PCR) the effects of nicotine for cytodifferentation of murine periodontal ligament (MPDL) cell and also its effect on mineralized nodule formation. The authors found that gene expression of extracellular matrices and osteoblastic transcription factors were reduced in nicotine-treated MPDL cells. In addition, mineralized nodule formation was inhibited in MPDL cells in the presence of nicotine and concluded that nicotine may negatively regulate the cytodifferentation and the mineralization of MPDL cells.

A recent study conducted by Ng et al. (2013) opened a new way to understand the mechanisms of interaction of nicotine with the healing process. The authors investigated the effect of nicotine regenerative potentials of human mesenchymal stem cells (MSC) and periodontal ligament-derived stem cells (PDLSC) through genetic and microRNA (miRNA) regulation. Nicotine reduced significantly MSC and PDLSC proliferation and also retarded the locomotion of these adult stem cells. Furthermore, gene expression showed the reduced osteogenic differentiation capabilities in the presence of nicotine. In addition, the miRNA profile of nicotine-treated PDLSC was altered. The authors concluded that the results suggested that miRNAs might play an important role in the nicotine effects on stem cells.

In summary it can be said that tobacco and several isolated components of tobacco are cytotoxic for periodontal cells and also change their physiological ability of differentiation and adhesion. In addition, the tobacco and its components increase the synthesis of prostaglandins, pro-inflammatory cytokines and metalloproteinases related to increased tissue damage. This can all lead to lower repair and regeneration of periodontal tissues. We provide a summary of the consequences of compounds in tobacco on cell types in Table 1.

3.2. In Vivo Studies

In scientific research, animal models must be used whenever there are any impeditive ethical issues to develop the methodology in humans due to risk, toxicity and death. These models are of great importance to better understand drug interaction with living tissues, regeneration models and tissue healing, as well as the physiological response to physical and chemical stimuli. Animal models have been widely used in medical science to assess the interaction of tobacco compounds with living tissues. Periodontology has been using this model to understand more deeply the physiological interaction of tobacco compounds in the periodontium.

Several studies evaluating the systemic impairment of cigarette smoke have been published. Terashima et al. (1997) studied the effect of cigarette smoke inhalation (CSI) in rabbits on the rate of production and the release of polymorphonuclear leukocytes (PMN) from the bone marrow into the peripheral blood circulation. The results showed that chronic exposure CSI promoted a significant reduction in PMN transit time through bone marrow into the peripheral circulation by reducing the transit time of the post-mitotic. However, in both pools mitotic and post-mitotic, there were significant increases in the number of PMN. The authors conclude that these changes contribute to the observation of leukocytosis in smokers. In another study, Vanscheeuwijcka et al. (2002) evaluated in rats the toxicity of CSI testing a mixture of primary cigarette smoke with the addition of manufactured compounds (experimental) and without the addition of these compounds (control). More than 333 manufactured ingredients used in tobacco, such as flavoring, colorants, menthol and liners were evaluated. The authors found that these elements were not capable of altering the toxicity of the smoke generated by cigarettes on PMN and the production of liver enzymes.

Low mechanical properties of bone exposed to CSI have been studied in the literature. Akhter et al. (2005) verified that mice exposed to CSI had low bone volume and trabecular thickness in femur and tibiae bones compared to control group and also had low strength properties. El-Zawawy et al. (2006) evaluated histologically, histometrically and radiographically a tibial fracture model in rats exposed to CSI. The authors found that the results suggest that animals exposed to CSI suffer a delay in bone remodeling compared to the control group and that the cigarette exposure delayed the chondrogenesis.

Other researchers have been studying the interference of CSI in periodontal impact and its cessation impairs in periodontal tissues. César-Neto et. al. (2006) histometrically evaluated the influence CSI on the alveolar bone of the furcation region in rats. The data showed that the animals that were continuously exposed to CSI had a lower proportion of mineralized tissues compared to the control group and CSI cessation, showing that the interruption of CSI exposure brings benefit to tissue mineralization. In another study of the same group, César-Neto et al. (2005a) observed that CSI increased furcation bone loss in rats with experimental periodontal disease induced by ligatures and negatively impacted in mandibular bone quality. Additionally, the authors found that CSI cessation seems to reverse its impact on mandibular bone, and, therefore, may be of clinical relevance. Benatti et al. (2005) evaluated the impact of CSI and the administration of nicotine injection (NI) on the periodontal healing process in the absence of biofilms in fenestration defects in rats, with root exposure and scaling of cementum and periodontal ligament. The authors found that the CSI group was associated with a lower bone density and a lower bone fill compared to the control group and NI, concluding that the CSI reduces the ability of periodontal healing.

Table 1. Cell response to tobacco compounds

Cell Type / Compound	Osteoblast	Osteoclast	Fibroblast	References
Nicotine	Inhibit	Stimulate	Inhibit	Ramp et al., 1991; Fang et al., 1991., Gullihorn et al., 2005 Tanaka et al., 2006; Tipton & Dabous, 1995; Gamal & Bayomy, 2002.
Acetaldehyde	-	-	Inhibit	Cataneo et al., 2000; Rota et al., 2001; Poggi et al., 2002.
Acrolein	-	-	Inhibit	Anand et al., 2011; Cataneo et al., 2000; Rota et al., 2001; Poggi et al., 2002.
Cigarette Smoke Condensate and Extract	Inhibit	-	Inhibit	Liu et al., 2001; Gullihorn et al., 2005; Zhang et al., 2009.

Table 2. Periodontal response in animal models to nicotine and cigarette smoke inhalation (CSI) in health, disease and occlusal trauma (OT)

Condition / Compound	Periodontal Health	Periodontal Diseases	Primary OT	Secondary OT	Periodontal Regeneration
Nicotine	-	-	Enhance bone loss	Enhance bone loss	-
CSI	Lower proportion of mineralized tissue	Enhance bone loss	Enhance bone loss and TRAP-positive cells	-	Low periodontal regeneration
References	César-Neto et al., 2006	César-Neto et al., 2005	Nogueira-Filho et al., 2004; Campos et al., 2013	Nogueira-Filho et al., 2004	Benatti et al., 2005; Corrêa et al., 2010

Another study observed the influence of CSI on regeneration technique in rats. Corrêa et al. (2010) used enamel matrix derivate (EMD) in non-infected fenestration defects in rats. The results showed that EMD may provide an increased defect fill and cementum formation in the presence or absence of CSI in the fenestration model. However, CSI produced a detrimental effect on bone healing when the density of newly formed bone was considered, showing that CSI negatively interfered with this periodontal regeneration technique.

Few studies show the negative impact of CSI and tobacco compounds on non-infectious periodontal lesions called primary occlusal trauma and now cigarette smoke rises as an indicator factor in the development of these lesions. Nogueira-Filho et al. (2004) verify histometrically the effect of peritoneal injections of nicotine in alveolar bone loss in lower molars of rats in which experimental occlusal trauma was developed by occlusal overload. These authors concluded that nicotine injection was able to worsen alveolar bone loss in teeth with primary and secondary occlusal trauma. Because there are other cytotoxic compounds in CSI besides nicotine, Campos et al. (2013) evaluated the impact of short-term CSI in experimental primary occlusal trauma (OT) in rats with a unilateral occlusal interference inducing experimental occlusal trauma. The authors concluded that CSI increases early bone loss and enhances TRAP-positive cells (osteoclasts) in association with OT, and the duration of CSI exposure negatively influences the periodontal parameters.

In summary, it can be concluded that nicotine and CSI can worsen periodontal parameters in infectious and non-infectious lesion and also interfere negatively with periodontal regeneration. Table 2 summarizes these findings.

3.3. Clinical Studies

In 1999, the American Academy of Periodontology classified smoking as one of the environmental conditions or exposures that may affect periodontitis (Armitage, 1999). As seen in this chapter, numerous *in vivo* and *in vitro* studies described the potential mechanisms whereby smoking tobacco may be a predisposition to periodontal diseases. Smoking may have a negative effect over the humoral immune, the cellular immune, and the inflammatory systems and also its cytotoxity has a negative impairment over periodontal tissue remodeling. Thus, the clinician should be alert to changes in radiographic and clinical periodontal parameters and also in the prognosis of the smoker patients within the proposed periodontal therapy. Table 3 present the effects of smoking on periodontal disease etiopathogenesis.

Radiographic studies in humans have been proposed to evaluate the negative influence of smoking on the alveolar bone. Bergström et al. (1991) evaluated the influence of smoking on alveolar crest height of patients with periodontal health using interproximal radiographic technique. Data showed that the distance of the cementum enamel junction (CEJ) to the interproximal septus was significantly higher in smokers, and that seemed to have a dose-dependent effect. Bolin et al. (1993) also observed significant marginal bone loss described as the ratio of "bone height/root length" measured in intraoral radiographs in smoking patients. These authors also found that smoking cessation had benefits in improving alveolar bone height among the patients. In a 20-year prospective study, Jansson and Lavstedt (2002) evaluated radiographs to assess proximal bone loss over these patients and found that smoking was significantly correlated to an increased marginal bone loss over 20 years and smoking cessation brought benefits to diminish marginal bone loss. In another prospective study, Baljoon et al., (2004) evaluated the presence and the extension of vertical bone loss using periapical radiographs in a 10-year study. After controlling for age, the severity of the vertical defects was also significantly associated with smoking. Rosa et al. (2008) evaluated the impact of smoking on alveolar bone loss in dental students without periodontitis through digital bitewing radiographs. All clinical criteria (plaque index, bleeding index, periodontal attachment level, gingival recession) that were assessed were significantly worse in smokers. Also, densitometry analysis and alveolar bone height were significantly lower in smokers even for those with low cigarette consumption. Thus, it can be concluded that cigarette consumption has a negative impact on alveolar bone.

Several authors have been examining the association between smoking and tooth loss rate. Krall et al. (1999) evaluated alveolar bone loss in cigar and pipe smokers and the measurements were assessed at each examination of intraoral periapical radiographs. The authors found that men who smoke cigars or pipes were at increased risk of experiencing tooth loss. In a retrospective study, Dannewitz et al. (2006) evaluated tooth loss in molars with furcation involvement (FI) and the prognostic factors for molar survival in patients underwent at least 5 years of supportive periodontal therapy. The authors found that smoking was one of the factors which increased tooth loss in patients with FI. Ando et al. (2013) assessed in a cohort study the number of teeth of middle-aged Japanese men who underwent health treatment. The authors concluded that smoking, low education level and poor nutritional status were associated with tooth loss among this population. In a cross-sectional study, Mai et al. (2013) found that in postmenopausal women, smoking was the major factor related to tooth loss due to periodontitis. Costa et al. (2013) also found that patients diagnosed with chronic moderate-severe periodontitis, who had finished active periodontal treatment and were in supportive therapy, found that smoking was one of the factors associated with tooth loss in regular compliers and irregular complier groups, showing that tooth prognosis can be altered in smokers.

Clinical studies have shown that periodontal parameters are worsened in smokers. In a clinical, radiographic and molecular study, Machtei et al. (1997) observed that smokers exhibited greater attachment loss (AL) and radiographic bone loss (BL) compared to non-smokers. The authors also verified that patients' cotinine level had direct correlation with outcomes of progressive periodontal breakdown. As in the previous study, Beck et al. (1997) also verify that patients who smoke had significantly more AL in a clinical 5-year survey. Machtei et al. (1999) demonstrated that current smokers exhibited mean annual attachment loss significantly greater than that of non-smokers, showing that smoking lead to a relevant disease progression. In another study, Albandar et al. (2000) observed that cigarette and cigar/pipe smokers had a higher prevalence of moderate and severe periodontitis and a higher prevalence and extent of AL and gingival recession (GR) than non-smokers and a multiple regression analysis showed that current tobacco smokers had an increased risk factor for periodontal disease. Authors also found deeper periodontal pockets depth (PPD) in smokers and a higher proportion of sites with a probing pocket depth of >5mm in all teeth (van der Weijden et al., 2001). Calsina et al. (2002) showed that smokers had 2.7 times and former smokers 2.3 times greater probabilities to have developed periodontal disease compared to non-smokers. Smokers also had greater PPD, GR and AL than former smokers or non-smokers. Shimazaki et al. (2006) discovered a higher proportion of teeth with PPD ≥4mm and a higher proportion of teeth with AL ≥ 5mm in smokers. Likewise, Haffajee and Socransky (2001a) concluded in a clinical study that current smokers had significantly more

AL, greater PPD and a higher number of missing teeth than non-smokers and also had greater AL than past smokers or those who never smoked. Even young smokers with an average age of 19.38 had a significant PPD compared to non-smokers (Machuca et al., 2000). In a Chinese population, Chen et al. (2001) also verified a greater increase in PPD and AL, as well as greater tooth loss among smoker patients of an earlier age.

Table 3. Smoke effect on periodontal disease etiopathogenesis

Etiology	Smoke effect
Periodontal physiology	Low levels of ICAM-1 Low levels of E-selectin Vasoconstrictive effect (controversial)
Periodontal immune response	Higher PMN count Higher level of M-CSF Higher level of PGE$_2$ Higher level of RANKL Higher level of MMPs Higher level of TNFsf Lower level of OPG
Periodontal microbiology	No effect on plaque volume No effect on bacterial virulence in gingivitis Increased virulence on subgingival samples in periodontitis

ICAM-1= intercellular adhesion molecule-1; E-selectin=endothelial selectin; PMN = polymorphonuclear; M-CSF=colony stimulated factor; PGE$_2$=prostaglandin E$_2$; RANKL=receptor activator of nuclear factor kappa-B ligand; MMPs=matrix metalloproteinases; TNFsf=tumor necrosis factor superfamily; OPG= osteoprotegerin.

Smokers have more sites with furcation lesions compared to non-smokers. Axselsson et al. (1998) showed that smokers had higher frequency of furcation lesions than non-smokers and the prevalence increases with age. Other studies evaluated periodontal status in 120 smokers and non-smokers showing that even smokers with regular hygiene have a higher prevalence and severity of periodontal disease in molar teeth and these teeth have more furcation involvement, attachment loss, gingival recession and tooth mobility compared to non-smokers (Kerdvongbundit & Wikesjö, 2002; Kerdvongbundit & Wikesjö, 2000).

Because of non-bleeding or slight gingiva bleeding, the gingival bleeding index or bleeding on probing in smoking patients can generate confusion in clinical evaluation and therefore gingival inflammation can be disguised. However, reduced gingival/periodontal bleeding in smokers is far from periodontal health. Most clinical studies show fewer sites exhibiting bleeding on probing in smokers compared to non-smokers (Haffajee & Socransky, 2001a,b; Chen et al., 2001; Shimazaki et al., 2006; Farina et al., 2013) and its major suppressive effect on gingival bleeding was found in heavy smokers (>10 cigarettes per day) showing a chronic and dose-dependent effect on gingival bleeding on probing (Dietrich et al., 2004). The mechanism for suppressing or reducing gingival bleeding in smokers is not yet well understood. It seems that interference of smoking is not directly caused by a vasoconstrictive action of nicotine, as can be found on laser flowmeter studies, but seems to be a result of a more profound influence on the vasculature and cellular metabolism (Palmer et al.1999; Meekin et al. 2000). Low levels of soluble intercellular adhesion molecule-1 (ICAM-1) and endothelial selection (E-selectin), a cell adhesion molecule expressed only on endothelial cells activated by cytokines, is verified in inflamed gingival tissue of smokers and can play an important role in bleeding diminishment (Rezavandi, 2002). But more studies are needed to confirm the biological process. Nonetheless, the patient must be notified that quitting smoking can increase gingival bleeding and thus it can be concluded that smoking affects the inflammatory response and that these changes are reversible (Nair et al., 2003).

It has been hypothesized that smokers had more calcium concentration in saliva and this fact could answer why higher amounts of supragingival calculus has been correlated with tobacco smoking (Bergström, 1999). But this information is still controversial and in a recent study (Sutej et al., 2012) authors did not find significant differences in salivary calcium levels in smokers compared to non-smokers, but they found a positive association between increased levels of salivary calcium and the development of periodontal disease.

There are still controversial findings in literature as to whether the virulence of plaque microbiota observed in smokers is higher than in non-smoking patients. In an experimental gingivitis study, Lie et al. (1998) could not find any differences in plaque composition between smokers and non-smokers, but the authors found that gingival bleeding in smokers in a 14-day experiment was significantly lower, showing that gingival inflammation could be due to other factors despite plaque virulence.

Another study could not find differences in subgingival samples of bacterial species *Porphyromonas gingivalis* (Pg), *Prevotella intermedia* (Pi), *Prevotella nigrescens* (Pn), *Tannerella forsythia* (Tf), *Agreggatibacter actinomycetemcomitans* (Aa), *Fusobacterium nucleatum* (Fn), *Treponema denticola* (Td), *Peptpstreptococcus micros* (Pm), *Campylobacter rectus* (Cr), *Eikenella corrodens* (Ec), *Selenomonas noxia* (Sn) and *Selenomonas intermedius* (Si) in smokers and non-smokers (Böstrom et al., 2001). However, Haffajee et al. (2001b) observed a greater prevalence of *Eubacterium nodatum*, *F. nucleatum ss vincentii*, Pi, Pm, Pn, *Bacteroides forsythus* (currently *Tannerella forsythia*), Pg and Td in subgingival plaque samples of smokers and Zambon et al. (1996) found greater relative risk of *B. forsythus* (currently *Tannerella forsythia*) infection in smokers. Besides plaque virulence, other cellular and immune responses are associated with more periodontal breakdown in smokers. Neutrophil apoptosis is significantly decreased in smokers which may explain the greater periodontal destruction (Shivanaikar et al., 2013). Metalloproteinase 8 (MMP-8), a collagen cleave enzyme, is also overexpressed in crevicular gingival fluid of smokers and is associated with lower periodontal parameters during maintenance patients (Leppilahti et al., 2013).

Higher levels of soluble receptor activators of nuclear-factor Kappa-B ligand (sRANKL), lead to osteoclast differentiation and tumor necrosis factor superfamily (TNFsf), which is a cytokine related to cell apoptosis, and lower levels of osteoprotegerin (OPG), a osteoclastogenesis inhibitory factor (Nile et al., 2013). All these dysfunctional marker levels lead to more periodontal destruction, worsening smoker prognosis.

Studies suggested that whether or not surgical, the periodontal basic therapy outcome for smoker patients is inferior to that of non-smoker patients and it leads to less reduction in PPD, less AL gain and more periodontal sites requiring re-treatment (Grossi et al., 1996; Papantonopoulos, 1999; Meulman et al., 2013). There are additional benefits in root coverage and regenerative procedures in smokers, but authors have shown less tissue stability, more residual gingival recession, more residual bone defect, deeper PPD, less complete root coverage after coronally advanced flaps with or without connective tissue graft due to tobacco smoke (Silva et al., 2006; Silva et al., 2007; Andia et al., 2008; Souza et al., 2008; Patel et al., 2012).

A recent systematic review with meta-analysis showed that smoking cessation can promote additional beneficial effects in reducing PPD and improving reduced attachment levels following non-surgical periodontal treatment (Chambrone et al., 2013). It can be concluded that smoker patients' response to any periodontal therapy is worse than that of non-smokers and that smoking cessation must be encouraged in the dental office not only for periodontal improvement but also for the patients' systemic health.

In summary, it can be concluded that smoking worsens periodontal parameters and the clinician should be alert to diagnose periodontal disease among smokers since they apparently have lower gingival bleeding (for a summary see Table 3 and Table 4).

4. THE INFLUENCE OF CIGARETTE SMOKE IN IMPLANTOLOGY

The long-term success of implant therapy has been reported by some authors (Albrektsson et al., 1986; Zarb & Schmitt, 1990). However, some patients have a higher number of implant failures. Some studies investigated the factors that could lead to implant loss (Lemmerman & Lemmerman, 2005). There are some conditions (local, behavioral and systemic) related with higher rates of failure, and smoking is the factor most frequently discussed (Lemmerman & Lemmerman, 2005).

Literature documented that smokers have higher rates of implant failure than non-smokers (De Bruyn & Collaert, 1994; Lambert et al., 2000) and higher incidence of peri-implant mucositis and peri-implantitis. These patients also have increased marginal bone loss around successfully integrated implants (Strietzel et al., 2007; Heitz-Mayfield, 2008; Roos-Jansaker et al., 2006). A meta-analysis evaluated 19 studies and concluded that the odds ratio of implant failure was significantly elevated when smokers were compared with non-smokers (Hinode et al., 2006). Furthermore, histological studies have documented the negative influence of smoking on bone healing around titanium implants inserted in rats (Nociti et al., 2002a, 2002b; Cesar-Neto et al.; 2003; Corrêa et al.; 2009).

The effects of nicotine on bone tissue are also documented. In cell cultures, nicotine seems to stimulate osteoclast differentiation and resorption of calcium phosphate (Henemyre et al., 2003) and inhibit proliferation of bone cells and extracellular matrix synthesis (Akmal et al., 2004). Silcox et al. (1995) suggested that the newly formed bone has inferior mechanical properties in the presence of systemic nicotine and Feitelson et al. (2003) stated that nicotine produces a chronic reduction in blood flow in the bone tissue.

In dentistry, several studies evaluated the effect of cigarette smoke inhalation in the bone tissue around dental implants. The intermittent cigarette smoke inhalation may impair bone quality around titanium implants placed in rats (Nociti et al., 2002b). César Neto et al. (2003) conducted a comparative study of the effects of nicotine administration and CSI around titanium implants and observed that cigarette smoke exerted a negative influence on bone-to-implant contact and bone area within the limits of the threads in both cortical and cancellous bone area. In contrast, nicotine administration reduced the bone area within the limits of the threads only in the cancellous bone area.

Table 4. Periodontal parameters in smokers and non-smokers. ATL= attachment loss; GR = gingival recession; PPD = probing pocket depth; GB = gingival bleeding

Parameters / Subjects	Alveolar bone height	Tooth loss	ATL	GR	PPD	Furcation lesion	GB	Calculus
Smoker	Lower	Enhanced tooth loss	Enhanced ATL	Enhanced	Deeper PPD	More sites	Diminished GB	Controversial
Non-smoker	Higher	Less tooth loss	Less ATL	Less GR	Shallow PPD	Less sites	Increased GB	Controversial
References	Bergstöm et al., 1991; Bolin et al., 1993; Jansson & Lavsted, 2002; Baljoon et al., 2004; Rosa et al., 2008.	Krall et al., 1999; Dannewitz et al., 2006; Ando et al., 2013; Mai et al., 2013; Costa et al., 2013.	Beck et al., 1997; Machtei et al., 1999; Albandar et al., 2000; Calsina et al., 2002.	Calsina et al., 2002; Kerdvongbundit & Wikesjö, 2000.	van der Weijden et al., 2001; Calsina et al., 2002; Simazaky et al., 2006; Haffajee & Sockransky, 2001.	Axselsson et al., 1998; Kerdvongbundit & Wikesjö, 2000; Kerdvongbundit & Wikesjö, 2002.	Haffajee et al., 2001; Chen et al., 2001; Shimazaky et al., 2006; Farina et al., 2013.	Sutej et al., 2012.

4.1. Mechanisms of Action on the Peri-Implant Tissues and on Osseointegration

4.1.1. In Vitro studies

Cigarette smoke and its components have negative effects on bone cell cultures. Ramp et al. (1991) studied the effect of nicotine on osteoblast type cells cultures. The results showed that nicotine inhibited alkaline phosphatase activity and collagen synthesis in a dose-dependent manner. Fang et al. (1991) examined the effects of nicotine on osteoblast proliferation and on alkaline phosphatase activity. It was observed that nicotine inhibited cell proliferation and stimulated phosphatase alkaline activity in a dose dependent manner. Gullihorn et al. (2005) compared the effects of nicotine and other components of cigarette smoke on osteoblasts. Strains of MC3T3-E1 osteoblasts were exposed to various doses of nicotine and cigarette smoke condensate. In this study, nicotine stimulated bone cells metabolism in a dose-dependent manner by increasing alkaline phosphatase activity and decreasing synthesis of total protein and collagen. These responses were observed even with nicotine doses (12.5ng/ mL) comparable to half the nicotine level circulating in smokers. Preparations of smoke condensate with equivalent nicotine concentrations reduced all indices of metabolic activity. Cell proliferation was stimulated by both nicotine (20-25%) and smoke condensates (38-46%). The results suggest that nicotine acts as a direct stimulant of bone cell metabolic activity, while the smoke condensates have an inhibitory effect.

Yuhara et al. (1999) evaluated nicotine influence on bone metabolism in cell cultures. Three cell lineages were used: osteogenic clonal rat calvaria (ROB-C26) pre-clonal mouse calvaria osteoblastic (MC3T3-E1) and osteoblast type cells taken from a co-culture of bone marrow cells of mice. The results showed that nicotine stimulated calcium deposition and alkaline phosphatase activity in ROB-C26 cells in a dose-dependent manner. Moreover, both activities were decreased in MC3T3-E1 cells, showing that nicotine affects osteoblast differentiation. It was also observed that nicotine affects osteoblast type cells differentiation. The authors concluded that nicotine can have a critical effect on bone metabolism.

In 2001, Liu et al. studied the direct action of cigarette smoke on human osteoprogenitor cells. Thus, bone marrow cells from normal individuals were isolated and cultured in monolayer and in three-dimensional type I collagen gel culture. In both culture conditions, cigarette smoke inhibited the proliferation of osteoprogenitor cells in a dose-dependent pattern. It was also observed that cigarette smoke inhibited the differentiation of osteoprogenitor cells into osteoblast-like cells and monolayer cultures were more susceptible to the adverse effects of cigarette smoke. Again, Liu et al. (2003) evaluated the ability of tobacco extracts to alter bone repair and remodeling responses of human osteoprogenitor cells and osteoblast-like cells. The chemotactic response and the contraction of the two types of cells were inhibited by cigarette smoke extract in a dose-dependent manner. Cigarette smoke extract also inhibited the production of fibronectin by both cells. The results demonstrated that cigarette smoke could interfere with the ability of bone cells to participate in the repair and remodeling processes.

Tanaka et al. (2005) investigated the effect of nicotine on cell proliferation, alkaline phosphatase activity (ALPase), formation of mineralized nodules and matrix-metalloproteinase expression in human osteosarcoma cells. The formation of mineralized nodules was suppressed by nicotine on day 10 of culture and calcium content on the 14th. The

ALPase activity, expression of type I collagen and osteopontin also decreased in the presence of nicotine after 5, 10 and 14 days of culture, respectively. In contrast, the amount of bone sialoprotein increased during the 14 days of culture with nicotine. These results suggest that nicotine suppresses osteogenesis by reducing the activity of ALPase and type I collagen production by osteoblasts. In another study, Tanaka et al. (2006) evaluated the effect of nicotine and LPS on the expression of macrophage stimulating colony factor (M-CSF), osteoprotegerin (OPG) and prostaglandin E2 (PGE2) in osteoblasts and the indirect effect of nicotine and LPS on the formation of osteoclast-like cells. Human osteoblasts were treated with nicotine alone and nicotine associated with LPS. M-CSF and PGE2 expression increased in cells cultured with LPS and nicotine compared to those grown only on nicotine. The expression of OPG increased in the early stage of culture with nicotine and LPS, but decreased in the final stage. The medium containing M-CSF and PGE2 produced by nicotine and LPS-treated human osteoblasts with soluble RANKL increased TRAP staining positive osteoclasts compared with that produced by nicotine treatment only. The results suggest that nicotine and LPS stimulate the formation of osteoclast-like cells by increased production of M-CSF and PGE2 and this association produces greater stimulation compared to the effect of nicotine alone.

Another study from 2006 conducted by Katono et al. evaluated the effects of nicotine on the expression of matrix metalloproteinases (MMPs), tissue inhibitors of matrix metalloproteinases (TIMPs), the plasminogen activation system including the component of tissue-type plasminogen activator (tPA), urokinase-type PA (uPA), and PA inhibitor type 1 (PAI-1), α7 nicotine receptor, and c-fos. The effect of the nicotine antagonist D-tubocurarine on nicotine-induced expression of MMP-1 was also analyzed. The treatment with nicotine resulted in the expression of MMP-1, 2, 3, and 13 but not MMP-14. In the presence of nicotine, the expression of uPA, PAI-1 or TIMP- 1, 2, 3, or 4 did not changed over the culture period, whereas the expression of PA increased significantly after day 7. Nicotine also increased α7 nicotine receptor and c-fos gene expression. The results suggest that nicotine stimulates bone matrix turnover by increasing the production of tPA and MMP- 1, 2, 3, and 13, and unbalancing the process of formation and resorption of bone matrix during the late process.

4.1.2. In Vivo studies

The literature shows several animal studies in which the negative effect of smoking is verified. Saldanha et al. (2004) evaluated in dogs the effect of administration of nicotine (2mg/kg 3 times/day - 4 months) on bone defects treated with guided bone regeneration. The results showed that nicotine was able to influence the area and density of new bone formation compared to the control group, which did not receive nicotine. The authors suggested that nicotine may influence, but does not prevent bone repair in defects treated by guided bone regeneration.

In order to study the full effect of smoking, César-Neto et al. (2003) compared the influence of nicotine administration 93mg/kg twice/ day) with the influence of cigarette smoke inhalation on bone healing around titanium implants (3 times/ day - 60 days). The results showed that CSI decreased the amount of bone-to-implant contact and bone area within the limits of the threads, in both the cortical and cancellous bone area. Nicotine influenced bone formation only in the cancellous bone area. The authors concluded that the negative impact of smoking is related to more than one molecule present in the cigarette smoke and not just nicotine.

Concerning the implant surface treatment, Stefani et al. (2002) evaluated the influence of nicotine administration on bone healing around titanium implants inserted in rabbits. In this study, a significant influence of the implant surface on the degree of bone-to-implant contact was detected in groups of higher nicotine doses (0.57mg/kg and 0.93mg/kg) for machined and Al2O3-blasted surfaces. The authors conclude that nicotine does not appear to influence the repair bone around titanium implants. In the same way, Corrêa et al. (2009) evaluated the influence of titanium surface treatment on osseointegration in animals that were exposed to CSI. Data analysis showed significant differences in implant surfaces in both zones for bone filling of the threads. CSI affected bone filling of the threads and bone density in both zones. No statistically significant differences were observed between surfaces in any of the groups for bone density. The authors concluded that this particular surface treatment may not be enough to overcome the negative effect of smoking on bone around titanium implants.

A study was conducted by Lima et al. (2013) to investigate the influence of recombinant human parathyroid Hormone (PTH 1-34) on reduction of the negative influence of cigarette smoke on bone around titanium implants. The authors used female Wistar rats that were divided in a control group (no CSI and subjected to injection of saline solution) and a group that was subjected to CSI and received subcutaneous injections of saline solution or intermittent doses of PTH (1-34) (3 times/week). The results are in accordance with the above discussed studies. Data analysis confirmed that CSI negatively affects bone around implants, since bone-to-implant contact and proportion of mineralized tissue were negatively influenced by CSI. Interestingly, in the presence of CSI, PTH (1-34) promoted the highest bone-to-implant contact in cortical and cancellous bone area and proportion of mineralized tissue in cancellous bone.

Kallala et al. (2013) recently reviewed the evidence of nicotine effect on bone and bone cells and fracture repair. In this study the authors included articles that specifically investigated the effects of nicotine on bone or fracture repair in animal or human models or in vitro effects on bone cells. *In vivo* studies of nicotine effects demonstrated widespread effects on bone including osteoneogenesis, osseointegration, steady-state skeletal bone and genes and cytokines relevant to bone cell physiology and bone homeostasis. In these studies, nicotine effects are mainly negative inhibiting bone cell metabolism and fracture repair.

4.1.3. Clinical Studies

Smoking has been known to be a predisposing factor for implant failure, especially in cases of multiple failures in the same individual. The implant survival rate ranges from 80 to 100% in smokers and 93 to 98% in non-smokers (De Bruyn & Collaert, 1994; Jones et al., 1999; Schwartz-Arad et al., 2002).

Jones and Triplett (1992) verified the tissue repair difficulty in patients who received bone grafts and dental implants. Fifteen patients were evaluated and 5 had graft and/or implant loss. Among these 5 patients, 4 reported a smoking habit in the pre-or post-operatory period. The authors established that smoking is a controllable factor, but highly related to problems in the process of tissue repair. Weyant (1994) evaluated the success of dental implants based on the failures and on the conditions of the peri-implant soft tissues. The success was related to the patients' general health, the surface coating material of the implant and implant surgical and healing complications. The health of peri-implant soft tissue was associated with smoking, surface coating material of the implant and implant provider's experience.

Noguerol et al. (2006) monitored the primary implant stability at first-stage surgery, and the variables associated with early implant failure. A 10-year retrospective study was conducted on 1084 Brånemark implants placed in 316 patients and early implant failure was significantly related to smoking habits, implant location, bone type, and implant features. Smoking habits were independently related to early failure. In 2006, DeLuca et al. conducted a long-term retrospective study to evaluate the survival of Brånemark endosseous dental implants in relation to cigarette smoking. The overall implant failure rate was 7.72%. Comparing smokers with non-smokers, the implant failure rate was higher in the first one (23.08% and 13.33%, respectively). Multivariate survival analysis showed early implant failure to be significantly associated with smoking at the time of stage 1 surgery and late implant failure to be significantly associated with a positive smoking history. Short implants and implant placement in the maxilla were additional independent risk factors for implant failure. Thus, smoking negatively influences both stages of implant placement. A retrospective study analyzed 136 patients who received dental implants in the posterior maxilla to identify predictors for implant failure in the posterior maxilla (Huynh-Ba et al., 2008). From 273 implants placed in the posterior maxilla, 14 implants failed (early and late failures combined), resulting in a 94.9% overall survival rate. Smoking and surgical complications had a statistically significant effect on implant failure. Once more, smoking clearly increased the risk for implant failure.

Alsaadi et al. (2007) conducted a retrospective study verifying the influence of local and systemic factors on the failure rate of implants. The global failure rate was 3.6% and factors such as smoking, osteoporosis, and Crohn's disease were associated with early implant failure. Regarding implant surface, Jones et al. (1999) compared the early failures of implants coated by plasma-spray titanium or hydroxyapatite and realized that 9% of non-smoker patients showed failure compared with 26% of smokers. The authors concluded that the history of cigarette smoking plays an important role in early implant failures, regardless of their surface characteristics. Once more, Alsaadi et al. (2008) evaluated the influence of local and systemic factors on the failure rate of implants with surfaces treated by electrochemical oxidation. There was an overall failure rate of 1.9% and there was a tendency for more failures for apical lesions, vicinity with natural dentition, smoking, hormone replacement therapy, gastric problems, Crohn's disease, diabetes mellitus type 1 and radical hysterectomy. An interesting prospective and controlled histologic study evaluated the impact of smoking on bone-to-implant contact, the bone density in the threaded area, and the bone density outside the threaded area around microimplants with anodized surface retrieved from human jaws (Shibli, et al. 2010). The authors included 24 smoker and non-smoker subjects who received one microimplant with oxidized surface at the same time as conventional implant surgery. Histomorphometric analysis revealed that 3 microimplants placed in smokers did not osseointegrate. Marginal bone loss, gap, and fibrous tissue were present around implants retrieved from smokers. Mean bone-to-implant contact and bone density were significantly reduced in smokers compared to non-smokers. This study shows the negative effects of smoking in the early stages of bone formation around dental implants. Implant survival was studied in periodontitis-susceptible smokers who received turned or oxidized surface oral implants (Sayardoust et al., 2013). In this way, smokers and never-smokers with previous advanced periodontitis, treated with implants were included in this study. Patients who never smoked had an implant survival rate of 96.9% and smokers, 89.6%. Turned implants failed more in the smokers group. The risk of smokers for implant failure was 4.68, for turned implants 6.40, and for oxidized implants 0. Based on the results, it can be suggested that oxidized surface implants are more suitable for periodontitis-susceptible patients who smoke.

Heitz-Mayfield and Huynh-Ba (2009) performed a review evaluating the history of treated periodontitis and smoking, both alone and combined, as risk factors for adverse dental implant outcomes. Implant survival rates for the history of treated periodontitis were > 90%. Most of the systematic reviews included in the study (three of four) considered smoking to be a significant risk for adverse implant outcome. Although implant survival rates in smokers were from 80% to 96%, survival rate of smokers is significantly lower than survival rate for non-smokers. The review suggested that the combination of treated periodontitis and smoking increases the risk of implant failure and peri-implant bone loss.

It is well known that systematic reviews and meta-analysis are the most reliable evidence and they are at the top of the evidence pyramid (Newman et al., 2003). To establish evidence on the effectiveness of interventions or treatments, systematic review and meta-analysis are the more suitable studies to answer these questions. Systematic reviews are useful to integrate information from a set of studies performed separately on specific therapeutic/intervention, which may present conflicting results and/or coincidence, and it is important to identify issues that require evidence, aiding orientation for future investigations (Linde & Willich, 2003). Following this statement, we discuss the evidence provided in some systematic reviews. These details are included below.

Klokkevold & Han (2007) evaluated the effect of smoking, diabetes, and periodontitis on the outcomes of implants. Regarding smoking, 19 were identified and one article met the criteria for both smoking and periodontitis. Implant survival and success rates were reported for smokers versus non-smokers. Survival and success rates were higher for non-smokers compared to smokers. When the bone quality was considered, there were greater differences between smokers and non-smokers, mainly for the trabecular bone. Strietzel et al. (2007) conducted a systematic literature review to investigate if smoking interferes with the prognosis of implants with and without accompanying augmentation procedures compared with non-smokers. Meta-analysis revealed a significantly enhanced risk for implant failure among smokers compared with nonsmokers, and for smokers receiving implants with accompanying augmentation procedures. The study indicated significantly enhanced risks of biologic complications among smokers. Five studies revealed no significant impact of smoking on the prognosis of implants with particle-blasted, acid-etched or anodic oxidized surfaces.

Abt (2009) conducted a systematic review and meta-analysis to evaluate failures of implant treatment or biological complication in smokers and nonsmokers. Meta-analysis revealed a significantly enhanced risk for implant failure in smokers with or without augmentation. The data analysis showed that in implants with particle-blasted, acid-etched or anodic oxidized surfaces, smoking had no significant impact. A recent systematic review was performed to evaluate the effects of smoking on the survival rate of dental implants placed in areas of maxillary sinus floor augmentation (Chambrone et al., 2013). Most of the selected studies (62.5%) established that smoking negatively affects implant survival in sites of sinus floor augmentation. When the pooled analysis was performed for the results of all studies included in the meta-analysis, it was observed that there is a statistically significant increased risk of implant failure in smokers. On the other hand, another analysis including only prospective studies (3 studies) did not find significant differences in implant failure between smokers and non-smokers. The review concludes that smoking is associated with implant failure in most individual studies, but when the prospective data was assessed in the meta-analysis, the detrimental effect of smoking was not confirmed. However, when this information is interpreted, it should be taken into consideration that there are very few prospective cohort studies focusing on the influence of smoking on grafted maxillary sinuses.

The results of the most important category of scientific publication are summarized in Table 5.

Table 5. Implant failure in smokers

Systematic Review	Meta-analysis	Results
Strietzel et al. (2007)	Yes	Risk factor for implant and augmentation procedures
Klokkevold & Han (2007)	-	Negative effect on implant survival and success, particularly in cancellous bone
Abt (2009)	Yes	Risk for implant failure in smokers, with or without augmentation. Particle-blasted, acid-etched or anodic oxidized surfaces: no impact.
Chambrone et al. (2013)	Yes	Associated with implant failure, but not in prospective studies

4.2. Influence on the Prevalence and Severity of Peri-Implant Diseases

Peri-implant diseases are defined as inflammatory lesions that develop in the tissues around implants. Following the classification of periodontal disease at teeth, peri-implant diseases are divided in peri-implant mucositis, (corresponding to gingivitis) and peri-implantitis (corresponding to periodontitis).

It is difficult to establish the prevalence of peri-implant diseases because clinical trials related to implant insertion frequently do not report the status of the peri-implant tissues. There are some systematic reviews and meta-analyses available in the literature concerning this issue. They will be discussed below.

Zitzmann & Berglundh (2008) conducted a review in order to verify the prevalence of peri-implant diseases including peri-implant mucositis and peri-implantitis. In this review, cross-sectional and longitudinal studies with 50 or more implant-treated subjects, with a function time of 5 years or more, were included. Unfortunately, only a few studies provided data on the prevalence of peri-implant diseases. Cross-sectional studies on implant-treated subjects are rare and data from only two study samples were available. The prevalence of mucositis was 80% for subjects and 50% for implants. Regarding the prevalence of peri-implantitis, it was 28% to 56% for subjects and from 12% to 43% for implant sites.

A recent retrospective study (De la Rosa et al., 2013) evaluated the predictors of peri-implant bone loss in a sample of patients treated with 10mm implants and single crowns. The patients included were systemically healthy and partially edentulous. Peri-implant bone loss was evaluated from data recorded at the most recent examination. Logistic regression analysis was performed to investigate associations between peri-implant bone loss and sex, duration of peri-implant maintenance, location and number of implants placed per patient, region of the mouth, smoking status, type of implant, and retention of restoration. The sample was composed of 104 subjects with four different types of dental implants and maintained for at least 3 years, totalizing 148 implants followed for an average period of continuing maintenance of 6 years (range, 3 to 15 years). From these 148 implants only one (1.8%) was lost. The outcomes of logistic regression analysis showed that the independent variables of smoking, retention of restoration (cemented vs. screw-retained), and type of implant (internal- or external-hex) were found to be correlated with peri-implant bone loss with odds ratios of 39.64, 4.85, and 0.04, respectively.

As discussed above, Sayardoust et al. (2013) studied the implant survival and peri-implant complication in periodontitis-susceptible smokers who received turned or oxidized surface oral implants. Thus, smokers and never-smokers with previous advanced periodontitis treated with implants were included in this study. In smokers, mean marginal bone loss at 5 years was 1.54 mm in turned implants and 1.16mm in oxidized implants. Patients who never smoked had significantly greater bone using oxidized implants, 1.26 mm, than with turned implants, 0.84 mm. Oxidized implants exposed similar bone loss between the groups. Turned implants lost significantly more bone in smokers.

The discussed animal and clinical studies show that smoking affects the survival of turned titanium implants and has less impact on the failure rate of rough surface implants. In the meantime, the effect on bone loss of rough surface implants should be taken into consideration. In this way, Vandeweghe and De Bruyn (2011) studied the effect of smoking on bone remodeling around moderately rough implants. The mean interproximal bone level was 1.36 mm. Smokers presented 60 implants that lost statistically significant more bone than the 303 implants in non-smokers and the higher bone loss was located in the maxilla.

As seen above, a systematic review and meta-analysis evaluated failures or biological complications of implant treatment in smokers and non-smokers (Abt, 2009). The systemic review showed significantly enhanced risks of peri-implant complications and bone loss in smokers.

Regarding the influence of smoking on peri-implant disease, there are only a few studies. Koldsland et al. (2011) assessed possible risk indicators for peri-implantitis at different levels of severity. History of periodontitis and peri-implant bone loss ≥ 2.0mm were associated with higher severity of peri-implantitis. No association was found between smoking and peri-implant disease in the present study population. The principal findings of this topic are summarized in Table 6.

4.3. Influence on Peri-Implant Disease Evolution

It has been shown through this chapter that smoking is reported as a significant determinant related to the peri-implant tissue changes and implant failure. Thus, certain aspects concerning current dental implant therapy should be considered for smokers in treatment planning, oral surgical procedures, and the maintenance phases of dental implant treatment. The initiation and early development of an inflammatory reaction in peri-implant tissues can be induced by bacterial metabolites as it occurs in periodontal tissues. However, there are some systemic and environmental situations, such as smoking, that can modify or intensify this response. Inflammatory cytokines in peri-implant tissues have an important role in regulating and amplifying the inflammatory response, as it happens in periodontal tissues.

The inflammatory cytokines such as interleukin (IL)-1β, tumor necrosis factor (TNF)-α, and prostaglandin (PG) E_2 are considered biochemical markers for peri-implant destruction because of their high crevicular concentrations in compromised implant sites (Graves & Cochran, 2003). IL-1β is released from various cells (macrophages, fibroblasts, and osteoblasts) to upregulate inflammatory reactions (Lachmann et al., 2007). PGE_2 is found in great quantity in peri-implantitis tissues and is considered to be proinflammatory, causing vasodilatation and enhancement of vascular permeability and activation of osteoclasts at the sites of inflammation, on peri-implant tissues (Basegmez et al., 2012). PGE_2 has also been associated with osteoclast-mediated bone resorption (Yalçn et al., 2005). Tatli et al. (2013), in a cross sectional study, evaluated the effects of smoking on peri-implant health status and inflammatory cytokines interleukin-1b, tumor necrosis factor-α, and prostaglandin E_2 levels in peri-implant crevicular fluid and analyzed their correlation with clinical parameters in well-maintained implant patients. All clinical parameters were significantly higher in the smoker group, except plaque scores. Significantly increased levels of cytokines were observed in the smoker group and the correlation between the cytokine levels and clinical parameters were more manifested in smokers. Thus, even in well maintained patients, the risk of complications in smokers is higher.

The long-term marginal implant bone loss, survival, and radiographic success of single dental implants among current, past smokers, and non-smokers were compared in Levin et al. (2008). From single implants, 4 implants failed and 2 of the failures were due to mechanical neck break and 2 resulted from peri-implantitis and bone loss. Current smokers had higher marginal bone loss during all time intervals than former smokers and both demonstrated higher marginal bone loss compared to non-smokers. These results reaffirm the relation between smoking and peri-implant bone loss. Therefore, it is evident that smoking reduces the success rate of implants as well as increasing the frequency failure and complications in the peri-implant tissues.

Table 6. Prevalence of peri-implant disease on smokers

Study	Meta-analysis	Prevalence of peri-implant disease
Zitzmann & Berglundh (2008)		Mucositis: 80% subjects; Peri-implantitis: 50% implants/ 28- 56% subjects; 12- 43% implant s
Atieh et al. (2013)	Yes	Peri-implant disease: 36.3% and 14.3% with supportive maintenance
De la Rosa et al. (2013)	-	More bone loss in smokers
Sayardoust et al. (2013)	-	Higher bone loss in smokers with turned implants
Vandeweghe & De Bruyn (2011)	-	More bone loss in smokers (60 x 303 implants in smokers x non-smokers)
Abt (2009)	Yes	Risk of peri-implant complications and bone loss in smokers
Koldsland et al. (2011)	-	No association between smoking and peri-implant disease

4.4. Influence on the Repair Process and Outcome of Therapy

Smoking affects various aspects of innate and adaptive immune responses such as changes in neutrophil function, antibody production, activity of fibroblasts and in the vascular factors, and in the inflammatory mediator production.

Fredriksson et al. (1999) observed increased blood white cell count and neutrophils in smokers. The authors found lower rates of hapatoglobin and alpha-1 antitrypsin in smoking patients. Furthermore, cigarette consumption also reduced IgG synthesis, especially IgG$_2$, which makes the antibody-dependent phagocytosis by neutrophils difficult. Similarly, Smith et al. (2003) observed a higher total number of white blood cells and granulocytes in the systemic circulation of smokers. Graswinckel et al. (2004) found lower levels of immunoglobulin G (IgG) in smokers compared with non-smokers. Furthermore, Apatzidou et al. (2005) found that smokers had less *Agregatibacter actinomycetemcomitans* (Aa) IgG than non-smokers. The total amount of IgG$_2$ (Graswinckel et al., 2004) and IgG$_2$ reactive with Aa were also reduced in smokers (Tangada et al., 1997). The reduction of these immunoglobulins could decrease the immune response in smokers. Loos et al. (2004) analyzed the number of T cells (CD3+) and its subsets (CD4+ and CD8+) and proliferative capacity of B and T cells (CD19+) in periodontitis in smokers and non-smokers. The collapse of the periodontium in smokers was associated with high numbers of CD3+ T CD4+ and CD8+ T cells and enhanced proliferation of T cells.

Peñarrocha et al. (2004) investigated peri-implant bone resorption around 108 dental implants 1 year after prosthetic loading using extraoral panoramic, conventional intraoral periapical, and digital radiologic techniques, considering smoking, implant location, and morphology. No significant association was observed in panoramic radiography. When periapical radiography was performed, there was positive linear association and when periapical radiographs were digital, the association found was significant. The implants located in the maxilla and those placed in patients who smoked 11 to 20 cigarettes per day were associated with significantly greater bone loss. Thus, smoking and implant location in the maxilla were associated with increased peri-implant marginal bone resorption.

Gruica et al. (2004) evaluated the impact of the IL-1 genotype and smoking status on the prognosis and development of complications of osseointegrated implants. From 292 implants, 51 had late infectious complications and 241 survived without any biologic complications. The population included 53 smokers and they were subdivided in accordance with the quantity of cigarettes smoked. From the total 180, 127 were never smokers. Sixty-four of 180 (36%) patients were tested positive for the IL-1 genotype polymorphism. The non-smoking group had no significant correlation between implant complications and a positive IL-1 genotype. At the same time, there was a relationship between the positive IL-1 genotype and implant complications for heavy smokers. An implant failure or a biologic complication during the follow-up period was identified in half of the heavy smokers and IL-1 genotype-positive patients. A retrospective study was conducted by Jansson et al. (2005) in order to evaluate the absolute failure rate of Brånemark implants installed over a 10-year period in patients treated for periodontal disease prior to implant treatment and under regular professional maintenance. The authors also verify the rate of interleukin-1 (IL-1) polymorphism in those patients who experienced at least one implant failure during the first year of function, and the prevalence of periodontal pathogens in dental and peri-implant sites with and without signs of inflammation. Some patients were clinically examined and were tested genetically for IL-1 genotypes. The absolute implant survival rate was 95.32%. Implant loss in the examined group was 32 of 106 (30.1%); 10 (45%) of the 22 patients were smokers, and 6 (27%) of the 22 patients were IL-1 genotype positive. IL-1 genotype did not lead to more implant loss; however, smoking presented a significant synergistic effect. Between patients who were IL-1 genotype positive and those who were IL-1 genotype negative, the differences in regard to bleeding on probing or periodontal pathogens did not reach statistical significance. Thus, a synergistic effect found between smoking and a positive IL-1 genotype resulted in a significantly higher implant loss.

Levin and Schwartz-Arad (2002) reported that the rate loss of marginal bone surrounding the implant is about three times higher in smokers. In addition, the incidence of postoperative complications is higher among smokers. This negative response seems to be associated with arterial vasoconstriction, decreased blood flow given by release of by-products such as nicotine, carbon monoxide and hydrogen, which increases cyano-platelet aggregation and leukocyte and fibroblasts dysfunction.

Charalampakis et al. (2011) performed a retrospective study to follow patients after peri-implantitis treatment. Two hundred and eighty-one patients were selected based on microbial analysis of bacterial samples taken from diseased implants. It was not possible to follow the peri-implantitis progression in 54.7% of the patients. Smoking, smoking dose and early disease development were found to be significantly correlated to failure of peri-implantitis treatment. Bone plastic surgery together with antibiotics was significantly associated with arrested lesions.

5. IMPORTANCE OF SMOKING CESSATION AND THE ROLE OF THE DENTIST

The beneficial effects of smoking cessation are shown in medicine and dentistry. A meta-analysis (Ward & Klesges, 2001) demonstrated that current smokers presented significantly reduced bone mass compared to former and never smokers and that former smokers presented bone mass that is intermediate or similar to never smokers. Glassman et al. (2000) reported that smoking cessation may present a beneficial effect on bone loss. Concerning bone healing, it was observed that patients who quit smoking for periods longer than 6 months, after instrumented spinal fusion presented nonunion rates similar to non-smokers. Considering lung disease, the time for recovery is longer. The reversibility of smoking effects has also been investigated in dentistry. In vitro studies observed a reversible condition promoted by cigarette compounds on periodontal cells (Cattaneo et al., 2000). Smoking cessation also exerted a beneficial effect on periodontal risk, decreasing the number of years since quitting. Lied et al. (1999) and Bergstrom et al. (2000) conducted longitudinal studies showing that patients who stopped smoking lost significantly less marginal bone than current smokers. Grossi et al. (1997) studied the effect of cessation on periodontal therapy and showed beneficial results with more healing and reduction of *Bacterioides forsythus* and *Phorphyromonas gingivalis*.

Quitting smoking is the most effective way to reduce the harmful effects of smoking. Bain (1996) evaluated a cessation protocol in which implant patients who smoked were encouraged to stop for 1 week before and 8 weeks after implant placement. The author found no difference in the failure rate between non-smoking controls and the smokers who quit the habit, whereas a significant difference was found between the continuing smokers and smokers who followed the cessation protocol. Histological studies have also shown a beneficial effect of both temporary and complete smoking cessation on bone around titanium implants inserted in the rat tibiae and on tooth-supporting bone (Cesar-Neto et al. 2005a, 2005b, 2006).

It is important and it is the responsibility of health professionals to advise the patients about the negative effects of smoking on implant therapy and in the treatment of peri-implant diseases. There is enough evidence concerning the positive effect of smoking cessation on peri-implant tissues.

Christen (2001) described the 20-year experience of the Faculty of Dentistry, University of Indiana (USA) in the smoking cessation program, where students have this program in their curriculum. The author describes the anti-smoking therapy protocol, which includes the technique of 5 A´s for simple interventions and nicotine replacement therapy and medications for patients with higher dependency. The author also highlights the importance of creating an environment free of cigarettes.

Dentists can apply the model of the 5 A's (Glynn Manley, 2008), following the steps described below:

1. ASK: question about tobacco use
2. ADVISE: Advised to stop smoking
3. ASSESS: evaluates the positive desire to stop smoking
4. ASSIST: assists during abstinence
5. ARRANGE: organizes control appointments to prevent relapse.

Some patients may need other techniques such as nicotine therapy replacement and medication. The professionals should be able to individualize and associate techniques to fit the needs of each patient. If the professionals do not feel prepared to prescribe drug therapy for the patients, the patients must be sent to a smoking control center, where usually a multidisciplinary team with doctors, psychologists and nurses treat these patients.

CONCLUSION

In the light of the discussed studies, it can be concluded that smoking negatively influences the progression of periodontitis and peri-implant diseases and also emerges as a possible risk indicator for non-infectious periodontal lesions such as primary occlusal trauma. However, cigarette smoking should not be an absolute contra-indication for periodontal and implant therapy, but patients should be informed that they will have less periodontal parameter improvements after non-surgical or surgical periodontal therapy and they are at a slightly greater risk of implant failure if they continue to smoke during the initial healing phase following implant insertion or if they have a significant smoking history. Thus, certain aspects concerning current periodontal and dental implant therapy should be considered for smokers in treatment planning, oral surgical procedures, and the maintenance phases of dental implant treatment. Due to the harmful systemic and local effects of tobacco, smoking cessation should be encouraged by the dentist.

REFERENCES

Abt, E. (2009). Smoking increases dental implant failures and complications. *Evid. Based Dent*, *10*, 79-80.

Akmal, M., Kesani, A., Anand, B., Singh, A., Wiseman, M. & Goodship, A. (2004). Effect of nicotine on spinal disc cells: a cellular mechanism for disc degeneration. *Spine*, *1*, 568-75.

Albandar, J. M., Streckfus, C. F., Adesanya, M. R. & Winn, D. M. (2000). Cigar, pipe, and cigarette smoking as risk factors for periodontal disease and tooth loss. *J. Periodontol*, *71*(12), 1874-81.

Albrektsson, T., Zarb, G. A., Worthington, P. & Ericsson, A. R. (1986). The long-term efficacy of currently used dental implants: a review and proposed criteria for success. *Int. J. Oral Maxillofac. Implants*, *1*, 11–25.

Alsaadi, G., Quirynen, M., Komárek, A. & van Steenberghe, D. (2007). Impact of local and systemic factors on the incidence of oral implant failures, up to abutment connection. *J. Clin. Periodontol.*, *34*, 610-7.

Alsaadi, G., Quirynen, M., Komárek, A. & van Steenberghe, D. (2008). Impact of local and systemic factors on the incidence of late oral implant loss. *Clin. Oral. Implants. Res.*, *19*, 670-6.

American Psychiatric Association. (2000). *Diagnostic and Statistical Manual of Mental Disorders*. 4th edition - text revision. American Psychiatric Association: Washington, DC.

Anand, N., Emmadi, P., Ambalavanan, N. & Ramakrishnan, T. (2011). Effect of a volatile smoke component (acrolein) on human gingival fibroblasts: an in vitro study. *J. Indian Soc. Periodontol.*, *15*(4), 371-5.

Andia, D. C., Martins, A. G., Casati, M. Z., Sallum, E. A. & Nociti, F. H. (2008). Root coverage outcome may be affected by heavy smoking: a 2-year follow-up study. *J. Periodontol.*, *79*(4), 647-53.

Ando, A., Ohsawa, M., Yaegashi, Y., Sakata, K., Tanno, K., Onoda, T., Itai, K., Tanaka, F., Makita, S., Omama, S., Ogasawara, K., Ogawa, A., Ishibashi, Y., Kuribayashi, T., Koyama, T. & Okayama, A. (2013). Factors related to tooth loss among community-dwelling middle-aged and elderly Japanese men. *J. Epidemiol.*, *23*(4), 301-6.

Armitage, G. C. (1999). Development of a classification system for periodontal diseases and conditions. *Ann. Periodontol.*, *4*(1), 1-6.

Axelsson, P., Paulander, J. & Lindhe, J. (1998). Relationship between smoking and dental status in 35-, 50-, 65-, and 75-year-old individuals. *J. Clin. Periodontol.*, *25*(4), 297-305.

Bain, C. A. (1996). Smoking and implant failure—benefits of a smoking cessation protocol. *Int. J. Oral. Maxillofac. Implants.*, *11*, 756-759.

Baljoon, M., Natto, S. & Bergstrom, J. (2004). The association of smoking with vertical periodontal bone loss. *J. Periodontol.*, *75*(6), 844-51.

Barnoya, J. & Glantz, S. A. (2005). Cardiovascular effects of secondhand smoke: nearly as large as smoking. *Circulation*, *111*, 2684-2698.

Basegmez, C., Yalcin, S., Yalcin, F., Ersanli, S. & Mijiritsky, E. (2012). Evaluation of peri-implant crevicular fluid prostaglandin E2 and matrix metalloproteinase-8 levels from health to peri-implant disease status: A prospective study. *Implant Dent.*, *21*, 306–310.

Beck, J. D., Cusmano, L., Green-Helms, W., Koch, G. G. & Offenbacher, S. (1997). A 5-year study of attachment loss in community-dwelling older adults: incidence density. *J. Periodontal Res.*, *32*(6), 506-15.

Beckers, S. & Camu, F. (1991). The anaesthetic risk of tobacco smoking. *Acta Anaesthesiol. Belg.*, *42*. 45-56.

Benatti, B. B., César-Neto, J. B., Gonçalves, P. F., Sallum, E. A. & Nociti, F. H. Jr. (2005). Smoking affects the self-healing capacity of periodontal tissues: a histological study in the rat. *Eur. J. Oral Sci.*, *113*(5), 400-3.

Benowitz, N. L. (1998). *Nicotine safety and toxicity*. Oxford Univ. Press: New York.

Benowitz, N. L. & Hennigfield, J. E. (1994). Establishing a nicotine threshold for addiction: the implications for tobacco regulation. *N. Eng. J. Med.*, *331*, 123.

Bergstrom, J., Eliasson, S. & Dock, J. (2000). A 10-year prospective study of tobacco smoking and periodontal health. *J. Periodontol*, *71*, 1338-1347.

Bergström, J. (1999). Tobacco smoking and supragingival dental calculus. *J. Clin. Periodontol*, *26*(8), 541-7.

Bergström, J., Eliasson, S. & Preber, H. (1991). Cigarette smoking and periodontal bone loss. *J. Periodontol*, *62*(4), 2, 42-6. Erratum in: *J. Periodontol*, 1991, *62*(12), 809.

Bolin, A., Eklund, G., Frithiof, L. & Lavstedt, S. (1993). The effect of changed smoking habits on marginal alveolar bone loss: a longitudinal study. *Swed. Dent. J.*, *17*(5), 211-6.

Boström, L., Bergström, J., Dahlén, G. & Linder, L. E. (2001). Smoking and subgingival microflora in periodontal disease. *J. Clin. Periodontol.*, *28*(3), 212-9.

Brasil. Ministério da Saúde, Instituto Nacional de Câncer (INCA), Pan American Health Organization (PAHO). (2010). *Global Adult Tobacco Survey - Brazil Report*. Rio de Janeiro: INCA.

Brunton, L. L., Chabner, B. A. & Knollmann, B. C. Goodman & Gillman: *The Pharmacological Basis of Therapeutics*. McGraw Hills. New York. 12 ed.

Calsina, G., Ramón, J. M. & Echeverría, J. J. (2002). Effects of smoking on periodontal tissues. *J. Clin. Periodontol.*, *29*(8), 771-6.

Campos, M. L., Corrêa, M. G., Junior, F. H., Casati, M. Z., Sallum, E. A. & Sallum, A. W. (2013). Cigarette smoke inhalation increases the alveolar bone loss caused by primary occlusal trauma in a rat model. *J. Periodontal. Res.*, May 16. [Epub ahead of print]

Cattaneo, V., Cetta, G., Rota, C., Vezzoni, F., Rota, M. T., Gallanti, A., Boratto, R. & Poggi, P. (2000). Volatile components of cigarette smoke: effect of acrolein and acetaldehyde on human gingival fibroblasts in vitro. *J. Periodontol*, *71*(3), 425-32.

César-Neto, J. B., Benatti, B. B., Manzi, F. R., Sallum, E. A., Sallum, A. W. & Nociti, F. H. (2005b). The influence of cigarette smoke inhalation on bone density. A radiographic study in rats. *Braz. Oral. Res.*, *19*, 47-51.

César-Neto, J. B., Benatti, B. B., Neto, F. H., Sallum, A. W., Sallum, E. A. & Nociti, F. H. (2005a). Smoking cessation may present a positive impact on mandibular bone quality and periodontitis-related bone loss: a study in rats. *J. Periodontol.*, *76*(4), 520-5.

César-Neto, J. B., Benatti, B. B., Sallum, E. A., Casati, M. Z. & Nociti, F. H. Jr. (2006). The influence of cigarette smoke inhalation and its cessation on the tooth-supporting alveolar bone: a histometric study in rats. *J. Periodontal. Res.*, *41*(2), 118-23.

César-Neto, J. B., Duarte, P. M., Sallum, E. A., Barbieri, D., Moreno Jr., H. & Nociti Jr, F. H. (2003). A comparative study on the effect of nicotine administration and cigarette smoke inhalation on bone healing around titanium implants. *J. Periodontol*, *74*, 1454–1459.

Chambrone, L., Preshaw, P. M., Rosa, E. F., Heasman, P. A., Romito, G. A., Pannuti, C. M. & Tu, Y. K. (2013). Effects of smoking cessation on the outcomes of non-surgical periodontal therapy: a systematic review and individual patient data meta-analysis. *J. Clin. Periodontol*, *40*(6), 607-15.

Charalampakis, G., Rabe, P., Leonhardt, A. & Dahlén, G. (2011). A follow-up study of peri-implantitis cases after treatment. *J. Clin. Periodontol.*, *38*, 864-71.

Chen, X., Wolff, L., Aeppli, D., Guo, Z., Luan, W., Baelum, V. & Fejeskov, O. (2001). Cigarette smoking, salivary/gingival crevicular fluid cotinine and periodontal status: a 10-year longitudinal study. *J. Clin. Periodontol.*, *28*(4), 331-9.

Christen, A. G. (2001) Tobacco cessation, the dental profession, and the role of dental education. *J. Dental Education.*, *65*, 368-374.

Corrêa, M. G., Campos, M. L., Benatti, B. B., Marques, M. R., Casati, M. Z., Nociti, F. H. Jr. & Sallum, E. A. (2010). The impact of cigarette smoke inhalation on the outcome of enamel matrix derivative treatment in rats: histometric analysis. *J. Periodontol.*, *81*(12), 1820-8.

Côrrea, M. G., Gomes Campos, M. L., César-Neto, J. B., Casati, M. Z., Nociti, F. H. & Sallum, E. A. (2009). Histometric evaluation of bone around titanium implants with different surface treatments in rats exposed to cigarette smoke inhalation. *Clin. Oral Implants Res.*, *20*, 588-93.

Costa, F. O., Lages, E. J., Cota, L. O., Lorentz, T. C., Soares, R. V. & Cortelli, J. R. (2013). Tooth loss in individuals under periodontal maintenance therapy: 5-year prospective study. *J. Periodontal Res.*, May 7. [Epub ahead of print].

Dannewitz, B., Krieger, J. K., Hüsing, J. & Eickholz, P. (2006). Loss of molars in periodontally treated patients: a retrospective analysis five years or more after active periodontal treatment. *J. Clin. Periodontol.*, *33*(1), 53-61.

De Bruyn, H. & Collaert, B. (1994). The effect of smoking on early implant failure. *Clin. Oral Implants. Res.*, *5*, 260–264.

De la Rosa, M., Rodríguez, A., Sierra, K., Mendoza, G. & Chambrone, L. (2013). Predictors of peri-implant bone loss during long-term maintenance of patients treated with 10-mm implants and single crown restorations. *Int. J. Oral Maxillofac Implants*, *28*, 798-802.

DeLuca, S., Habsha, E. & Zarb, G. A. (2006). The effect of smoking on osseointegrated dental implants. Part I: implant survival. *Int. J. Prosthodont*, *19*, 491-8.

Dietrich, T., Bernimoulin, J. P. & Glynn, R. J. (2004). The effect of cigarette smoking on gingival bleeding. *J. Periodontol*, *75*(1), 16-22.

El-Zawawy, H. B., Gill, C. S., Wright, R. W. & Sandell, L. J. (2006). Smoking delays chondrogenesis in a mouse model of closed tibial fracture healing. *J. Orthop. Res.*, *24*(12), 2150-8.

Fang, M. A., Frost, P. J., Iida-Klein, A. & Hahn, T. J. (1991). Effects of nicotine on cellular function in UMR 106-01 osteoblast-like cells. *Bone*, *12*(4), 283-6.

Farina, R., Tomasi, C. & Trombelli, L. (2013). The bleeding site: a multi-level analysis of associated factors. *J. Clin. Periodontol, 40*(8), 735-42.

Feitelson, J. B., Rowell, P. P., Roberts, C. S. & Fleming, J. T. (2003). Two week nicotine treatment selectively increases bone vascular constriction in response to norepinephrine. *J. Orthop. Res., 21*, 497-502.

Focchi, G. R. A. (2003). Tobacco use: a review. *Psychiatry On-Line Brazil, 8*, available at: http://www.polbr.med.br/arquivo/artigo0303_2.htm. Retrieved Out 10, 2008.

Fredriksson, M. I., Figueredo, C. M., Gustafsson, A., Bergström, K. G. & Asman, B. E. (1999). Effect of periodontitis and smoking on blood leukocytes and acute-phase proteins. *J. Periodontol, 70*, 1355-60.

Furtado, R. D. (2002). Implicações anestésicas do tabagismo. *Rev. Bras. Anestesiol., 52*, 354-67.

Gamal, A. Y. & Bayomy, M. M. (2002). Effect of cigarette smoking on human PDL fibroblasts attachment to periodontally involved root surfaces in vitro. *J. Clin. Periodontol,* 29(8), 763-70.

Genco, R. J. (1996). Current view of risk factors for periodontal diseases, *J. Periodontol,* 67(Suppl.), 1041-1049.

Giannopoulou, C., Geinoz, A. & Cimasoni, G. (1999). Effects of nicotine on periodontal ligament fibroblasts in vitro. *J. Clin. Periodontol, 26*(1), 49-55.

Glassman, S. D., Anagnost, S. C., Parker, A., Burke, D., Johnson, J. R. & Dimar, J. R. (2000). The effect of cigarette smoking and smoking cessation on spinal fusion. *Spine, 25*, 2608-2615.

Glynn, T. J. & Manley, M. W. (2008). *How to help your patients stop smoking. A National Cancer Institute Manual for Physicians.* US Department of Health and Human Services: Washington.

Grafström, R. C., Dypbukt, J. M., Sundqvist, K., Atzori, L., Nielsen, I., Curren, R. D. & Harris, C. C. (1994). Pathobiological effects of acetaldehyde in cultured human epithelial cells and fibroblasts. *Carcinogenesis, 15*(5), 985-90.

Graswinckel, J. E., van der Velden, U., van Winkelhoff, A. J., Hoek, F. J. & Loos, B. G. (2004). Plasma antibody levels in periodontitis patients and controls. *J. Clin. Periodontol, 31*, 562-8.

Graves, D. T. & Cochran, D. (2003). The contribution of interleukin-1 and tumor necrosis factor to periodontal tissue destruction. *J. Periodontol, 74*, 391–401.

Grossi, S. G., Skrepcinski, F. B., De Caro, T., Zambon, J. J., Cummins, D. & Genco, R. J. (1996). Response to periodontal therapy in diabetics and smokers. *J. Periodontol, 67*, 1094–102.

Grossi, S. G., Zambon, J., Machtei, E. E., Schifferle, R., Andreana, S., Genco, R. J., Cummins, D. & Harrap, G. (1997). Effects of smoking and smoking cessation on healing after mechanical periodontal therapy. *J. Am. Dent. Assoc., 128*, 599- 607.

Gruica, B., Wang, H. Y., Lang, N. P. & Buser, D. (2004). Impact of IL-1 genotype and smoking status on the prognosis of osseointegrated implants. *Clin. Oral Implants. Res., 15*, 393-400.

Gullihorn, L., Karpman, R. & Lippielo, L. (2005). Differential effects of nicotine and smoke condensate on bone cell metabolic activity. *J. Orthop. Trauma., 19*(1), 17-22.

Haffajee, A. D. & Socransky, S. S. (2001a). Relationship of cigarette smoking to attachment level profiles. *J. Clin. Periodontol., 28*, 283–295.

Haffajee, A. D. & Socransky, S. S. (2001b). Relationship of cigarette smoking to the subgingival microbiota. *J. Clin. Periodontol.*, 28, 377–388.

Hanes, P. J., Schuster, G. S. & Lubas, S. (1991). Binding, uptake, and release of nicotine by human gingival fibroblasts. *J. Periodontol.*, 62(2), 147-52.

Haverstoch, B. D. & Mandrachia, V. J. (1998). Cigarette smoking and wound healing: implications in foot and ankle surgery. *J. Foot Ankle Surg.*, 31(1), 69-74.

Heitz-Mayfield, L. J. & Huynh-Ba, G. (2009). History of treated periodontitis and smoking as risks for implant therapy. *Int. J. Oral Maxillofac. Implants*, 24 Suppl, 39-68.

Heitz-Mayfield, L. J. A. (2008). Peri-implant diseases: diagnosis and risk indicators. *J. Clin. Periodontol*, 35, 292–304.

Henemyre, C. L., Scales, D. K., Hokett, S. D., Cuenin, M. F., Peacock, M. E., Parker, M. H., Brewer, P. D. & Chuang, A. H. (2003). Nicotine stimulates osteoclast resorption in a porcine marrow cell models. *J. Periodontol*, 74, 1440-6.

Hinode, D., Tanabe, S., Yokoyama, M., Fujisawa, K., Yamauchi, E. & Miyamoto, Y. (2006). Influence of smoking on osseointegrated implant failure: a meta-analysis. *Clin. Oral Implants Res.*, 17, 473–478.

Huynh-Ba, G., Friedberg, J. R., Vogiatzi, D. & Ioannidou, E. (2008). Implant failure predictors in the posterior maxilla: a retrospective study of 273 consecutive implants. *J. Periodontol*, 79, 2256-61.

James, J. A., Sayers, N. M., Drucker, D. B. & Hull, P. S. (1999). Effects of tobacco products on the attachment and growth of periodontal ligament fibroblasts. *J. Periodontol.*, 70(5), 518-25.

Jansson, H., Hamberg, K., De Bruyn, H. & Bratthall, G. (2005). Clinical consequences of IL-1 genotype on early implant failures in patients under periodontal maintenance. *Clin. Implant Dent. Relat. Res.*, 7, 51-9.

Jansson, L. & Lavstedt, S. (2002). Influence of smoking on marginal bone loss and tooth loss - a prospective study over 20 years. *J. Clin. Periodontol.*, 29(8), 750-6.

Jones, J. D., Lupori, J., Van Sickels, J. E. & Gardner, W. (1999). A 5-year comparison of hydroxyapatite-coated titanium plasma-sprayed and titanium plasma-sprayed cylinder dental implants. *Oral Surg. Oral Med. Oral Pathol. Oral Radiol. Endod.*, 87, 649-52.

Jones, J. K. & Triplett, R. G. (1992). The relationship of cigarette smoking to impaired intraoral wound healing: a review of evidence and implications for patient care. *J. Oral Maxillofac. Surg.*, 50, 237-9, discussion 239-40.

Kallala, R., Barrow, J., Graham, S. M., Kanakaris, N. & Giannoudis, P. V. (2013). The in vitro and in vivo effects of nicotine on bone, bone cells and fracture repair. *Expert Opin. Drug Saf.*, 12, 209-33.

Katono, T., Kawato, T., Tanabe, N., Suzuki, N., Yamanaka, K., Oka, H., Motohashi, M. & Maeno, M. (2006). Nicotine treatment induces expression of matrix metalloproteinases in human osteoblastic Saos-2 cells. *Acta. Biochim. Biophys. Sin.* (Shanghai), 38, 874-82.

Kerdvongbundit, V. & Wikesjö, U. M. (2000). Effect of smoking on periodontal health in molar teeth. *J. Periodontol*, 71(3), 433-7.

Kerdvongbundit, V. & Wikesjö, U. M. (2002). The prevalence and severity of periodontal disease at mandibular molar teeth in smokers with regular oral hygiene habits. *J. Periodontol.*, 73(7), 735-40.

Klokkevold, P. R. & Han, T. J. (2007). How do smoking, diabetes, and periodontitis affect outcomes of implant treatment? *Int. J. Oral Maxillofac. Implants.*, 22 Suppl, 173-202.

Koldsland, O. C., Scheie, A. A. & Aass, A. M. (2011). The association between selected risk indicators and severity of peri-implantitis using mixed model analyses. *J. Clin. Periodontol*, *38*, 285-92.

Krall, E. A., Garvey, A. J. & Garcia, R. I. (1999). Alveolar bone loss and tooth loss in male cigar and pipe smokers. *J. Am. Dent. Assoc.*, *130*(1), 57-64.

Lachmann, S., Kimmerle-Müller, E., Axmann, D., Scheideler, L, Weber, H. & Haas, R. (2007). Associations between peri-implant crevicular fluid volume, concentrations of crevicular inflammatory mediators, and composite IL-1A-889 and IL-1b +3954 genotype. A cross-sectional study on implant recall patients with and without clinical signs of peri-implantitis. *Clin. Oral Implants Res.*, *18*, 212–223.

Lemmerman, K. J. & Lemmerman, N. E. (2005). Osseointegrated dental implants in private practice: a long-term case series study. *J. Periodontol.*, *76*, 310–319.

Leppilahti, J. M., Kallio, M. A., Tervahartiala, T., Sorsa, T. & Mäntylä, P. (2013). Gingival Crevicular Fluid (GCF) Matrix Metalloproteinase -8 Levels Predict Treatment Outcome Among Smoking Chronic Periodontitis Patients. *J. Periodontol.*, May 9. [Epub ahead of print].

Levin, L., Hertzberg, R., Har-Nes, S. & Schwartz-Arad, D. (2008). Long-term marginal bone loss around single dental implants affected by current and past smoking habits. *Implant Dent.*, *17*, 422-9.

Lie, M. A., van der Weijden, G. A., Timmerman, M. F., Loos, B. G., van Steenbergen, T. J. & van der Velden, U. (1998). Oral microbiota in smokers and non-smokers in natural and experimentally-induced gingivitis. *J. Clin. Periodontol.*, *25*(8), 677-86.

Liede, K. E., Haukka, J. K, Hietanen, J. H., Mattila, M. H., Ronka, H. & Sorsa, T. (1999). The association between smoking cessation and periodontal status and salivary proteinase levels. *J. Periodontol*, *70*, 1361-1368.

Lima, L. L., César Neto, J. B., Cayana, E. G., Nociti, F. H. Jr., Sallum, E. A. & Casati, M. Z. (2013). Parathyroid hormone (1-34) compensates the negative effect of smoking around implants. *Clin. Oral Implants Res.*, *24*, 1055-9.

Linde, K. & Willich, S. N. (2003). How objective are systematic reviews? Differences between reviews on complementary medicine. *J. R. Soc. Med.*, *96*, 17-22.

Lindquist, L. W. & Carlsson. G. E. (1985). Long terms effects on chewing with mandibular fixed prostheses on osseointegrated implants. *Acta Odontolol. Scandinavica.*, *43*, 39–45.

Liu, X., Kohyama, T., Kobayashi, T., Abe, S., Kim, H. J., Reed E. C. & Rennard S. I. (2003). Cigarette smoke extract inhibits chemotaxis and collagen gel contraction mediated by human bone marrow osteoprogenitor cells and osteoblast-like cells. *Osteoporos. Int.*, *14*(3), 235-42.

Liu, X. D., Zhu, Y. K., Umino, T., Spurzem, J. R., Romberger, D. J., Wang, H., Reed, E. & Rennard, S. I. (2001). Cigarette smoke inhibits osteogenic differentiation and proliferation of human osteoprogenitor cells in monolayer and three-dimensional collagen gel culture. *J. Lab. Clin. Med.*, *137*(3), 208-19.

Loos, B. G., Roos, M. T., Schellekens, P. T., van der Velden, U. & Miedema, F. (2004). Lymphocyte numbers and function in relation to periodontitis and smoking. *J. Periodontol*, *75*, 557-64.

Machtei, E. E., Dunford, R., Hausmann, E., Grossi, S. G., Powell, J., Cummins, D., Zambon, J. J. & Genco, R. J. (1997). Longitudinal study of prognostic factors in established periodontitis patients. *J. Clin. Periodontol.*, *24*(2), 102-9.

Machtei, E. E., Hausmann, E., Dunford, R., Grossi, S., Ho, A., Davis, G., Chandler, J., Zambon, J. & Genco, R. J. (1999). Longitudinal study of predictive factors for periodontal disease and tooth loss. *J. Clin. Periodontol*, *26*(6), 374-80.

Machuca, G., Rosales, I., Lacalle, J. R., Machuca, C. & Bullón, P. (2000). Effect of cigarette smoking on periodontal status of healthy young adults. *J. Periodontol*, *71*(1), 73-8.

Mai, X., Wactawski-Wende, J., Hovey, K. M., La Monte, M. J., Chen, C., Tezal, M. & Genco. R. J. (2013). Associations between smoking and tooth loss according to the reason for tooth loss: the Buffalo OsteoPerio Study. *J. Am. Dent. Assoc.*, *144*(3), 252-65.

Martin, T. (2008). Hydrogen cyanide in cigarette smoke. Available at: http://quitsmoking.about.com/cs/nicotineinhaler/a/cyanide.htm. Retrieved Out 20, 2008.

Meekin, T. N., Wilson, R. F., Scott, D. A., Ide, M. & Palmer, R. M. (2000). Laser Doppler flow meter measurement of relative gingival and forehead skin blood flow in light and heavy smokers during and after smoking. *J. Clin. Periodontol*, *27*(4), 236-42.

Meulman, T., Giorgetti, A. P., Gimenes, J., Casarin, R. C., Peruzzo, D. C. & Nociti, F. H. Jr. (2013). One stage, full-mouth, ultrasonic debridement in the treatment of severe chronic periodontitis in smokers: a preliminary, blind and randomized clinical trial. *J. Int. Acad. Periodontol*, *15*(3), 83-90.

Nair, P., Sutherland, G., Palmer, R. M., Wilson, R. F. & Scott, D. A. (2003). Gingival bleeding on probing increases after quitting smoking. *J. Clin. Periodontol*, *30*, 435–437.

Newman, M. G., Caton, J. G. & Gunsolley, J. C. (2003). The use of the evidence-based approach in a periodontal therapy contemporary science workshop. *Ann. Periodontol*, *8*, 1-11.

Ng, T. K., Carballosa, C. M., Pelaez, D., Wong, H. K., Choy, K. W., Pang, C. P. & Cheung, H. S. (2013). Nicotine alters MicroRNA expression and hinders human adult stem cell regenerative potential. *Stem Cells Dev.*, *22*(5), 781-90.

Nile, C. J., Sherrabeh, S., Ramage, G. & Lappin, D. F. (2013). Comparison of circulating tumour necrosis factor superfamily cytokines in periodontitis patients undergoing supportive therapy: a case-controlled cross-sectional study comparing smokers and non-smokers in health and disease. *J. Clin. Periodontol*, *40*(9), 875-82.

Nociti, F. H. Jr., Cesar Neto, J. B., Carvalho, M. D., Sallum, E. A. & Sallum, A. W. (2002a). Intermittent cigarette smoke inhalation may affect bone volume around titanium implants in rats. *J. Periodontol*, *73*, 982-7.

Nociti, F. H. Jr., Cesar Neto, J. B., Carvalho, M. D. & Sallum, E. A. (2002b). Bone density around titanium implants may be influenced by intermittent cigarette smoke inhalation: a histometric study in rats. *Int. J. Oral Maxillofac. Implants*, *17*, 347-52.

Nogueira-Filho, G. R., Froes Neto, E. B., Casati, M. Z., Reis, S. R., Tunes, R. S. & Tunes, U. R. (2004). Nicotine effects on alveolar bone changes induced by occlusal trauma: a histometric study in rats. *J. Periodontol*, *75*(3), 348-52.

Noguerol, B., Muñoz, R., Mesa, F., de Dios Luna, J. & O'Valle, F. (2006). Early implant failure. Prognostic capacity of Periotest: retrospective study of a large sample. *Clin. Oral Implants Res.*, *17*, 459-64.

Oberg, M., Jaakkola, M. S., Woodward, A., Peruga, A. & Prüss-Ustün, A. (2011). Worldwide burden of disease from exposure to second-hand smoke: a retrospective analysis of data from 192 countries. *Lancet*, *377*, 139-46.

Organización Panamericana de la Salud. World Bank. (2000). *La epidemia del tabaquismo: los gobiernos y los aspectos ecnoômicos del control del tabaco*. Washington, DC.

Page, R. C. & Kornman, K. S. (1997). The pathogenesis of human periodontitis: an introduction. *Periodontol, 2000, 14*, 9-11.

Palmer, R. M., Scott, D. A., Meekin, T. N., Poston, R. N., Odell, E. W. & Wilson, R. F. (1999). Potential mechanisms of susceptibility to periodontitis in tobacco smokers. *J. Periodontal Res., 34*(7), 363-9.

Papantonopoulos, G. H. (1999). Smoking influences decision making in periodontal therapy: a retrospective clinical study. *J. Periodontol, 70*, 1166–73.

Patel, R. A., Wilson, R. F. & Palmer, R. M. (2012). The effect of smoking on periodontal bone regeneration: a systematic review and meta-analysis. *Periodontol, 83*, 143-155.

Peñarrocha, M., Palomar, M., Sanchis, J. M., Guarinos, J. & Balaguer, J. (2004). Radiologic study of marginal bone loss around 108 dental implants and its relationship to smoking, implant location, and morphology. *Int. J. Oral Maxillofac. Implants, 19*, 861-7.

Poggi, P., Rota, M. T. & Boratto, R. (2002). The volatile fraction of cigarette smoke induces alterations in the human gingival fibroblast cytoskeleton. *J. Periodontal Res., 37*(3), 230-5.

Ramp, W. K., Lenz, L. G. & Galvin, R. J. (1991). Nicotine inhibits collagen synthesis and alkaline phosphatase activity, but stimulates DNA synthesis in osteoblast-like cells. *Proc. Soc. Exp. Biol. Med., 197*, 36-43.

Raupach, T., Schäfer, K., Konstantinides, S. & Andreas, S. (2006). Secondhand smoke as an acute threat for the cardiovascular system: a change in paradigm. *Eur. Heart. J., 27*(4), 386-92.

Rezavandi, K., Palmer, R. M., Odell, E. W., Scott, D. A. & Wilson, R. F. (2002). Expression of ICAM-1 and E-selectin in gingival tissues of smokers and non-smokers with periodontitis. *J. Oral Pathol. Med., 31*, 59-64.

Robbers, J. E., Speedie, M. K. & Tyler, V. E. (1996). Pharmacognosy and Pharmacobiotechnology. Williams and Wilkins, Baltimore, MD.

Robertson, C. R. & Richard, H. D. (1998). Health law and ethics. Prying open the door to the tobacco industry's secret about nicotine: The Minnesota tobacco trial. *JAMA., 280*, 1173.

Roos-Jansaker, A. M., Renvert, H., Lindahl, C. & Renvert, S. (2006). Nine to fourteen-year follow-up of implant treatment. Part III: Factors associated with peri-implant lesions. *J. Clin. Periodontol., 33*, 296-301.

Rosa, G. M., Lucas, G. Q. & Lucas, O. N. (2008). Cigarette smoking and alveolar bone in young adults: a study using digitized radiographs. *J. Periodontol, 79*(2), 232-44.

Rota, M. T., Poggi, P. & Boratto, R. (2001). Human gingival fibroblast cytoskeleton is a target for volatile smoke components. *J. Periodontol, 72*(6), 709-13.

Saldanha, J. B., Pimentel, S. P., Casati, M. Z., Sallum, E. A., Barbieri, D., Moreno, H. J. & Nociti, F. H. (2004). Guided bone regeneration may be negatively influenced by nicotine administration: a histologic study in dogs. *J. Periodontol, 4*, 565-71.

Sayardoust, S., Gröndahl, K., Johansson, E., Thomsen, P. & Slotte, C. (2013). Implant Survival and Marginal Bone Loss at Turned and Oxidized Implants in Periodontitis-Susceptible Smokers and Never-Smokers: A Retrospective, Clinical, Radiographic Case-Control Study. *J. Periodontol.* [Epub ahead of print]

Schwartz-Arad, D., Samet, N. & Samet, N. (2002). Mamlider, A. Smoking and complications of endosseous dental implants. *J. Periodontol, 73*, 153-7.

Shibli, J. A, Piattelli, A., Iezzi, G., Cardoso, L. A., Onuma, T., de Carvalho, P. S., Susana D., Ferrari, D. S., Mangano, C. & Zenóbio, E. G. (2010). Effect of smoking on early bone healing around oxidized surfaces: a prospective, controlled study in human jaws. *J. Periodontol*, *81*, 575-83.

Shimazaki, Y., Saito, T., Kiyohara, Y., Kato, I., Kubo, M., Iida, M. & Yamashita, Y. (2006). The influence of current and former smoking on gingival bleeding: the Hisayama study. *J. Periodontol.*, *77*(8), 1430-5.

Shivanaikar, S. S., Faizuddin, M. & Bhat, K. (2013). Effect of smoking on neutrophil apoptosis in chronic periodontitis: an immunohistochemical study. *Indian J. Dent. Res.*, *24*(1), 147.

Silcox, D. H., Daftari, T., Boden, S. D., Schimandle, J. H., Hutton, W. C. & Whitesides, T. E. Jr. (1995). The effect of nicotine on spinal fusion. *Spine*, *20*, 1549-53.

Silva, C. O., de Lima, A. F., Sallum, A. W. & Tatakis, D. N. (2007). Coronally positioned flap for root coverage in smokers and non-smokers: stability of outcomes between 6 months and 2 years. *J. Periodontol.*, *78*(9), 1702-7.

Silva, C. O., Sallum, A. W., de Lima A. F. & Tatakis, D. N. (2006). Coronally positioned flap for root coverage: poorer outcomes in smokers. *J. Periodontol*, *77*(1), 81-7.

Silverstein, P. (1992). Smoking and wound healing. *Am. J. Med.*, *93*, 22-24.

Souza, S. L., Macedo, G. O., Tunes, R. S., Silveira e Souza, A. M., Novaes, A. B. Jr., Grisi, M. F., Taba, M. Jr., Palioto, D. B. & Correa, V. M. (2008). Subepithelial connective tissue graft for root coverage in smokers and non-smokers: a clinical and histologic controlled study in humans. *J. Periodontol*, *79*(6), 1014-21.

Stark, M. J., Rohde, K., Maher, J. E., Pizacani, B. A., Dent, C. W., Bard., R., Carmella, S. G., Benoit, A. R., Thomson, N. M. & Hecht, S. S. (2007). The impact of clean indoor air exemptions and preemption policies on the prevalence of a tobacco-specific lung carcinogens among nonsmoking bar and restaurant workers. *American Journal of Public Health*, *97*(8), 1457-63.

Stavropoulos, A., Mardas, N., Herrero, F. & Karring, T. (2004). Smoking affects the outcome of guided tissue regeneration with bioresorbable membranes: a retrospective analysis of intrabony defects. *J. Clin. Periodontol.*, *31*, 945–950.

Stefani, C. M., Nogueira, F., Sallum, E. A., de Toledo, S., Sallum, A. W. & Nociti, F. H. Jr. (2002). Influence of nicotine administration on different implant surfaces: a histometric study in rabbits. *J. Periodontol*, *2*, 206-12.

Strietzel, F. P., Reichart, P. A., Kale, A., Kulkarni, M., Wegner, B., Kuchler, I. (2007). Smoking interferes with the prognosis of dental implant treatment: a systematic review and meta-analysis. *J. Clin. Periodontol*, *34*, 523–544.

Sutej, I., Peros, K., Benutic, A., Capak, K., Basic, K. & Rosin-Gorget, K. (2012). Salivary calcium concentration and periodontal health of young adults in relation to tobacco smoking. *Oral Health Prev. Dent.*, *10*(4), 397-403.

Tanaka, H., Tanabe, N., Shoji, M., Suzuki, N., Katono, T., Sato, S., Motohashi, M. & Maeno, M. (2006). Nicotine and lipopolysaccharide stimulate the formation of osteoclast-like cells by increasing macrophage colony-stimulating factor and prostaglandin E2 production by osteoblasts. *Life Sci.*, *78*(15), 1733-40.

Tanaka, H., Tanabe, N., Suzuki, N., Shoji, M., Torigoe, H., Sugaya, A., Motohashi, M. & Maeno, M. (2005). Nicotine affects mineralized nodule formation by the human osteosarcoma cell line Saos-2. *Life Sci.*, *77*, 2273-84.

Tangada, S. D., Califano, J. V., Nakashima, K., Quinn, S. M., Zhang, J. B., Gunsolley, J. C., Schenkein, H. A. & Tew, J. G. (1997). The effect of smoking on serum IgG2 reactive with Actinobacillus actinomyce-temcomitans in early-onset periodontitis patients. *J. Periodontol*, *68*, 842-50.

Tatli, U., Damlar, I., Erdoğan, O. & Esen, E. (2013). Effects of smoking on periimplant health status and IL-1β, TNF-α, and PGE2 levels in periimplant crevicular fluid: a cross-sectional study on well-maintained implant recall patients. *Implant. Dent.*, *22*, 519-24.

Terashima, T., Wiggs, B., English, D., Hogg, J. C. & van Eeden, S. F. (1997). The effect of cigarette smoking on the bone marrow. *Am. J. Respir. Crit. Care Med.*, *155*(3), 1021-6.

Tipton, D. A. & Dabbous, M. K. (1995). Effects of nicotine on proliferation and extracellular matrix production of human gingival fibroblasts in vitro. *J. Periodontol*, *66*(12), 1056-64.

Tonetti, M. S. (1998). Cigarette smoking and periodontal disease: etiology and management of disease. *Ann. Periodontol*, *3*, 88-101.

van der Weijden, G. A., de Slegte, C., Timmerman, M. F. & van der Velden, U. (2001). Periodontitis in smokers and non-smokers: intra-oral distribution of pockets. *J. Clin. Periodontol*, *28*(10), 955-60.

Vandeweghe, S. & De Bruyn, H. (2011). The effect of smoking on early bone remodeling on surface modified Southern Implants®. *Clin. Implant. Dent. Relat. Res.*, *13*, 206-14.

Vanscheeuwijck, P. M., Teredesai, A., Terpstra, P. M., Verbeeck, J., Kuhl, P., Gerstenberg, B., Gebel, S. & Carmines, E. L. (2002). Evaluation of the potential effects of ingredients added to cigarettes. Part 4: subchronic inhalation toxicity. *Food Chem. Toxicol.*, *40*(1), 113-31.

Weyant, R. J. (1994). Characteristics associated with the loss and peri-implant tissue health of endosseous dental implants. *Int. J. Oral Maxillofac. Implants.*, *9*, 95-102.

World Health Organization. (1992). *The ICD-10: Classification of mental and behavioural disorders: clinical descriptions and diagnostic guidelines*. World Health Organization: Geneva.

World Health Organization. (2000). *Air quality guidelines for Europe*. World Health Organization: Copenhagen.

World Health Organization. (2003). *Tobacco Free Initiative*. World Health Organization: Geneva.

World Health Organization. (2007). *Protection from exposure to second-hand tobacco smoke. Policy recommendations*. World Health Organization: Geneva. Available at: http://www.who.int/tobacco/resources/publications/wntd/2007/pol_recommendations/en/index.html. Retrieved Out 20, 2008.

World Health Organization. (2008). *Report on the global tobacco epidemic*. World Health Organization: Geneva.

World Health Organization. (2012). *WHO global report: mortality attributable to tobacco*. World Health Organization: Geneva.

Yalçn, S., Basegmez, C., Mijiritsky, E., Yalçn, F., Isik, G. & Onan, U. (2005). Detection of implant crevicular fluid prostaglandin E2 levels for the assessment of peri-implant health: a pilot study. *Implant. Dent.*, *14*, 194–200.

Yanagita, M., Kojima, Y., Kawahara, T., Kajikawa, T., Oohara, H., Takedachi, M., Yamada, S. & Murakami, S. (2010). Suppressive effects of nicotine on the cytodifferentiation of murine periodontal ligament cells. *Oral Dis.*, *16*(8), 812-7.

Yuhara, S., Kasagi, S., Inoue, A., Otsuka, E., Hirose, S. & Hagiwara, H. (1999). Effects of nicotine on cultured cells suggest that it can influence the formation and resorption of bone. *Eur. J. Pharmacol.*, *383*, 387-93.

Zambon, J. J., Grossi, S. G., Machtei, E. E., Ho, A. W., Dunford, R. & Genco, R. J. (1996). Cigarette smoking increases the risk for subgingival infection with periodontal pathogens. *J. Periodontol*, *67*(10 Suppl), 1050-4.

Zarb, G. A. & Schmitt, A. (1990). The longitudinal clinical effectiveness of osseointegrated dental implants: The Toronto study. Part II: the prosthetic results. *J. Prosthet. Dent.*, *64*, 53–61.

Zhang, W., Song, F. & Windsor, L. J. (2009). Cigarette smoke condensate affects the collagen-degrading ability of human gingival fibroblasts. *J. Periodontal Res.*, *44*(6), 704-13.

Zitzmann, N. U. & Berglundh, T. (2008). Definition and prevalence of peri-implant diseases. *J. Clin. Periodontol*, *35*(8) Suppl, 286-91.

Chapter 9

HEALTH AND ENVIRONMENTAL PITFALLS AND FALLACIES OF SMOKING

Dr. Sona B. Nair[*]
Research Scientist, National Institute of Immunohaematology
K. E. M. Hospital Campus, Mumbai, India

ABSTRACT

Smoking is evolving as one of the main addictions and risk factors responsible for major health problems in addition to other risk factors such as stress, unhealthy eating habits, lack of proper rest and sleep. A large body of literature has shown smoking to be one of the major risk factors in the development of chronic obstructive lung disease, stroke, peripheral vascular diseases, and cancer of lungs, larynx, mouth, urinary bladder kidney and pancreas. Though cigarette smoking is one of the common methods, tobacco chewing, hookah, bidi, cigars are other forms of tobacco consumption which are all equally harmful to health causing serious health problems.

Many factors like the pattern of inhalation of smoke, the brands of cigarette used, duration of smoking play a major role in the development of disease. Tobacco smoke contains over 7,000 different chemicals and chemical compounds which go from the lungs to blood and from there to tissues thus affecting all the organs in the body causing cellular changes and increasing the blood viscosity and decreasing the oxygen carrying capacity of the blood.

Second hand smoke or passive smoking causes similar serious health hazards as direct smoking due to high levels of toxic chemicals present in the environment of smokers. The habit of smoking and tobacco consumption also causes air and water pollution. The cigarette butts when thrown on the streets are washed into rivers and sea by rain water and the chemicals present in them are released in to the water. The smoke and the particulate matter released from the burning end of the cigarette smoke and the smoke released by the smoker remains in the air for a long time which when inhaled by people cause severe health problems.

Thus it is extremely important to make people understand how smoking and tobacco use not only harms them but also the surrounding people and environment.

---

[*] Phone :091 22 4138518/19, email :sonabnair@yahoo.com

INTRODUCTION

Smoking is a leading cause of preventable death worldwide today. There is a famous quote on smoking by an unknown author "A cigarette is a pipe with a fire at one end and a fool at the other".

This quote aptly describes the current scenario in the world where people bogged down by stress and anxieties are trying to resort to easy ways of relief from their problems. Cigarette smoking is one of the common methods of consuming tobacco. Tobacco is often mixed with additives to enhance the addictive potency and to increase the effects of smoke on the mind and body so that the craving to smoke increases once the feel good factor weans off. More and more youngsters in the age group of 15 to 35 years are reporting in hospitals with major cardiac problems and respiratory problems. Smoking is one of the main common factors seen among them.

Some of them start smoking to impress their peers and some start smoking to get over their stress and tension (Hoffman et al. 2006). They believe that casually smoking one or two cigarettes will not lead to addiction. But the fact is that serious symptoms of addiction such as having strong urges to smoke, feeling anxious or irritable appear among youths within weeks or only days after occasional smoking first begins (Di Franza et al. 2007, Doubeni et al. 2010). Every day, an additional 3,500 kids try their first cigarette and about 1,000 other kids less than 18 years old become new regular daily smokers (Di Franza et al. 2000).

Smoking is one of the main risk factors for a number of chronic diseases affecting coronary, peripheral and cerebral arteries especially in young individuals. Smoking cigarettes with high nicotine content causes rise in blood pressure, heart rate, left ventricular and diastolic pressure and coronary sinus. It increases arterial and venous carbon monoxide levels simultaneously causing a decrease in coronary sinus and in arterial and venous oxygen partial pressure levels with a partial recovery within 30minutes. A large volume of work has been done in the past both on acute and chronic smokers showing these results (Wilbert and Aronow 1974, Hawkins 1972, Mehta and Mehta 1982, Madsen and Dyerberg 1984, Nair et al. 2001, Sutherland 2011, Xu et al. 2006).

The purpose of this chapter is therefore to bring to light the already known and unknown facts about smoking and its effects on human life and society at large. This chapter explains in simplified way the harmful effects of the chemicals that constitute the cigarette smoke and how it damages our body. Thus smoking does not in any way alleviate our problems but in fact we are paying money to buy more problems for ourselves in the form of bad health and thus adding on to our sufferings and economic burden. It adds to the stress level and anxiety of the smokers thinking about the extra economic burden added due to treatment and medicines (Oster et al. 1984, Behan et al. 2005). Smoking also puts at risk the health of others who don't smoke but are forced to become passive smokers due to the environmental pollution caused due to smoking.

Constituents of Tobacco Smoke and Its Inhalation Patterns

Tobacco leaves are harvested and cured to allow for the slow oxidation and degradation of carotenoids in tobacco leaf. Tobacco smoke contains over 7,000 different chemicals which includes 69 known carcinogens and chemical compounds which have diversified adverse effects on the body (International Agency for Research on Cancer [IARC] 2004, Rodgman and Perfetti 2009). They go from the lungs to blood and from there to tissues thus affecting all the organs in the body causing cellular changes (Peto et al. 1992). Tobacco contains nicotine, tar, polynuclear aromatic hydrocarbons, phenol, cresol and N-nitrosonornide, benzol in particulate phase while the gaseous phase contains carbon monoxide, hydrocyanide, ammonia acetaldehyde, various oxides of nitrogen and acrolein (Kar and Das, 1989).

The main components of cigarette smoke can be listed as follows:

- carbon monoxide found in car exhaust and nicotine which is the main addictive component of the cigarette and the main product of cigarette smoke
- formaldehyde which is found as by product of cigarette smoke is used to embalm dead bodies and preserve them
- ammonia used to increase the absorption rate of nicotine is used to clean toilets and for sewage and waste water treatment and is a main ingredient of liquid fertilizer
- arsenic which is used as pesticide on tobacco plants, remains on it and is inhaled as a part of cigarette smoke
- acetone is another by product from cigarette smoke which is used to remove nail polish and as cleaner
- propylene glycol added to cigarettes to prevent it from drying up, and it actually speeds up the delivery of nicotine to the brain
- turpentine which is used to flavor menthol cigarettes is used as a thinner in paints and varnish
- benzene which is another by product of cigarette smoke is used in pesticides and gasoline
- cadmiumis a metallic compound that tobacco plants take up from soil and then it remains in smoke is used in making batteries
- hydrogen cyanide, lead and nickel are other compounds found in smoke

A burning cigarette is a complex system consisting of many chemical and physical processes. There are two main regions in the burning region of the cigarette viz a combustion zone and a pyrolysis/distillation zone. Each mechanism and its interaction have a great effect on the levels of chemical constituents of the smoke inhaled by the smoker which ultimately has different effects on them. In the *combustion zone* oxygen reacts with carbonized tobacco producing gaseous products and in the *pyrolysis zone* the smoke cools down and forms the aerosols (Baker 2006). Thus when a smoker inhales a bolus of smoke that is formed it mainly contains two fractions (i) particulate matter containing nicotine produced when the smoke cools down in the cooler pyrolysis zone which reaches the lungs (ii) gaseous phase containing carbon monoxide and other gases produced when oxygen reacts with carbonized tobacco in combustion zone (Arnson et al. 2010).

A burning cigarette produces 3 kinds of smoke (a) mainstream smoke which is inhaled by the smoker and then exhaled (b) side-stream smoke which is produced from the burning end of the cigarette (c) smoke exhaled to the general atmosphere by smokers. Thus the environmental factors also influence the effect of smoking on smokers (Szponar et al. 2012).

Studies have shown that the risk of developing a disease due to cigarette smoking not only depends on the number of cigarettes smoked by an individual per day but also on several other factors like the brand of the cigarette smoked, the method of smoke inhalation (if superficial inhalation or deep inhalation of smoke) and the duration of smoking (Reddy and Shaikh 2008, Conolly et al. 2007, Nair and Ghosh 2013). The contents of cigarette and their quantity also vary between different brands of cigarettes and so will their effects on individuals using those (Lee 2001, Baker et al. 2007). The additives that are added to enhance the flavour and effect of nicotine on the smoker have a great role to play in the choice of cigarette a smoker gets addicted to. A new study published in the *British Medical Journal* shows that cigarettes packaged in plain unappealing packs make the smokers think about the urgency to quit smoking. Novelty packing with different shapes and the way packs open have been found to attract youngsters more (Ford 2013).

Different studies conducted in the U.S., Japan and India have shown varying contents of nicotine concentrations in the cigarettes (Winn et al. 1981, Greer et al. 1986, Maher et al. 1994). Plant variety, cultivation, curing methods, the presence or absence of filter, the type of wrapper used for wrapping tobacco to make cigarettes are known to influence the formation and levels of toxic chemicals in tobacco and tobacco smoke (Kozlowski et al. 1988, Fukumota et al. 1981). The hazard of smoking greatly depends on the way of puffing and inhalation and also on the number of cigarettes smoked per day (Helmut and Ehrly 1981).

Bidi is a thin cigarette found in South Asia and is commonly used by lower income workers (Kamboj 2008, Agrawal et al. 2013).They are made by filling and wrapping the tobacco flakes in tendu leaves and with a string tied at one end. Bidis are not in any way safer than cigarettes. The nicotine content of bidis was found to be much higher than that in cigarettes (Maher et al. 1994, Kozlowski 1988). They produce higher levels of carbon monoxide, nicotine and tar than cigarettes. Moreover smokers who smoke bidis generally prefer deep inhalations which contribute to an increased risk of development of disease (Reddy et al. 2008).

Cigars, pipes, hookahs are other forms of smoking tobacco. Chewing of tobacco is also a very hazardous form of tobacco consumption because tobacco remains in contact with the mouth cells and tissues for a longer time increasing the risk of oral cancer.

How Smoke Travels in the Body after Smoking

When a person smokes he/she ingests a large amount of chemicals and carcinogens with each puff. The first thing that happens in first few seconds is that a mix of gases is released which enters the throat and lungs. The ciliary hair present in nose and lungs are paralyzed by the chemicals in the smoke and they are no longer capable of protecting the body from the smoke. Once the smoke reaches the lungs it damages the alveoli. The smoke then turns into tar and sticks on the throat and lungs killing the healthy lung cells.

Cigarettes with filter does reduce the amount of tar entering the body to some extent but the smoker then has to inhale deeply to get the required amount of nicotine in the body that makes him feel good. Ultimately the person ingests the same amount of smoke with or without filter. The smoke then reaches other parts of the body and damages it. In the long run a continuous smoker loses his sense of smell and taste due to the tar that gets coated on this tongue and inside his nose.

Health Hazards of Tobacco Smoking

The pharmacological response seen in the smoker is primarily due to nicotine (Kelly et al. 1984). Nicotine is a very strong and addictive drug and its effect on the body is further increased due to the additives added to tobacco to enhance flavour and effects of the smoke. Nicotine causes physical and psychological dependency. It is an alkaloid, whose inhalation is known to trigger the secretion of vasopressin, a potent vasoconstrictor hormone with a possible action on coronary arteries. It also stimulates sympathoneural and sympathoadrenal activity and influences systolic blood pressure, heart rate and platelet aggregation (U.S. Department of Health and Human Services 2010).

Smoking cigarettes with high nicotine content causes rise in blood pressure, heart rate, left ventricular end diastolic pressure and coronary sinus. It increases arterial and venous carbon monoxide levels, simultaneously causing a decrease in coronary sinus and in arterial and venous oxygen partial pressure levels with a partial recovery within 30 minutes (Wilbert and Aronow 1974, U.S. Department of Health and Human Services 2010). The addictive power of nicotine is due to its immediate and direct effects on brain. Smoking actually alters the brain chemistry and increases stress levels in smokers. Smoking does not relieve stress. In fact the feelings of relaxation that they experience during smoking are temporary and return to the stressed level once they stop smoking (Modesto-Lowe and Chmielewska 2013, Leventhal et al. 2013).

Smokers have fewer dopamine receptors, a specific cell receptor found in the brain that is believed to play a role in addiction. The release of dopamine gives one a feeling of relaxation. One of the leading hypothesis regarding the mechanism of addiction states that nicotine exposure initially increases dopamine transmission, but subsequently decreases dopamine receptor function and number. The initial increase in dopamine activity from nicotine results initially in pleasant feelings for the smoker, but the subsequent decrease in dopamine leaves the smoker craving more cigarettes. Regular doses of nicotine leads to changes in the brain which then leads to nicotine withdrawal symptoms when the supply of nicotine reduces.

Smoke contains several carcinogenic and pyrolytic products that bind to DNA and cause genetic mutations. It has been reported that nicotine suppresses the death of lung cancer cells by affecting the signaling pathways (Mai et al. 2003, Jin et al. 2005). Apoptosis or cell death is a controlled, naturally occurring process in the body that is very important to remove injured or genomically unstable cells to prevent the surrounding normally occurring cells from damage (Rich et al. 2000). DNA damaging agents from tobacco smoke act to bring about inactivation of apoptosis by interfering the pathway of apoptosis (Reed 2000). Cigarette smoke contains benzene in large quantities and the exposure to which causes myelogenous leukemia in humans (IARC 1983).

Smokers have 3 to 4 times higher risk of developing heart attack compared to nonsmokers. Smoking increases the risk to the entire cardiovascular system. The fact that cigarette smoking affects flow behavior of blood has been well documented (Yong 1990). Tobacco smoke also increases the blood coagulability which is contributing to the cause of heart attack. Due to more viscous blood there is a state of stagnation and deficient oxygen supply to the tissues leading to hypoxia (Wasserman 1989). This reduced oxygen supply leads to lowered redox state, rapid glycogen utilization, increased osmolality and swelling of cells and metabolic acidosis. Metabolic acidosis has a very strong negative effect on the structure and functions of red blood cells. The slower the blood flow in the capillaries, the greater is the internal viscosity of the red blood cells and the greater the chances of breakdown of haemodynamic mechanisms at macro and microcirculatory levels. This further decreases the oxygen supply to the tissues, leading to hypoxia and further decrease in pH. Hypoxia stimulates the production of red blood cells i.e. increase in hematocrit. Hematocrit is one of the strong determinants of blood viscosity. Increase in hematocrit coupled with blood viscosity has serious effects on organ perfusion (Gagnon et al. 1994). Thus, a vicious circle sets in which leads to further deterioration of blood flow, making smokers more susceptible to development of vascular disorders.

Carbon monoxide from tobacco smoke which has an affinity 245 times greater than oxygen combines with haemoglobin and reduces the oxygen supply to the tissues thus leading to heart attack, stroke and peripheral vascular disease. This risk is 20 times if the carboxyhaemoglobin (COHb) level is 5% or more (U.S. Department of Health and Human Services1979, 2010).

Smoking is also an important cause of stroke. Stroke is a disease that affects the arteries leading to and within the brain. Stroke can be caused either by a clot obstructing the flow of blood to the brain (called an ischemic stroke) or by a blood vessel rupturing and preventing blood flow to the brain (hemorrhagic stroke).

When a stroke occurs that part of the brain does not get the blood supply and the nutrients and oxygen it needs and the brain cells die. That part of the brain which controls a particular body functions will be affected leading to paralysis of that part of the body. Cigarette smoke greatly aggravates and speeds up the formation of atherosclerosis (term used for hardening and thickening of arteries) in coronary artery aorta and arteries of legs. Smoking also can cause peripheral vascular disease by reduction of blood supply to the legs. The blood vessels narrow often resulting in gangrene and amputation of the limb.

Tobacco smoke both mainstream and second hand smoke aggravates the asthmatic attacks in known asthma patients. Some studies have shown a higher prevalence of asthma in adults who were exposed to cigarette smoke since childhood (Larsson et al. 2001).

Chronic bronchitis produced by smoking inflames the lungs and airways resulting in increased mucous production. Emphysema destroys the air sacs of the lungs which cannot readily absorb oxygen. In intrinsic airway narrowing the airway and the lungs become narrow due to inflammation of the walls and muscle contraction (Gerrard et al. 1980, Maloet al. 1982, Buczkoet al. 1984, Taylor 1985, Behrman 2000, Fitzpatrick and Blair 2000). Cigarette smoke also has been reported to affect the natural and adaptive immune defense mechanisms of the body (Sopori 2002). Tobacco smoke interferes with drug breakdown, or drug metabolism which is very important to drug effectiveness and safety (Desai 2001, Eke 2002).

Patients with sickle cell anemia who smoke and are exposed to environmental smoke are known to have increased incidence of Acute Chest Syndrome, a condition that presents with severe chest pain, and is a life-threatening emergency (Young et al. 1992).

Cigarette smoking also makes diabetes difficult to control and also harms reproduction and children's health (U.S. Department of Health and Human Services 2010). Tobacco use causes miscarriages in pregnant women, premature birth and low birth weight (Noakes et al. 2003, Committee on Drugs, 2000-2001). It has been shown that tobacco use can lead to cancer of mouth, throat, lungs, larynx, oesophagus, urinary bladder, kidney, pancreas and possibly cervix and liver.

Smoking and chewing of tobacco also known as smokeless tobacco also causes cancer of the mouth and lungs and the incidence has been found to be higher in people who chew tobacco (Fant et al. 1999, Shah et al. 1998, Sawyer et al. 1992, Kampangsri et al. 2013, Patil et al. 2013).

Smoking can cause premature graying of hair and hair loss (Trueb 2003) and the main culprits are nicotine and carbon monoxide present in cigarette smoke. Smoking also causes premature ageing (Trueb 2003). *Smokers face* is a term used by doctors to describe the facial changes in smokers due to smoking for long time. Deep dark lines around the eyes and corners of the mouth, wrinkles and skin appears grey in colour. Nearly half of all the smokers get smokers face (Model 1985, Koh et al. 2002).

Nicotine constricts the blood vessels and the blood flow to the shaft is affected thus reducing the supply of oxygen. Carbon monoxide binds to hemoglobin instead of oxygen and thus affects the oxygen carrying capacity of the blood and its ability to remove toxins from the body. These factors prevent the oxygenation of hair tissue and skin and the effective removal of free radicals from the body thus aggravating the problem of hair loss, graying and premature aging.

Green tobacco sickness (GTS) is an occupational illness associated with tobacco farming (Ballard et al. 1995, Mc Knight and Spiller 2005). It is also called *nicotine poisoning* or *Green Monster,* which is caused due to the nicotine that is absorbed into the body through the pores of the skin. When a high amount of nicotine is absorbed into the body due to continuous handling of tobacco leaves, it causes nicotine poisoning.

The symptoms include headache, nausea, vomiting, weakness, abdominal cramps, dizziness, difficulty in breathing (Ballard et al. 1995). In some countries children from poor families are employed in tobacco farming to add to the family income. These children are vulnerable to *green tobacco sickness* (Browning et al. 2003).

Second Hand or Passive Smoking

Second hand smoke is the smoke that fills any closed spaces with many people like hotels and offices when a smoker burns any tobacco product like cigarettes or bidi. It is a mixture of smoke from the burning end of a cigarette, pipe or cigar and the smoke exhaled from the lungs of the smokers. Second hand smoke causes the same effects in the body that a smoker has. It can cause bronchitis, pneumonia, ear infections, viscosity of the blood increases and platelets become sticky causing blood clots leading to heart attacks and thrombosis (Enga et al. 2012, Barua and Ambrose 2013).

LPS and ergosterol present in tobacco smoke contribute to inflammation and airway diseases. It has been found recently that the levels of ergosterol present in the cigarette smoke were significantly higher in rooms with ongoing smoking than in rooms without smoking (Szponar et al. 2012).

Thus the smoker is not only at the risk of disease due to his own smoking but the risk is constantly aggravated when he is constantly exposed to smoke exhaled from other smokers in the vicinity. Children are very vulnerable to second hand smoke because their body defense mechanism is still developing and therefore have the greatest risk of developing damaging health effects.

Smoking and Its Effects on Environment

Cigarette smoking also affects the environment in a variety of ways. The cigarette butts that are thrown on the streets are equally harmful. They contain the same chemicals that cigarette smoke contains. Cigarette butts are toxic and non-bio degradable and take up to twelve years to degrade. That is because filters are made up of cellulose acetate which is a form of plastic and plastics don't decompose easily (Novotony and Zhao 1999). They are washed in to the beaches, rivers and other sources of water supply during rain. The chemicals in these butts get released in to the water and affecting the water quality. This water becomes poisonous to the marine life also to humans when such contaminated water is supplied for drinking purpose. The marine animals ingest these cigarette butts and are killed (County of Fairfax 2008).

The processing of tobacco produces huge amounts of toxic solid liquid and gaseous wastes (Novotony and Zhao 1999). Curing or drying of tobacco leaves requires huge amounts of woods which leads to cutting down of trees and causing deforestation. The packing of tobacco also requires paper which also needs wood and leads to deforestation.

Cigarette smoke produces fine particulate matter which is the most dangerous cause of air pollution and affecting human health (Invernizzi 2004). When a smoker smoke, a large amount of smoke is inhaled which is called the mainstream smoke and a part of this inhaled smoke is exhaled as processed mainstream smoke. A major part of the pollutants are released from the burning end of the cigarette called the side stream smoke. The dangerous particles in the second hand smoke can linger in the air for hours or even longer. This air when inhaled aggravates the problem of bronchitis, asthma and other respiratory problems in individuals.

CONCLUSION

Smoking is thus an extremely hazardous and very costly affair with respect to one's own health and the health of ones close ones and the environment. Not only the smokers themselves but the people in their close vicinity are forced to inhale the smoke from cigarette and have serious health consequences for no fault of theirs. Smoking is extremely addictive habit. So if one thinks that if he or she will smoke a couple of cigarettes just to have fun and to impress their peers and then quit, it is very difficult. Because the addictive properties of cigarette smoke and its pseudo make good feeling and its false relieving effect from stress makes one crave to get back to smoking.

Cigarettes of different brands itself are costly depending upon their additives and nicotine content. In addition to the cost of buying tobacco products, smokers would face additional cost in the form of additional utilization of healthcare services as consequences of smoking. Therefore, it would be better to abstain from smoking and not to get carried away by peer pressure or the illusions of having a stress and anxiety free time during smoking.

REFERENCES

Agrawal, S., Karan, A., Selvaraj, S., Bhan, N., Subramanian, S.V., Millet, C., (2013).Socio economic patterning of tobacco use in Indian states. *Int. J. Tuberc. Lung Dis.* 17(8),1110-1117.

Arnson, Y., Shoenfeld, Y., Amital, H., (2010). Effects of tobacco smoke on immunity, inflammation and autoimmunity. *Journal of Autoimmunity.* 34(3), J258-J265.

Baker, R. R., Pereire da Silva, J. R., Smith, G., (2004).The effect of tobacco ingredients on smoke chemistry and toxicity. Part I: Flavourings and additives. *Food and Chemical Toxicology.* 42,3-37.

Baker, R.R., (2006). Smoke generation inside a burning cigarette: Modifying combustion to develop cigarettes that may be less hazardous to health. *Progress in Energy and Combustion Science.* 32(4), 373-385.

Ballard T., Ehlers J., Fruend E., Auslander M., Brandit V., Halperin W., (1995). Green Tobacco Sickness: Occupational nicotine poisoning in tobacco workers. *Arch. Environ.Health.* 50,384-389.

Barua, R.S., Ambrose, J.A., (2013) Mechanisms of coronary thrombosis in cigarette smoke exposure. *Arteriosclerosis, Thrombosis and Vascular Biology.* 33,1460-1467.

Behan, D.F., Eriksen, M.P., Lin, Y., (2005).Economic Effects of Environmental Tobacco Smoke Report. Schaumburg, IL: Society of Actuaries.1-95. Available athttp://www.soa.org/files/research/projects/ets report final draft(final-3)

Behrman, (2000). *Nelson Textbook of Pediatrics, Sixteenth Edition*, Copyright W.B. Saunders Company.

Browning, S.R., Westneat,S.C., Donnelly, C., Reed, D., (2003). Agricultural tasks and injuries among Kentucky farm children: results of Farm Family Health and Hazard Surveillance Project. *South Med. J.* 96,1203 -1212.

Buczko, G.B., Day, A., Vanderdoelen, J.L., Boucher, R., Zamel, N., (1984). Effects of cigarette smoking and short term smoking cessation on airway responsiveness to inhaled methacholine. *Am. Rev. Respir. Dis.* 129,12-4.

Committee on Drugs, 2000-2001., (2001).The transfer of drugs and other chemicals into human milk. *Pediatrics.* 108(3),776-789.

County of Fairfax, V.A.Don't be a litterbug: You're your butt where it belongs! (2008). Available at http://www.fairfaxcounty.gov/nvswcd/newsletter/buttlitter.htm.

Dagher, A., Bleicher, C., Aston, A.D.J., Gunn, R.N., Clarke, P.B.S., Cumming, P., (2001) Reduced dopamine D1 receptor binding in the ventral striatum of cigarette smokers. *Synapse.* 42(1), 48-53.

Desai, H.D., Seabolt, J., Jann, M. W., (2001).Smoking in patients receiving psychotropic medications. *C.N.S. Drugs.* 15(6),469-494.

Di Franza, Jr., Savageau, J.A., Fletcher, K., O'Loughlin, J., Pbert, L., Ockene, J.K., et al. (2007). Symptoms of tobacco dependence after brief intermittent use: The development and assessment of nicotine dependence in Youth-2 study. *Archives of Pediatrics and Adolescent Medicine.* 161(7),704-710.

DiFranza, J.R., Eddy, J..J, Brown, L.F., Ryan, J.L., Bogojavlensky, A., (1994).Tobacco Acquisition and Cigarette Brand Selection among Youth. *Tobacco Control.* 3,334-338.

Doubeni, C.A., Reed, G., Di Franza, Jr., (2010). Early course of nicotine dependence in adolescent smokers. *Pediatrics*. 125(6),1127-1133.

Eke, B.C., Iscan, M., (2002). Effects of cigarette smoke with different tar contents on hepatic and pulmonary xenobiotic metabolizing enzymes in rats. *Human & Experimental Toxicology*. 21(1),17-23.

Enga, K.F., Braekkan, S.K., Hansen-Kronje, I.J., Cessie, L.E. S., Rosendaal, F.R., Hansen, J.B., (2012). Cigarette smoking and the risk of venous thromboembolism: The Tromso Study. *Journal of Thrombosis and Haemostasis*. 10,2068-2074.

Fant, R.V., Henningfield, J.E., Nelson, R.A., Pickworth, W.B., (1999). Pharmacokinetics and pharmacodynamics of moist snuff in humans. *Tobacco Control*. 8,387-392.

Fitzpatrick, T.M., Blair, E.A., (2000). Smoking and pulmonary and Cardiovascular Disease: Upper Airway Complications of Smoking. *Clinics in Chest Medicine*. 21(1),147-157.

Ford, A., Mackintosh, A. M., Moodie, C., Richardson, S., Hastings, C., (2013). Cigarette pack design and adolescent smoking susceptibility: a cross sectional survey. *B.M.J. open*. 3(9), e003282.

Gamberino, W.C., Gold, M.S., (1999). Neurobiology of Tobacco Smoking & Other Addictive Disorders. *The Psychiatric Clinics of North America*. 22(2),301-312.

Gerrard, J.W., Cockcroft, D.W., Mink, J.T., Cotton, D.J., Poonawala, R., Dosman, J., (1980) Increased non-specific bronchial reactivity in cigarette smokers with normal lung function. *Am. Rev. Respir. Dis.* 122,577-581.

Greer, R.O., Poulson, T.C., Boone, M. E., Lindemuth, J.E., Crosby, L., (1986). Smokeless tobacco associated oral changes in juvenile, adult and geriatric patients. Clinical and histomorphologic features. *Geriodontics*. 2,87-98.

Hawkins, R. I., (1972). Smoking, platelets and thrombosis. *Nature*. 236(5348), 450-452.

Hoffman, B.R., Sussman, S., Unger, J.B., Valente, T., (2006).Peer influences on adolescent cigarette smoking: A theoretical review of literature. *Substance Use and Misuse*. 41(1),103-155.

Hogan, M. J., (2000). Adolescent Medicine: Diagnosis & Treatment of Teen Drug Use. *The Medical Clinics of North America*. 84(4), 927-966.

International Agency for Research on Cancer *IARC (2004). Monographs on the Evaluation of the Carcinogenic Risks to Humans: Tobacco Smoke and Involuntary Smoking*. Vol. 83. Lyon (France): International Agency for Research on Cancer.

International Agency for Research on Cancer. *IARC (1983). Monographs on the Evaluation of Carcinogenic Risks of Chemicals to Humans: Polynuclear Aromatic Compounds, Part 1: Chemical, Environmental and Experimental Data*. Vol. 32. Lyon (France): International Agency for Research on Cancer.

Invernizzi, G., (2004). Paticulate matter from tobacco versus diesel car exhaust: an educational perspective. *Tobacco Control*. 13, 219-221.

Jin, Z., Xin, M., Deng, X., (2005). Survival function of protein kinase $C\iota$ as a novel nitrosamine 4-(methylnitrosamino)-1-(3-pyridyl)-1-butanone-activated Bad kinase. *Journal of Biological Chemistry*. 280(16),16045–16052.

Kamboj, M., (2008). Bidi Tobacco. *British Dental Journal*. 205(12), 639.

Kampangsri, W., Vatanasapt, P., Kamsa-Ard, S., Suwanrungruang, K., Promthet, S., (2013).Betel quid chewing and user aero- digestive tract cancers : a prospective cohort study in khonkaen, Thailand. *Asian Pac. J. Cancer*. 14(7),4335-4338.

Koh, J.S., Kang, H., Choi, S.W., Kim, H.O., (2002).Cigarette smoking associated with premature facial wrinkling: image analysis of facial skin replicas. *Int. J. Dermatol.* 41(1), 21-27.

Larsson, M.L., Frisk, M., Hallstrom, J., Kiviloog, J., Lundback, B., (2001). Environmental Tobacco Smoke Exposure During Childhood is Associated With Increased Prevalence of Asthma in Adult. *Chest.* 120(3),711-717.

Lee, P.N., (2001). Lung Cancer and type of cigarette smoked. *Inhal. Toxicol.* 13(11), 951-76.

Leventhal, A.M., Ameringer, K.J., Osborn, E., Zvolensky, M.J., Langdon, K.J., (2013). Anxiety and depressive symptoms and affective patterns of tobacco withdrawal. *Drug Alcohol Depend.* doi:pii: S0376-8716(13)00234-2.

Madsen, H., Dyerberg, J., (1984). Cigarrete smoking and its effects on platelet vessel wall interaction. *Scand. J. Clin. Lab. Invest.* 44,203-206.

Maher, R., Lee, A.T., Warnakulasurfa, K.A., Lewis, J.A., Johnson, N.W., (1994). Role of areca nut in causation of oral submucous fibrosis: A case control study in Pakistan. *J. Oral Pathol. Med.* 23,65-69.

Mai, H., May, W.S., Gao, F., Jin, Z., Deng, X., (2003). A functional role for nicotine in Bcl2 phosphorylation and suppression of apoptosis. *Journal of Biological Chemistry.* 278(3),1886–1891.

Malo, J.L., Filiatrault, S., Martin, R.R., (1982). Bronchial responsiveness to inhaled methacholine in young asymptomatic smokers. *J. Appl. Physiol.* 52,1464-1470.

Mc Knight, R.H., Spiller, H.A., (2005). Green tobacco sickness in children and adolescents. *Public Health Rep.* 120(6), 602-606.

Mehta, P., Mehta, J., (1982). Effects of smoking on platelets and on plasma thromboxane-prostacyclin balance in man. *Prostaglandines, Leukotrienes and Medicine.* 9,141-150.

Model, D., (1985). Smoker's face: an underrated clinical sign? *Br. Med. J.* (Clin. Res. Ed.). 291,1760-1762.

Modesto-Lowe, V., Chmielewska, A., (2013). Coping with urges to smoke: What is a Clinician to do? *Conn. Med.* 77(5), 289-294.

Nair, S., Ghosh, K., (2013). The myriad effects of cigarette smoke. *Journal of Thrombosis and Haemostasis.*11,1-2.

Nair, S., Kulkarni, S.,Camoens, H.M.T., Ghosh, K., Mohanty, D., (2001).Changes in platelet glycoprotein receptors after smoking – a flow cytometric study. *Platelets.*12,20-26.

Noakes, P. S., Holt, P. G., Prescott, S.L.,(2003). Maternal smoking in pregnancy alters neonatal cytokine responses. *Allergy.* 58,1053-1058.

Nonovotony, T.E., Zhao, F., (1999). Consumption and production waste: another externality of tobacco use. *Tobacco Control.* 8,75-80.

Oster, G., Colditz, G. A., Kelly, N.L., (1984). The economic costs of smoking and benefits of quitting for individual smokers. *Prev. Med.* 13(4), 377-389.

Patil, P.B., Bathi, R.,Chaudhari, S., (2013).Prevalence of oral mucosal lesions in dental patients with tobacco smoking, chewing and mixed habits: A cross sectional study in South India. *J. Family Community Medicine.* 20(2),130-135.

Peto, R., Lopez, A.D., Borcham, J., Thun, M., Heath, C. Jr., (1992). Mortality from tobacco in developed countries: Indirect estimation from National and Vital Statistics. *Lancet.* 339,1268-1278.

Reddy, S.S., Shaik Hyder Ali, K.H., (2008). Estimation of nicotine content in popular Indian brands of smoking and chewing tobacco products. *Indian J. Dent. Res.*19(2), 88-91.

Reed, J.C., (2000) Mechanisms of apoptosis. *American Journal of Pathology.* 157(5),1415–1430.

Rich, T., Allen, R.L., Wyllie, A.H., (2000). Defying death after DNA damage. *Nature.* 407(6805), 777–783.

Rodgman, A., Perfetti, T.A.(2009). *The Chemical Components of Tobacco and Tobacco Smoke.* Boca Raton (FL): CRC Press, Taylor & Francis Group.

Sawyer, D.R., Wood, N.K., (1992). Oral Cancer: Etiology recognition and management. *Dent. Clin. North. Am.* 30, 919-944.

Shah, N., Sharma, P.P., (1998). Role of chewing and smoking habits in the etiology of oral submucous fibrosis: A case control study. *J. Oral Pathol. Med.* 27, 475-479.

Sopori, M., (2002). Effects of cigarette smoke on the immune system. *Nature Reviews Immunology.* 2(5),372–377.

Sutherland, M.T., Ross, T.J., Shakleya, D.M., Huestis, M.A., Stein, E.A., (2011).Chronic smoking, but not acute nicotine administration, modulates neural correlates of working memory. *Psychopharmacology (Berl.).* 213(1), 29-42.

Szponar, B., Pehrson, C., Larsson, L., (2012). Bacterial and fungal markers in tobacco smoke. *Sci. Total Environ.*438, 447-451.

Taylor R.G., Joyce H., Gross, E., Holland, F., Pride, N.B., (1985). Bronchial reactivity to inhaled histamine and annual rate of decline in FEV in male smokers and ex-smokers. *Thorax.*40, 9-16.

Trueb, R.M., (2003). Association between smoking and hair loss: another opportunity for health education against smoking? *Dermatology.* 206(3),189-191.

U.S. Department of Health and Human Services, (2010). How Tobacco smoke causes disease: the biology and behavioral basis for smoking attributable disease: A report of the Surgeon General, Atlanta G.A., Centers for Disease Control and Prevention, National Center for Chronic Disease Prevention and Health Promotion, Office on Smoking and Health, Available at http://www.surgeongeneral.gov/library

U.S. Department of Health and Human Services. (1979) *Smoking and Health: A Report of the Surgeon General.* Washington: U.S. Department of Health, Education, and Welfare, Public Health Service, Office of the Assistant Secretary for Health, Office on Smoking and Health. DHEW Publication No. (PHS) 79-50066.

Wilbert, S. and Aronow, M.D., (1974). Tobacco and Heart. *J.A.M.A.* 229(13),1799-1800.

Winn, D.M., Blot, W.J., Shy, C.M., Pickle, L.W., Toledo, A., Fraumeni J.F. Jr., (1981). Snuff dipping and oral cancer among women in the Southern United states. *N. Engl. J. Med.* 304,745-749.

Xu, J., Mendrek, A., Cohen, M.S., Monterosso, J., Simon, S., Body, A.L., Jarvik, M., Rodriguez, P., Ernst, M., London, E.D., (2006). Effects of acute smoking on brain activity vary with abstinence in smokers performing the N-Back task: a preliminary study. *Psychiatry Res.* 148 (2-3),103-109.

Young, Jr. R.C., Rachal, R.E., Hackney, Jr. R.L., Uy, C.G., Scott, R.B., (1992). Smoking is a factor in Causing Acute Chest Syndrome in Sickle Cell Anemia. *Journal of the National Medical Association.* 84(3), 267-271.

In: Smoking Restrictions
Editor: Nazmi Sari

ISBN: 978-1-63321-148-3
© 2014 Nova Science Publishers, Inc.

Chapter 10

ASSESSMENT OF CIGARETTE SMOKING TOXICITY USING CANCER STEM CELLS

Kanda Yasunari[*]
*Division of Pharmacology, National Institute of Health Sciences,
Setagaya, Japan*

ABSTRACT

Growing evidence suggests that cigarette smoking is associated with the development and promotion of various human cancers. Cigarette smoke is well known to contain thousands of molecules, including carcinogens. Although nicotine, the main addictive component, is not carcinogenic, nicotine is able to induce proliferation, migration, and angiogenesis of various cancer cells. Moreover, nicotine was recently shown to expand cancer stem cells via its nicotinic acetylcholine receptor. This review summarizes the novel role of nicotine in cancer stem cells. The findings provide new insights into the assessment of cigarette smoking toxicity.

INTRODUCTION

The World Health Organization (WHO) estimates over 5 million premature deaths are attributable to cigarette smoking annually worldwide (WHO 2008a). Around half of all regular smokers will die from smoking in middle age (Peto 1994). Cigarette smoke contains over 4,000 different chemicals, many of which are toxic and carcinogenic in a variety of cells and related to increased risks of various cancers (Hoffmann et al. 2001). However, limited experimental data support direct links between cigarette smoking and cancer.

Growing evidence suggests that tumors are organized in a hierarchy of heterogeneous cell populations and initiated from a small population of stem/stem-like cells called cancer stem cells (CSCs) or tumor-initiating cells (Visvader et al. 2008). CSCs exhibit self-renewal, drug

---

[*] Address: 1-18-1, Kamiyoga, Setagaya 158-8501, Japan. Phone: +81-3-3700-9704, Fax: +81-3-3700-9704, E-mail: kanda@nihs.go.jp

resistance, and high tumorigenicity. Only genetic mutation–induced CSCs can form tumors. There are several protocols for isolating and characterizing CSCs from diverse tumors and established cell lines. Aldehyde dehydrogenase (ALDH), a detoxifying enzyme responsible for the oxidation of intracellular aldehydes, is a functional marker of CSCs; its expression is correlated with poor prognosis, increased metastasis, and chemotherapy resistance in patients (Ginestier et al. 2007, Jiang et al. 2009, van den Hoogen et al. 2010). However, the effect of cigarette smoking on CSCs has not been fully understood.

Nicotine, a major component of cigarette smoke, contributes to the growth, progression, and metastasis of a variety of cancers (Egleton et al. 2008). Recent studies suggest that nicotine has the ability to induce the CSC phenotype in several types of cancer (Hirata et al. 2010, Yu et al. 2012). Furthermore, the CSC phenotype is mediated by crosstalk between nicotine and the stem cell pathway. Thus, the nicotine-mediated CSC phenotype may be involved in the progression of cancer.

This review highlights CSCs in cigarette smoking research. The findings may provide important insights into carcinogenesis caused by cigarette smoking.

CIGARETTE SMOKING IS A MAJOR RISK FACTOR FOR MANY TYPES OF CANCER

Cigarette smoking is well established as a major risk factor associated with the development and progression of various cancers (Burns 2003, Vineis et al 2004). There is sufficient evidence for a causal association between cigarette smoking and various cancers, such as cancers of the upper digestive tract, oral cavity, pharynx, esophagus, stomach, liver, pancreas, lungs, and kidneys (Gandini et al.2008). However, evidence linking smoking to breast cancer is insufficient. Several epidemiological studies suggest there is no overall association between active smoking and breast cancer risk (Palmer et al. 1993, Terry et al. 2002). In contrast, recent cohort studies suggest an increased risk of breast cancer for women who start smoking at a young age (Al-Delaimy et al. 2004). It has been proposed that the breasts should be added to the list of target organs of tobacco-related carcinogenicity (Collishaw et al. 2009).

As mentioned above, cigarette smoke contains over 4,000 chemicals, many of which are toxic and carcinogenic in a variety of cells (Hoffmann et al. 2001). For example, nicotine, a major component in cigarette smoke, can induce cancer cell proliferation (Shin et al. 2004, Ye et al. 2004). Polycyclic aromatic hydrocarbons and nicotine-derived nitrosamines have been identified as the major and potent carcinogens in lung cancer (Hecht 1999, Hecht 2002). Although cigarette smoking has been studied extensively, limited experimental data support the direct link between cigarette smoking and cancer.

CSC CONCEPT

Growing evidence suggests that many types of cancer are initiated from a small population of CSCs (Visvader et al. 2008). The CSC concept was first proposed in the mid-1990s (i.e. Lapidot et al. 1994). In their study, Lapidot et al. found that the most subtypes of acute myeloid leukemia could be engrafted in immunodeficient mice; however, engraftment could be initiated from only $CD34^+CD38^-$ fractions. Moreover, this xenotransplantation assay revealed that the frequency of CSCs was in the order of 1 per 1,000,000 tumor cells (Bonnet et al. 1997). Therefore, very rare populations are believed to have the ability to self-renew and produce heterogeneous tumors.

Flow cytometry and xenotransplantation have revealed CSCs in solid tumors in organs such as brain, breast, colon, pancreas, prostate, and ovaries (Al-Hajj et al. 2003, Singh et al. 2004, Collins et al. 2005, Ponti et al. 2005, Dalerba et al. 2007, Curley et al. 2009). Due to technical difficulties in the purification of rare CSCs, current methods aim to enrich CSCs; these methods include the sphere formation, surface marker, side population, and ALDEFLUOR assay (see Figure 1). CSCs in established cancer cell lines are considered good in vitro models. These CSCs can be easily prepared by the protocols as shown in Figure 1.

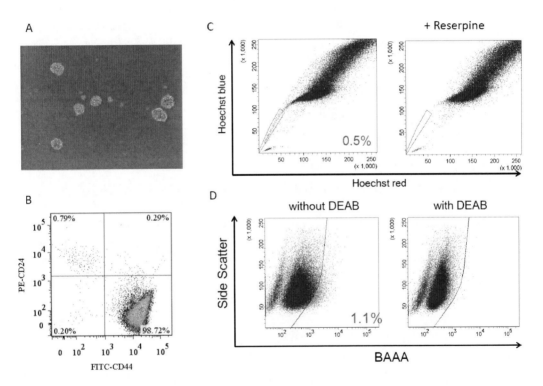

Figure 1. Isolation of CSCs from various tumors and cell lines. Current methods for enriching CSCs. Cancer cell line has some CSC population that is identified by (A) Sphere formation, (B) surface marker, (C) side population, (D) and ALDEFLUOR assays.

The sphere culture technique was originally developed to isolate neural stem cells (Reynolds et al. 1992). Neural stem cells can be expanded in serum-free DMEM/F12 media supplemented with N_2 supplement and 20 ng/mL basic fibroblast growth factor using non-adherent dishes. The non-adherent culture conditions are then applied to enrich CSCs in solid tumor (Dontu et al. 2003). To date, many types of cancer cells have been found to be capable of forming spheres.

CSCs have been isolated by various cell surface markers from many types of cancers. For example, $CD34^+CD38^-$ cell population has been identified as a cell surface marker of leukemic CSCs (Bonnet et al. 1997). Meanwhile, CD44⁺CD24⁻ cell population has been identified as a marker of breast CSCs (Al-Haji et al. 2003). CD133 has been used to enrich CSCs from colon, prostate, and pancreas (Richardson et al. 2004, Hermann et al. 2007, O'Brien et al. 2007). Thus, the choice of markers is dependent on tissues.

The side population and ALDEFLUOR assays were developed as direct functional markers of CSCs. These methods overcome the barrier of diverse surface markers, replacing them with more direct functional markers. The side population assay is based on the efficient and specific efflux of the fluorescent DNA-binding dye, Hoechst 33342, by an ATP-binding cassette transporter (Goodell et al. 1996). The ALDEFLUOR assay is based on the finding that human hematopoietic stem cells have increased ALDH activity, which oxidizes intracellular aldehydes and results in the oxidation of retinol to retinoic acid (Hess et al. 2004).

Although increasing evidence supports the CSC concept, it is still unclear how CSCs are generated in cancer. It is speculated that CSCs are generated by malignant transformation including genetic and epigenetic mutations in normal stem cells (Visvader et al. 2008). It should be determined whether the malignant transformation occurs only in CSCs. In addition, recent studies suggest conversion between CSCs and non-CSCs (Chaffer et al. 2011, Gupta et al, 2011). The authors of these studies demonstrate the possibility that the dedifferentiation of transformed malignant cells results in CSC generation. This plasticity may account for the current inconsistencies observed in the CSC model.

NOVEL ROLE OF NICOTINE IN CSC REGULATION

As mentioned above, the CSC concept is very attractive for understanding the complex tumorigenicity process. Cigarette smoking might affect CSCs, which develop tumors in various tissues including the breasts. It is well known that nicotine, which is the active component of cigarette smoke, elicits many responses, such as proliferation, migration, and angiogenesis in various cancer cells (see Figure 2).

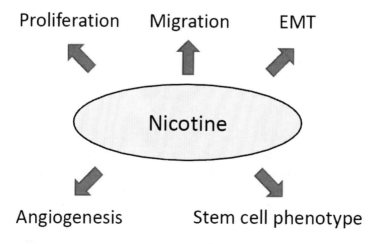

Figure 2. Various nicotine-mediated responses in cancer. Nicotine induces multiple responses, such as proliferation, migration, and angiogenesis in many typos of cancer.

For example, nicotine stimulates the proliferation of various cancer cells such as gastric tumor cells and colon cancer cells (Shin et al. 2004, Ye et al. 2004). Moreover, nicotine stimulates invasion and epithelial–mesenchymal transition (EMT), which is a process associated with the enhancement of tumor cell migration and metastasis, in a variety of human cancer cell lines such as MCF-7 and A549 (Dasgupta et al. 2009). Furthermore, nicotine can produce vascular endothelial growth factor, a major contributor to angiogenesis, thus inducing abnormal vessel formation (Heeschen et al. 2002, Cooke et al. 2004, Kanda et al. 2007).

We recently found that nicotine, whose concentrations are comparable to that reported in the plasma of cigarette smokers, increases ALDEFLUOR-positive breast CSCs (Hirata et al. 2010). Consistent with these data, nicotine is capable of increasing the CSC phenotype in the head and neck squamous cell carcinoma cell lines UMSCC-10B and HN-1 (Yu et al. 2012). These results suggest that nicotine plays a critical role in the development of cigarette smoking–induced cancers by regulating the CSC phenotype.

The neuronal nicotinic acetylcholine receptor (nAChR) signaling pathway plays a critical role in cancer (Egleton et al. 2008). nAChRs possesses ligand-gated ion channels and are composed of a heteropentamer or homopentamer of 5 subunits enclosing a central ion channel. Although the physiological ligand of nAChR is acetylcholine, cigarette smoke components such as nicotine and 4-(methylnitrosamino)-1-(3-pyridyl)-1-butanone (NNK) are known to be agonists of nAChRs (Lindstrom et al. 1996). The nAChR that contains α7 subunits (α7-nAChR), which possesses the distinctive feature of being homomeric, has been found to induce the breast CSC phenotype. CSC maintenance and proliferation are reported to be correlated with EMT (Mani et al. 2008). Furthermore, EMT is mediated via α7-nAChR in A549 lung cancer cells (Dasgupta et al. 2009). Therefore, it would be also of great interest to consider the effects of α7-nAChR on CSC populations in other tumor types. A finding suggesting α7-nAChR is involved in CSC maintenance would pave the route to elucidation of the effects of nicotine on tumor progression.

As several lines of evidence suggest a direct link between nicotine and CSCs, attempts have been made to elucidate the molecular mechanisms by which nicotine induces CSC proliferation. As CSCs are considered to have molecular similarities to embryonic and normal adult stem cells, their self-renewal behavior is reported to be mediated by several signaling pathways (Takebe et al. 2010). Signaling pathways, such as Notch, Wnt and Hedgehog, play a role in the self-renewal and differentiation of normal stem cells. Alterations in genes that encode signaling molecules belonging to these pathways have been found in human tumor samples (Lobo et al. 2007, Sánchez-García et al. 2007), suggesting that they are involved in CSC regulation. Notably, Notch signaling has been identified to mediate nicotine-induced breast CSCs (Hirata et al. 2010). As shown in Figure 3, nicotine has been shown to induce the Notch activation in breast cancer. Nicotine induces the expression of the Notch target gene *Hes1* and the nicotine-induced increase in ALDEFLUOR-positive CSCs is blocked by DAPT, which prevents Notch signaling by inhibiting cleavage of the activated Notch receptor by γ-secretase. Another study suggests stimulation with nicotine leads to the induction of stem cell markers such as Oct-4, Nanog, and CD44 (Yu et al. 2012). Thus, it has become clear that nicotine affects stem cell function. However, the mechanisms underlying the nicotine-mediated stem cell pathway activation remain to be determined.

ROLES OF OTHER COMPONENTS OF CIGARETTE SMOKE IN CSCS

Cigarette smoke components promote carcinogenesis via a multistep process that involves exposure to and the activation of carcinogens. A recent study has shown that the airway basal cells in smokers' lungs gain human embryonic stem cell (hESC) genes, suggesting a relationship between cigarette smoke and lung CSCs (Shaykhiev et al 2013). This study suggests that the acquirement of the stem cell phenotype by smoking might develop tumors in human. As hESC-related genes are overexpressed in breast cancer and associated with poor prognosis (Ben-Porath et al 2008), it is possible that elements of the reprogramming are acquired by healthy adult tissues chronically exposed to carcinogens in cigarette smoke.

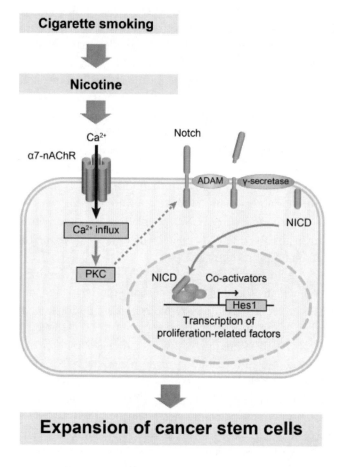

Figure 3. Crosstalk between α7-nAChR and Notch signaling. Nicotine binds to α7-nAChR and activates the Notch signaling pathway via intracellular Ca^{2+} influx and protein kinase C (PKC). Notch is then cleaved by ADAM and γ-secretase to release the Notch intracellular domain (NICD). NICD translocates to the nucleus and activates the transcription of genes such as *Hes1*, thereby promoting stem cell proliferation and self-renewal.

Cigarette smoke is a complex mixture of chemicals. Cigarette smoke extract is widely used to mimic cigarette smoking (Nakamura et al 1995, Nishio et al 1998). It has been shown to promote the expansion of CSC-like side population (An et al 2012). Among the multiple components of cigarette smoke, nitrosamines such as NNK and polyaromatic hydrocarbons (PAHs) such as benzo[α]pyrene are known to lead to the formation of DNA adducts. These chemicals are believed to be major factors in smoking-induced carcinomas (Hecht 1999). As CSCs are possibly modulated by genetic changes, these DNA adducts might regulate the CSC phenotype in cancer.

The WHO Study Group on Tobacco Product Regulation published an expert advice paper on smoke component regulation (WHO 2008b). Based on Hoffmann et al. (2001), a comprehensive list of priority toxicants was proposed. In addition to nitrosamines and PAHs, the list includes carbonyl compounds (e.g., acetaldehyde, acrolein, and formaldehyde), formaldehyde, benzene, 1,3-butadiene, and carbon monoxide. Future studies should be performed to determine which components promote CSC proliferation in various cancers.

The risk of cigarette smoking-related diseases appears to be dependent on dose (Hatsukami et al. 2007). Reducing the concentrations of important toxicants is expected to lower the risks related to tobacco smoking. In addition, reduced toxicant prototype cigarettes with substantially reduced levels of cigarette smoke toxicants have recently been developed (Shepperd et al. 2013). As evaluating tobacco-related diseases is time consuming and needs a lot of cost, the CSC concept might elucidate the most important toxicants in cigarette smoke and contribute to the development of reduced toxicant prototype cigarettes.

CONCLUSION

Growing evidence suggests that CSCs play a critical role in cancer development. CSCs in established cancer cell lines are easily isolated by the protocols and are good in vitro models. Although the contribution of CSCs to cancer development still remains unclear, it is an attractive notion that the CSC model is used for evaluation of the risk of cigarette smoke in cancer. Notably, nicotine has an ability to mediate the CSC phenotype by utilizing the stem cell pathway. Since cigarette smoke is a complex mixture of chemicals, other component might promote CSC proliferation in various cancers. In the future, it is expected to identify specific components in cigarette smoke involved in tumorigenesis via "stemness" in many types of cancer.

CONFLICT OF INTEREST

The authors declare that there are no cwasonflicts of interest.

ACKNOWLEDGMENTS

This work was supported by the Advanced research for medical products Mining Programme of the National Institute of Biomedical Innovation (NIBIO, #09-02), a Grant-in-Aid for Scientific Research from the Ministry of Education, Culture, Sports, Science, and

Technology, Japan (#26670041), a Health and Labour Sciences Research Grant from the Ministry of Health, Labour and Welfare, Japan.

REFERENCES

Al-Delaimy, W.K., Cho, E., Chen, W.Y., Colditz, G., Willet, W.C., (2004). A prospective study of smoking and risk of breast cancer in young adult women. *Cancer. Epidemiol. Biomarkers. Prev.* 13, 398-404.

Al-Hajj, M., Wicha, M.S., Benito-Hernandez, A., Morrison, S.J, Clarke, M.F., (2003). Prospective identification of tumorigenic breast cancer cells. *Proc. Natl. Acad. Sci .USA.* 100, 3983-3988.

An, Y., Kiang, A., Lopez, J.P., Kuo, S.Z., Yu, M.A., Abhold, E.L., Chen, J.S., Wang-Rodriguez, J., Ongkeko, W.M., (2012). Cigarette smoke promotes drug resistance and expansion of cancer stem cell-like side population. *PLoS ONE.* 7, e47919.

Ben-Porath, I., Thomson, M.W., Carey, V.J., Ge, R., Bell, G.W., Regev, A., Weinberg R.A., (2008). An embryonic stem cell-like gene expression signature in poorly differentiated aggressive human tumors. *Nat. Genet.* 40, 499-507.

Bonnet, D., Dick, J.E., (1997). Human acute myeloid leukemia is organized as a hierarchy that originates from a primitive hematopoietic cell. *Nat. Med.* 3, 730-737.

Burns, D.M. (2003). Tobacco-related diseases. *Seminars in Oncology Nursing.* 19, 244–249.

Chaffer, C.L., Brueckmann, I., Scheel, C., Kaestli, A.J., Wiggins, P.A., Rodrigues, L.O., Brooks, M., Reinhardt, F., Su, Y., Polyak, K., Arendt, L.M., Kuperwasser, C., Bierie, B., Weinberg R.A., (2011). Normal and neoplastic nonstem cells can spontaneously convert to a stem-like state. *Proc. Nat. Acad. Sci. USA*. 108, 7950-7955.

Cooke, J.P., Bitterman, H., (2004). Nicotine and angiogenesis: a new paradigm for tobacco-related diseases. *Ann. Med.* 36, 33-40.

Collins, A.T., Berry, P.A., Hyde, C., Stower, M.J., Maitland, N.J., (2005). Prospective identification of tumorigenic prostate cancer stem cells. *Cancer. Res.* 65, 10946-10951.

Collishaw, N.E., Boyd, N.F., Cantor, K.P., Hammond, S.K., Johnson, K.C., Millar, J., Miller, A.B., Miller, M., Palmer, J.R., Salmon, A.G., Turcotte, F.(2009). Canadian Expert Panel on Tobacco Smoke and Breast Cancer Risk., Available at http://otru.org/wp-content/uploads/2012/06/Expert-Panel-Executive-Summary-EN.pdf

Curley, M.D., Therrien, V.A., Cummings, C.L., Sergent, P.A., Koulouris, C.R., Friel, A.M., Roberts, D.J., Seiden, M.V., Scadden, D.T., Rueda, B.R., Foster, R., (2009). Cd133 expression defines a tumor initiating cell population in primary human ovarian cancer. *Stem. Cells.* 27, 2875-2883.

Dalerba, P., Dylla, S.J., Park, I.K., Liu, R., Wang, X., Cho, R.W., Hoey, T., Gurney, A., Huang, E.H., Simeone, D.M., Ricci-Vitiani, L., Lombardi, D.G., Pilozzi, E., Biffoni, M., Todaro, M., Peschle, C. and De Maria, R., (2007). Identification and expansion of human colon-cancer-initiating cells. *Nature* 445, 111-115.

Dasgupta, P., Rizwani, W., Pillai, S., Kinkade, R., Kovacs, M., Rastogi, S., Banerjee, S., Carless, M., Kim, E., Coppola, D., Haura, E., Chellappan, S., (2009). Nicotine induces cell proliferation, invasion and epithelial-mesenchymal transition in a variety of human cancer cell lines. *Int. J. Cancer.* 124, 36-45.

Dontu, G., Abdallah, W.M., Foley, J.M., Jackson, K.W., Clarke, M.F., Kawamura, M.J., Wicha, M.S., (2003). In vitro propagation and transcriptional profiling of human mammary stem/progenitor cells. *Genes. Dev.* 17, 1253-1270.

Egleton, R.D., Brown, K.C., Dasgupta P., (2008). Nicotinic acetylcholine receptors in cancer: multiple roles in proliferation and inhibition of apoptosis. *Trends. Pharmacol. Sci.* 29, 151-158.

Gandini, S., Botteri, E., Iodice, S., Boniol, M., Lowenfels, A.B., Maisonneuve, P., Boyle, P., (2008). Tobacco smoking and cancer: a meta-analysis. *Int. J. Cancer.* 122, 155-164.

Ginestier, C., Hur, M.H., Charafe-Jauffret, E., Monville, F., Dutcher, J., Brown, M., Jacquemier, J., Viens, P., Kleer, C.G., Liu, S., Schott, A., Hayes, D., Birnbaum, D., Wicha, M.S., Dontu, G., (2007). ALDH1 is a marker of normal and malignant human mammary stem cells and a predictor of poor clinical outcome. *Cell. Stem. Cell.* 1, 555–567.

Goodell M.A., Brose, K., Paradis, G., Conner, A.S., Mulligan, R.C., (1996). Isolation and functional properties of murine hematopoietic stem cells that are replicating in vivo. *J. Exp. Med.* 183, 1797-1806.

Gupta, P.B., Fillmore, C.M., Jiang, G., Shapira, S.D., Tao, K., Kuperwasser, C., Lander, E.S., (2011). Stochastic state transitions give rise to phenotypic equilibrium in populations of cancer cells. *Cell.* 146, 633-644.

Hatsukami, D.K., Joseph, A.M., Lesage, M., Jensen, J., Murphy, S.E., Pentel, P.R., Kotlyar, M., Borgida, E., Le, C., Hecht, S.S., (2007). Developing the science base for reducing tobacco harm. *Nicotine. Tob. Res.* 9, S537-53.

Heeschen, C., Weis, M., Aicher, A., Dimmeler, S., Cooke, J.P., (2002). A novel angiogenic pathway mediated by non-neuronal nicotinic acetylcholine receptors. *J. Clin. Invest.* 110, 527-536.

Hermann, P.C., Huber, S.L., Herrler, T., Aicher, A., Ellwart, J.W., Guba, M., Bruns, C.J., Heeschen, C., (2007). Distinct populations of cancer stem cells determine tumor growth and metastatic activity in human pancreatic cancer. *Cell. Stem. Cell.* 1, 313-323.

Hecht, S.S., (1999). Tobacco smoke carcinogens and lung cancer. *J. Natl. Cancer. Inst.* 91, 1194-1210.

Hecht, S.S., (2002). Cigarette smoking and lung cancer: chemical mechanisms and approaches to prevention. *Lancet. Oncol.* 3, 461-469.

Hess, D.A., Meyerrose, T.E., Wirthlin, L., Craft, T.P., Herrbrich, P.E., Creer, M.H., Nolta, J.A., (2004). Functional characterization of highly purified human hematopoietic repopulating cells isolated according to aldehyde dehydrogenase activity. *Blood.* 104, 1648-1655.

Hirata, N; Sekino, Y; Kanda, Y., (2010). Nicotine increases cancer stem cell population in MCF-7 cells. *Biochem. Biophys. Res. Commun.* 403, 138–143.

Hoffmann, D., Hoffmann, I., El-Bayoumy, K., (2001). The less harmful cigarette: a controversial issue. a tribute to Ernst L. *Wynder. Chem. Res. Toxicol.* 14, 767–790.

van den Hoogen, C., van der Horst, G., Cheung, H., Buijs, J.T., Lippitt, J.M., Guzmán-Ramírez, N., Hamdy, F.C., Eaton, C.L., Thalmann, G.N., Cecchini, M.G., Pelger, R.C., van der Pluijm, G., (2010). High aldehyde dehydrogenase activity identifies tumor-initiating and metastasis-initiating cells in human prostate cancer. *Cancer. Res.* 70, 5163–5173.

Jiang, F., Qiu, Q., Khanna, A., Todd, N.W., Deepak, J., Xing, L., Wang, H., Liu, Z., Su, Y., Stass, S.A., Katz, R.L., (2009). Aldehyde dehydrogenase 1 is a tumor stem cell-associated marker in lung cancer. *Mol. Cancer Res.* 7, 330–338.

Kanda, Y., Watanabe Y., (2007). Nicotine-induced vascular endothelial growth factor release via the EGFR-ERK pathway in rat vascular smooth muscle cells. *Life Sci.* 80, 1409 - 1414.

Lapidot, T., Sirard, C., Vormoor, J., Murdoch, B., Hoang, T., Caceres-Cortes, J., Minden, M., Paterson, B., Caligiuri, M.A., Dick, J.E., (1994). A cell initiating human acute myeloid leukaemia after transplantation into SCID mice. *Nature.* 367, 645-648.

Lindstrom, J., Anand, R., Gerzanich, V., Peng, X., Wang, F., Wells G., (1996). Structure and function of neuronal nicotinic acetylcholine receptors. *Prog. Brain. Res.* 109, 125-137.

Lobo N.A., Shimono Y., Qian D., Clarke M.F. (2007). The biology of cancer stem cells. *Annu. Rev. Cell. Dev. Biol.* 23, 675-699.

Mani, SA; Guo, W; Liao, MJ; Eaton, EN; Ayyanan, A; Zhou, AY; Brooks, M; Reinhard, F; Zhang, CC; Shipitsin, M; Campbell, LL; Polyak, K; Brisken, C; Yang, J; Weinberg RA. The epithelial-mesenchymal transition generates cells with properties of stem cells. *Cell* 2008;133:704-15.

Nakamura, Y., Romberger, D.J., Tate, L., Ertl, R.F., Kawamoto, M., Adachi, Y., Mio, T., Sisson, J.H., Spurzem, J.R., Rennard, S.I., (1995). Cigarette smoke inhibits lung fibroblast proliferation and chemotaxis. *Am. J. Respir. Crit. Care. Med.* 151, 1497-1503

Nishio, E., Watanabe, Y., (1998). Cigarette smoke extract is a modulator of mitogenic action in vascular smooth muscle cells. *Life. Sci.* 62, 1339-1347.

O'Brien, C.A., Pollett, A., Gallinger, S., Dick, J.E., (2007). A human colon cancer cell capable of initiating tumour growth in immunodeficient mice. *Nature.* 445, 106-110.

Palmer, J.R., Rosenberg, L., (1993). Cigarette smoking and the risk of breast cancer. *Epidemiol. Rev.* 15, 145-156.

Peto, R., (1994). Smoking and death: the past 40 years and the next 40. *BMJ.* 309, 937-939.

Ponti, D., Costa, A., Zaffaroni, N., Pratesi, G., Petrangolini, G., Coradini, D., Pilotti, S., Pierotti, M.A., Daidone M.G., (2005). Isolation and in vitro propagation of tumorigenic breast cancer cells with stem/progenitor cell properties. *Cancer. Res.* 65, 5506-5511.

Reynolds, B.A., Weiss, S., (1992). Generation of neurons and astrocytes from isolated cells of the adult mammalian central nervous system. *Science.* 255, 1707-1710.

Richardson, G.D., Robson, C.N., Lang, S.H., Neal, D.E., Maitland, N.J., Collins, A.T., (2004). CD133, a novel marker for human prostatic epithelial stem cells. *J. Cell. Sci.* 117, 3539-3545.

Sánchez-García I., Vicente-Dueñas C. and Cobaleda C. (2007). The theoretical basis of cancer-stem-cell based therapeutics of cancer: can it be put into practice? *Bioessays.* 29, 1269-1280.

Shaykhiev, R., Wang, R., Zwick, R.K., Hackett, N.R., Leung, R., Moore, M.A., Sima, C.S., Chao, I., Downey, R.J., Strulovici-Barel, Y., Salit, J., Crystal R.G., (2013). Airway basal cells of healthy smokers express an embryonic stem cell signature relevant to lung cancer stem cells. *Stem. Cells.* 31, 1992–2002.

Shepperd, C.J., Eldridge, A., Camacho, O.M., McAdam, K., Proctor, C.J., Meyer, I., (2013). Changes in levels of biomarkers of exposure observed in a controlled study of smokers switched from conventional to reduced toxicant prototype cigarettes. *Regul. Toxicol. Pharmacol.* 66, 147-62.

Shin, V.Y., Wu, W.K., Ye, Y.N., So, W.H., Koo, M.W., Liu, E.S., Luo, J.C., Cho, C.H., (2004). Nicotine promotes gastric tumor growth and neovascularization by activating extracellular signal-regulated kinase and cyclooxygenase-2. *Carcinogenesis.* 25, 2487-2495.

Singh, S.K., Hawkins, C., Clarke, I.D., Squire, J.A., Bayani, J., Hide, T., Henkelman, R.M., Cusimano, M.D, Dirks, P.B., (2004). Identification of human brain tumour initiating cells. *Nature.* 432, 396-401.

Takebe, N., Ivy, S.P., (2010). Controversies in cancer stem cells: targeting embryonic signaling pathways. *Clin. Cancer. Res.* 16, 3106-3112.

Terry, P.D., Rohan T.E., (2002). Cigarette smoking and the risk of breast cancer in women: a review of the literature. *Cancer. Epidemiol. Biomarkers. Prev.* 11, 953-971.

Vineis, P., Alavanja, M., Buffler, P., Fontham, E., Franceschi, S., Gao, Y.T., Gupta, P.C., Hackshaw, A., Matos, E.,; Samet, J., Sitas, F., Smith, J., Stayner, L., Straif, K., Thun, M.J., Wichmann, H.E., Wu, A.H., Zaridze, D, Peto, R., Doll R., (2004). Tobacco and cancer: recent epidemiological evidence. *J. Natl. Cancer. Inst.* 96, 99-106.

Visvader, J.E., Lindeman, G.J., (2008). Cancer stem cells in solid tumours: accumulating evidence and unresolved questions. *Nat. Rev. Cancer.* 8, 755–768.

WHO., (2008a). WHO Report on the Global Tobacco Epidemic: The MPOWER Package, Available at http://www.who.int/tobacco/ mpower/mpower_report_full_2008.pdf

WHO., (2008b). The Scientific Basis of Tobacco Product Regulation; Second Report of a WHO Study Group Technical Report Series. Available at http://www.who.int/tobacco /global_interaction/tobreg/publications/9789241209519.pdf

Ye, Y.N., Liu, E.S., Shin, V.Y., Wu, W.K., Luo, J.C., Cho, C.H., (2004). Nicotine promoted colon cancer growth via epidermal growth factor receptor, c-Src, and 5-lipoxygenase-mediated signal pathway. *J. Pharmacol. Exp. Ther.* 308, 66-72.

Yu, M.A., Kiang, A., Wang-Rodriguez, J., Rahimy, E., Haas, M., Yu, V., Ellies, L.G., Chen, J., Fan, J.B., (2012). Brumund, KT; Weisman, RA; Ongkeko, WM. Nicotine promotes acquisition of stem cell and epithelial-to-mesenchymal properties in head and neck squamous cell carcinoma. *PLoS One.* 7, e51967.

INDEX

#

20th century, vii, 5, 7
21st century, 7, 16

A

access, 22, 25, 37, 58, 74, 136
acetaldehyde, 136, 137, 141, 163, 165, 175, 191
acetone, 175
acetylcholine, 185, 189, 193, 194
acid, 119, 155, 156, 188
acidosis, 177
active type, 137
activity level, 40, 41
acute myeloid leukemia, 187, 192
ADAM, 190
additives, 119, 137, 174, 176, 177, 180, 181
adhesion, 140, 141, 142, 148
adiposity, 112
adolescents, 75, 78, 113, 132, 183
adult smoking, 14, 18, 24, 31, 36, 37
adult stem cells, 142, 189
adults, vii, 23, 24, 29, 37, 63, 74, 81, 133, 139, 163, 178
adverse effects, 13, 135, 142, 151, 175
advertisements, 4, 12, 13, 16, 24, 25
advertising bans, vii, 3, 9, 11, 13, 16, 17, 19, 20, 24
aerosols, 175
affective disorder, 127, 128, 129
Africa, 5, 7
age, 12, 16, 18, 36, 37, 38, 39, 40, 43, 46, 47, 48, 49, 50, 56, 60, 66, 69, 70, 71, 79, 80, 84, 85, 86, 87, 88, 90, 91, 92, 94, 95, 96, 98, 99, 109, 110, 130, 137, 146, 147, 174, 185, 186
agencies, 3, 4, 12, 26
agriculture, 97
airflow obstruction, 124

airports, 24
airway responsiveness, 181
airways, 178
alcohol consumption, 40, 41, 131, 132
alcohol dependence, 130
alcohol use, 130, 131
alcoholics, 131, 132, 133
alcoholism, 128, 130, 131, 132
aldehydes, 138, 186, 188
alkaloids, 138
alters, 66, 168, 177, 183
alveoli, 176
American Psychiatric Association, 137, 162
amine, 137
ammonia, 137, 175
amputation, 178
angiogenesis, 185, 188, 189, 192
annual rate, 184
antibody, 159, 165
anticholinergic, 123
antidepressants, 129
anti-smoking policies, vii, 3, 4, 5, 9, 16
anxiety, 127, 128, 129, 130, 132, 133, 174, 180
anxiety disorder, 129, 130, 133
aorta, 178
apoptosis, 148, 170, 177, 183, 184, 193
appointments, 161
aromatic hydrocarbons, 137, 175, 186
arsenic, 175
artery(s), 178
Asia, 4, 82, 110
assessment, 25, 132, 171, 181, 185
asthma, 39, 83, 139, 178, 180
astrocytes, 194
asymptomatic, 183
atherosclerosis, 178
atmosphere, 175
ATP, 188

attachment, 135, 136, 140, 142, 146, 147, 149, 150, 163, 165, 166
attitudes, 75
Australia, 5, 7, 10, 11, 12, 16, 21, 22, 23, 24, 25, 26, 27, 28, 29, 30, 31
Austria, 5, 7, 10, 11, 19
autoimmunity, 181
avoidance, 25
awareness, 16, 22

B

ban, 3, 4, 9, 10, 11, 13, 14, 15, 16, 17, 18, 19, 20, 76
Bangladesh, 139
barriers, 24
base, 4, 40, 42, 50, 55, 193
batteries, 175
Beck Depression Inventory, 129, 131
behavioral aspects, vii
behavioral disorders, 137
behaviors, 61, 62, 84, 85, 97, 98, 110, 111, 132
Belgium, 5, 7, 10, 119
benchmarks, 82
beneficial effect, 127, 128, 149, 160, 161
benefits, 21, 23, 36, 124, 133, 145, 148, 162, 183
benzene, 175, 177, 191
bias, 54, 81, 82, 83, 91
binge drinking, 40, 41, 54, 58
biomarkers, 120, 194
bipolar disorder, 127, 128
birth weight, 4, 80, 178
bleeding, 146, 147, 148, 149, 150, 160, 164, 165, 168, 170
blood, 66, 112, 120, 125, 137, 138, 149, 159, 160, 165, 168, 173, 174, 175, 177, 178, 179
blood circulation, 66
blood clot, 179
blood flow, 149, 160, 168, 177, 178, 179
blood pressure, 112, 174, 177
blood stream, 66
blood supply, 178
blood vessels, 178, 179
blood-brain barrier, 137
bloodstream, 137
bone(s), 135, 136, 139, 140, 141, 143, 144, 145, 146, 148, 149, 150, 151, 152, 153, 154, 155, 156, 157, 158, 159, 160, 161, 162, 163, 164, 165, 166, 167, 168, 169, 171
bone cells, 149, 151, 153, 166
bone form, 152, 154
bone marrow, 140, 143, 151, 167, 171
bone mass, 160
bone resorption, 141, 158, 159

bone volume, 143, 168
bowel, 39
brain, 128, 175, 177, 178, 184, 187
brain activity, 184
brain chemistry, 177
Brazil, 5, 6, 8, 10, 11, 135, 139, 163, 165
breakdown, 128, 146, 148, 178
breast cancer, 186, 189, 190, 192, 194, 195
breastfeeding, 85
breathing, 138, 179
bronchitis, vii, 3, 4, 39, 178, 179, 180
bronchodilator, 123
building blocks, 26
businesses, 14
butadiene, 191
by-products, 160

C

calcium, 148, 149, 151, 170
calculus, 148, 163
calvaria, 151
campaigns, 3, 4, 5, 12, 20, 24, 25, 26, 29, 31
Canadian Tobacco Monitoring Surveys, 65, 66, 76
cancer, vii, 3, 4, 22, 23, 39, 65, 66, 86, 98, 124, 125, 136, 139, 173, 176, 178, 184, 185, 186, 187, 188, 189, 191, 192, 193, 194, 195
cancer cells, 185, 187, 188, 189, 193
cancer death, 23
cancer stem cells (CSCs), 185, 193
cannabis, 23, 26, 29
carbon, 66, 71, 117, 118, 120, 125, 137, 138, 160, 174, 175, 176, 177, 179, 191
carbon dioxide, 137
carbon monoxide, 66, 71, 117, 118, 120, 137, 138, 160, 174, 175, 176, 177, 179, 191
carcinogen, 4, 139
carcinogenesis, 186, 190
carcinogenicity, 186
cardiovascular disease(s), 4, 23, 118, 119, 122, 139
cardiovascular system, 139, 169, 177
carotenoids, 174
categorization, 117, 118, 122
category a, 129
causal relationship, 37, 97, 98
causality, 41, 54
causation, 183
CDC, 4, 14, 17, 36, 61, 66, 118, 123, 139
cell culture, 149, 151
cell death, 141, 177
cell line(s), 151, 170, 186, 187, 189, 191, 192
cell metabolism, 140, 141, 153
cell surface, 187

cellulose, 180
census, 81, 86
central nervous system (CNS), 133, 137, 194
cerebral arteries, 174
cervix, 178
challenges, 28, 30
chemical(s), 37, 58, 65, 66, 71, 77, 122, 128, 135,
    136, 138, 143, 173, 174, 175, 176, 180, 181, 185,
    186, 190, 191, 193
chemotaxis, 142, 167, 194
chemotherapy, 186
Chicago, 62
child bearing, 96
childhood, 26, 62, 178
children, vii, 7, 13, 15, 24, 25, 75, 79, 80, 81, 83, 84,
    86, 90, 92, 93, 95, 96, 97, 99, 110, 113, 139, 178,
    179, 181, 183
Chile, 5, 8, 10
China, 139
chinese women, 125
chronic diseases, vii, 4, 39, 43, 50, 58, 174
chronic illness, 41, 54, 55
chronic obstructive pulmonary disease (COPD), 23,
    39, 118, 119, 123, 125
cigarette smoke, 117, 118, 119, 120, 121, 122, 123,
    124, 125, 138, 140, 141, 142, 143, 144, 145, 149,
    151, 152, 153, 163, 164, 168, 169, 173, 174, 175,
    176, 178, 179, 180, 181, 182, 183, 184, 186, 188,
    189, 190, 191
cigarette smokers, 181, 182, 189
cigarette smoking, 4, 17, 19, 20, 74, 76, 77, 78, 113,
    118, 122, 125, 133, 154, 161, 162, 164, 165, 166,
    168, 171, 173, 176, 177, 181, 182, 185, 186, 189,
    190, 191
circulation, 143, 159
city(s), 12, 18, 21, 22, 23, 25, 29
citizens, 22
classes, 35, 50, 51, 53, 54, 55, 56
classification, 50, 136, 156, 162
cleavage, 189
climate, 28
climate change, 28
clinical trials, 156
coastal region, 22
cocaine, 137
cognition, 127, 128
cognitive abilities, 113
collagen, 140, 141, 142, 148, 151, 152, 167, 169, 172
college students, 14, 17
colon, 187, 188, 189, 192, 194, 195
colon cancer, 189, 194, 195
combined effect, 22
combustion, 138, 175, 181

commercial, 24, 51
common law, 40
communication, 97
community(s), 22, 23, 24, 25, 26, 28, 30, 37, 84, 109,
    110, 131, 162, 163
community service, 22
compensation, 117, 122, 125
complications, 135, 136, 153, 154, 155, 157, 158,
    159, 160, 162, 169
composition, 138, 148
compounds, 135, 136, 137, 138, 140, 141, 142, 143,
    144, 145, 160, 173, 175, 191
computing, 87
conception, 82, 83
condensation, 142
connective tissue, 141, 148, 170
consensus, 91
constituents, 118, 119, 120, 124, 175
construction, 38, 58
consumers, 12, 41, 120
consumption, 3, 4, 5, 6, 7, 9, 12, 13, 14, 15, 16, 17,
    19, 20, 36, 38, 39, 40, 58, 63, 67, 69, 73, 74, 146,
    159, 173, 176
contaminated water, 180
contamination, 139
control condition, 140
control group, 142, 143, 152, 153
controlled studies, 130
controversial, 125, 136, 147, 148, 193
cooperation, 80
copyright, 181
coronary arteries, 177
coronary heart disease, 66, 119, 125
coronary thrombosis, 181
correlation(s), 14, 120, 121, 122, 146, 158, 159
cost, 7, 8, 9, 22, 23, 24, 63, 77, 180, 191
cost of living, 63
cost of smoking, 7
cotinine, 109, 110, 112, 113, 138, 140, 142, 146, 164
counseling, 130, 131
covering, 82
craving, 132, 133, 174, 177
crises, 9
cross-sectional study, 109, 112, 113, 146, 158, 167,
    168, 171, 183
crown(s), 156, 164
CSCs, 185, 186, 187, 188, 189, 190, 191
CSF, 141, 147, 152
cultivation, 176
culture, 25, 141, 151, 152, 167, 187
culture conditions, 151, 187
curriculum, 161
CVD, 119

cyanide, 138, 168
cycles, 37
cyclooxygenase, 195
cytochrome, 138
cytokines, 142, 148, 153, 158, 168
cytometry, 187
cytoskeleton, 141, 169
cytotoxicity, 140, 142
Czech Republic, 5, 6, 8, 10

D

Daily Smoker, 5, 6, 46, 47, 48, 49, 60, 69
damages, 65, 174, 176
data analysis, 155
data availability, 74
data gathering, 6
data set, 13, 14, 74, 81, 86
death rate, 7, 22, 29
deaths, 3, 4, 7, 30, 35, 66, 110, 137, 138
debridement, 168
decreasing returns, 13
defects, 143, 145, 146, 152, 170
deficit, 21, 22, 30
deforestation, 180
degradation, 174
Delta, 88, 89, 90
Denmark, 5, 6, 8, 10, 11
dental implants, 149, 153, 154, 155, 157, 158, 159, 162, 164, 166, 167, 169, 171, 172
dentist, 135, 162
Department of Health and Human Services, 78, 80, 113, 177, 178, 184
dependent variable, 86, 87
deposition, 123, 124, 151
depression, 5, 127, 128, 129, 132, 133
depressive symptoms, 129, 131, 183
depth, 146, 150
destruction, 140, 141, 148, 158, 165
detection, 138
developed countries, 13, 66, 136, 183
developing countries, vii, 17, 18, 136, 137
deviation, 82
diabetes, 4, 39, 83, 111, 154, 155, 166, 178
Diagnostic and Statistical Manual of Mental Disorders, 137, 162
diastolic pressure, 174, 177
dichotomy, 53
diet, 62
direct action, 151
direct cost(s), 7, 8
disease progression, 146

diseases, 4, 16, 36, 118, 120, 136, 137, 139, 156, 161, 166, 172, 179, 191, 192
disorder, 39, 111, 128, 137
displacement, 3, 13, 15, 16
displacement effect, 3, 13, 15, 16
distillation, 175
distribution, 4, 124, 137, 171
dizziness, 179
DNA, 125, 140, 169, 177, 184, 188, 191
DNA damage, 125, 184
doctors, 123, 161, 179
dogs, 152, 169
donors, 140
dopamine, 137, 177, 181
dopaminergic, 137
draft, 181
drought, 28
drug addict, 137
drug addiction, 137
drug interaction, 143
drug metabolism, 178
drug resistance, 186, 192
drug therapy, 161
drugs, 130, 140, 181
drying, 175, 180

E

East Asia, 5, 7
economic policy, 28
economic status, 25
economic welfare, 78
economics, 16, 73, 77
ecosystem, 28
education, 22, 23, 24, 25, 28, 35, 36, 37, 38, 39, 40, 41, 50, 51, 52, 53, 54, 55, 56, 57, 58, 62, 63, 73, 83, 84, 86, 146, 164, 184
educational attainment, 28
Egypt, 139
elementary school, 111
elucidation, 189
e-mail, 117
embryogenesis, 120
embryonic stem cells, 124
emergency, 178
emphysema, vii, 3, 4, 39
employment, 85
enamel, 145, 164
endogeneity, 86
endothelial cells, 148
endothelium, 139
energy, 40
energy expenditure, 40

England, 81, 109
environment(s), 24, 25, 28, 29, 38, 39, 63, 65, 139, 161, 173, 180
environmental conditions, 145
environmental factors, 37, 58, 175
Environmental Protection Agency, 4
environmental tobacco, 75, 77, 113, 138
enzyme(s), 148, 182, 186
epidemic, 16, 20, 63, 171
epidemiologic, 109, 132
epidemiology, 110, 124
epithelial cells, 165
equality, 26
equilibrium, 193
equity, 28
esophagus, 186
Estonia, 6, 8, 10
ethanol, 138
ethical issues, 143
ethics, 169
etiology, 139, 171, 184
Europe, 5, 7, 17, 29, 81, 82, 83, 95, 118, 124, 171
European Commission, 4, 17
European Parliament, 118
European Union (EU), 14, 17
everyday life, 27
evidence, vii, viii, 4, 5, 9, 16, 19, 21, 22, 23, 24, 25, 26, 29, 37, 38, 39, 53, 63, 66, 74, 75, 76, 78, 79, 92, 97, 109, 117, 118, 120, 122, 125, 129, 153, 155, 161, 166, 168, 185, 186, 188, 189, 191, 195
expected tar ratio, 122
expenditures, 14, 15, 17, 18, 19
exposure, 7, 15, 16, 19, 25, 37, 58, 62, 75, 77, 79, 80, 83, 110, 112, 113, 117, 120, 122, 138, 139, 143, 145, 168, 171, 177, 181, 190, 194
externalities, 16
extracellular matrix, 149, 171
extracts, 125, 151

F

families, 179
family income, 179
family members, 75, 80, 98
feelings, 177
femur, 143
fibroblast growth factor, 187
fibroblast proliferation, 194
fibroblasts, 138, 141, 142, 158, 159, 160, 162, 163, 165, 166, 171, 172
fibrosis, 183, 184
fibrous tissue, 154
filters, 119, 180

financial, 27
fine particulate matter, 180
Finland, 6, 8, 10
fires, 77
fixed effect model, 13
flavour, 119, 175, 176, 177
flexibility, 11
flights, 24
fluctuations, 91, 92
fluid, 148, 158, 163, 164, 167, 171
fluoxetine, 131
food, 28, 38
force, 9, 31, 50
Ford, 81, 110, 176, 182
formaldehyde, 137, 175, 191
formation, 140, 141, 142, 145, 151, 152, 170, 171, 176, 178, 187, 189, 191
Framework Convention on Tobacco Control, 9, 20, 23, 31
France, 6, 8, 10, 83, 111, 182
free radicals, 179
funding, 14, 22

G

gambling, 11
gangrene, 178
GATS, 139
gel, 151, 167
gender differences, 109
gene expression, 142, 152, 192
genes, 153, 189, 190
genetic mutations, 177
genotype, 159, 165, 166, 167
Germany, 6, 8, 10
gestation, 81
gingival, 141, 146, 147, 148, 149, 150, 162, 163, 164, 166, 168, 169, 170, 171, 172
gingivitis, 141, 147, 148, 156, 167
glycogen, 177
glycol, 175
governance, 26
governments, 28, 73
graduate students, viii
graph, 41, 70
Great Britain, 20
Great Depression, vii
Greece, 6, 8, 10
growth, 142, 166, 186, 189, 194, 195
growth factor, 189, 194, 195
guidelines, 6, 8, 9, 11, 171

H

hair, 58, 176, 179, 184
hair loss, 179, 184
half-life, 137, 138
harmful effects, vii, viii, 80, 92, 160, 174
hazards, vii, 138, 173
headache, 179
healing, 141, 142, 143, 145, 149, 152, 153, 160, 161, 163, 164, 165, 170
health and environmental effects, vii
Health and Human Services, 78, 113
health care, 11, 22, 27, 30, 36, 37, 38, 58
health care costs, 36
health condition, 41, 58
health education, 184
health effects, vii, 3, 4, 5, 13, 15, 16, 23, 25, 29, 66, 73, 75, 179
health information, 37, 38, 58
health problems, 3, 4, 41, 65, 66, 71, 173
health promotion, 22, 28
health risks, 79, 117, 120
health services, 22, 24, 28
health status, 22, 29, 35, 38, 39, 40, 41, 43, 50, 51, 53, 54, 56, 58, 86, 158, 171
heart attack, 23, 66, 177, 178, 179
heart disease, vii, 3, 4, 35, 39, 66, 119, 125, 128, 139
heart failure, 119
heart rate, 174, 177
heavy particle, 117, 121
height, 85, 145, 150
hematocrit, 178
hematopoietic stem cells, 188, 193
hemoglobin, 138, 179
hemorrhagic stroke, 178
heroin, 137
heterogeneity, 62
high school, 37, 38, 41, 50, 51, 52, 53, 54, 56
high school diploma, 38, 41, 56
higher education, 38, 54, 83
histamine, 184
history, 124, 129, 130, 131, 132, 133, 154, 155, 161
homelessness, 23
homeostasis, 153
homes, 13, 15, 26
Hong Kong, 124
hormone(s), 137, 154, 167, 177
hospitality, 30
host, 139
hotel(s), 18, 179
hotspots, 125
house, 89
household income, 85, 99
housing, 80, 89, 98, 99
human, 26, 62, 118, 122, 137, 138, 141, 142, 151, 153, 154, 162, 163, 165, 166, 167, 168, 169, 170, 171, 172, 174, 180, 181, 185, 188, 189, 190, 192, 193, 194, 195
human body, 137
human brain, 195
human capital, 62
human exposure, 118
human health, 118, 122, 180
human milk, 181
human right(s), 26
Hungary, 6, 8, 10
husband, 80, 86, 89, 97, 99
hydrocarbons, 138, 191
hydrogen, 124, 137, 160, 175
hydrogen cyanide, 137, 175
hydrogen peroxide, 124
hydroxyapatite, 154, 166
hygiene, 147, 166
hypothesis, 36, 129, 177
hypoxia, 138, 177

I

ICAM, 147, 148, 169
Iceland, 6, 7, 8, 10
identification, 192
iliac crest, 140
illusions, 180
image(s), 24, 183
image analysis, 183
imagery, 27
immune defense, 178
immune response, 140, 147, 148, 159
immune system, 184
immunity, 181
immunoglobulin(s), 159
implant failures, 149, 154, 162, 166
implant placement, 154, 160
implants, 136, 149, 152, 153, 154, 155, 156, 157, 158, 159, 160, 161, 164, 165, 166, 167, 168
improvements, 161
in vitro, 140, 145, 153, 162, 163, 165, 166, 171, 187, 191, 194
in vivo, 140, 145, 166, 193
incidence, 119, 135, 142, 149, 160, 162, 163, 178
income, 5, 7, 19, 23, 25, 28, 35, 36, 37, 38, 39, 40, 41, 43, 50, 51, 52, 53, 54, 55, 56, 57, 58, 74, 84, 85, 86, 98, 99, 110, 176, 179
income inequality, 110
incomplete combustion, 138
independent variable, 157

India, 139, 173, 176, 183
Indigenous, 21, 22, 26, 27, 28, 29, 30, 31
indirect effect, 15, 16, 25, 152
individual character, 85
individual characteristics, 85
individuals, 7, 12, 13, 15, 16, 36, 37, 38, 39, 40, 41, 74, 76, 85, 86, 129, 131, 133, 137, 141, 151, 162, 164, 174, 176, 180
Indonesia, 82, 109
indoor smoking bans, 5, 14, 16
induction, 189
industry(s), 4, 12, 14, 15, 97, 118, 123, 124, 137, 169
inequality, 28
inequity, 30
infants, 83, 85, 92, 110
infarction, 133
infection, 148, 172
inflammation, 120, 125, 139, 141, 147, 148, 158, 159, 178, 179, 181
inflammatory mediators, 167
infrastructure, 22, 73
ingest, 180
ingredients, 119, 143, 171, 181
inhibition, 141, 142, 193
inhibitor, 152
initiation, 76, 77, 78, 97, 109, 157
injections, 145
injury(s), 22, 141, 181
insecticide, 138
insertion, 135, 136, 156, 161
institutions, 85
integration, 135, 136
integrity, 141
intercellular adhesion molecule, 147, 148
interdependence, 22
interference, 140, 143, 145, 147
intervention, 27, 30, 84, 119, 123, 131, 132, 155
intestine, 137
ion channels, 189
Ireland, 6, 7, 8, 10
iron, 138
irritability, 129
Israel, 6, 8, 10
issues, 26, 28, 29, 73, 75, 140, 155
Italy, 6, 8, 10, 13, 18, 127

J

Japan, vii, 5, 6, 7, 8, 10, 79, 80, 81, 82, 84, 90, 96, 97, 99, 109, 110, 111, 112, 113, 176, 185, 192
Japanese women, 80, 82, 87, 96, 98, 99, 100

K

kidney(s), 137, 173, 178, 186
kill, 35
Korea, 6, 8, 10, 82, 97, 109

L

lactic acid, 138
larynx, 173, 178
laws, 13, 14, 17, 18, 20, 25, 75, 77, 78
lead, 4, 37, 83, 140, 142, 146, 148, 149, 160, 174, 175, 178, 191
leadership, 26
learning, 82
legislation, 117, 118, 122
legs, 178
leisure, 40
leisure time, 40
lesions, 139, 145, 147, 154, 156, 160, 161, 169, 183
leukemia, 177, 187
leukocytes, 143, 165
leukocytosis, 143
level of education, 39, 58
life course, 63, 112
life expectancy, 16, 22, 26, 31, 62
life experiences, 27
lifetime, 129, 133
ligament, 141, 142, 143, 165, 166, 171
ligand, 141, 147, 148, 189
light, 68, 69, 71, 72, 73, 76, 118, 123, 124, 161, 168, 174
liver, 137, 143, 178, 186
liver enzymes, 143
local community, 26
localization, 142
longitudinal study, 63, 109, 113, 163, 164
low-tar, vii, 117, 118, 120, 121, 122
lung cancer, vii, 3, 4, 23, 35, 98, 118, 124, 125, 128, 139, 177, 186, 189, 193, 194
lung disease, 128, 139, 160
lung function, 182
Luo, 195
Luxemburg, 20

M

Mackintosh, 182
macrophages, 158
magazines, 9
mainstream smoke, 118, 122, 123, 175, 180
major depression, 129, 131, 132

major depressive disorder, 129
majority, 37, 53, 71, 82, 98
malignant cells, 188
man, 183
management, 26, 30, 97, 123, 171, 184
manual workers, 97
manufacturing, 15, 117, 118, 119
marginal costs, 13
marijuana, 132
marital life, 97
marital status, 38, 40, 43, 46, 47, 48, 49, 58, 80, 85, 86, 96, 97, 99
market share, 12
marketing, 23
married couples, 97, 109, 110
married women, 96, 97
marrow, 143, 166
mass, 5, 25, 29, 31, 117, 118, 120, 122, 160
mass media, 25, 29, 31
maternal smoking, 109, 113
matrix, 142, 145, 147, 151, 152, 163, 164, 166
matrix metalloproteinase, 142, 147, 152, 163, 166
matter, 28, 51, 53, 54, 55, 119, 173, 175, 180, 182
maxilla, 154, 157, 159, 166
maxillary sinus, 155
measurement(s), 6, 91, 112, 113, 121, 122, 125, 146, 168
mechanical properties, 143, 149
media, 9, 13, 24, 25, 29, 187
median, 67
medical, 4, 7, 15, 16, 66, 82, 85, 91, 143, 191
medical science, 143
Medicare, 22, 24
medication, 161
medicine, 111, 160, 167
Mediterranean, 5
mellitus, 111, 154
membranes, 170
mental disorder, 128
mental health, 22, 23, 28, 86, 127, 128
merchandise, 4
mesenchymal stem cells, 142
messages, 12, 20, 23, 24, 25, 82
meta-analysis, 27, 129, 132, 149, 155, 157, 160, 164, 166, 169, 170, 193
metabolic, 177
metabolic acidosis, 177
metabolism, 138, 140, 141, 147, 151
metabolites, 138, 157
metabolized, 137
metabolizing, 182
metalloproteinase, 151
metastasis, 186, 189, 193

meter, 168
methodology, 40, 143
metropolitan areas, 22
Mexico, 6, 7, 8, 10, 139
mice, 125, 143, 151, 187, 194
microbiota, 148, 166, 167
microRNA, 142
Middle East, 7
migration, 185, 188, 189
mineralization, 142, 143
minimum wage, 39
Ministry of Education, 79, 191
Minneapolis, 132
miscarriages, 178
mitochondria, 138
MMP(s), 142, 147, 148, 152
models, 36, 76, 143, 144, 153, 166, 187, 191
modernization, 4
molecules, 185, 189
monolayer, 151, 167
monopoly, 80
morbidity, 36, 77, 122, 128, 139
morphology, 159, 169
mortality, 36, 61, 62, 63, 83, 118, 119, 122, 124, 125, 128, 132, 139, 171
motivation, 135
mucous membrane(s), 137
multidimensional, 27
multiple regression, 146
multiple regression analysis, 146
muscle contraction, 178
mutation(s), 186, 188
myocardial infarction, 125, 139
myosin, 137

N

nail polish, 175
narratives, 25
National Survey, 79
natural resources, 22
nausea, 91, 179
necrosis, 158, 168
negative effects, 92, 96, 128, 151, 154, 161
negative mood, 129, 131
negative relation, 65, 73
neglect, 121
neovascularization, 195
nervous system, 137
nervousness, 129
Netherlands, 5, 6, 8, 10, 117, 119
networking, 28
neurons, 194

neutrophils, 159
New England, 63
New Zealand, 6, 7, 8, 10, 110
nickel, 175
Nile, 148, 168
nitrates, 137
nitrogen, 137, 175
nitrosamines, 137, 186, 191
nodules, 151
non-OECD, 19
nonsmokers, 41, 53, 54, 55, 138, 155, 177
non-smokers, vii, 13, 14, 15, 16, 26, 51, 53, 74, 86, 136, 139, 140, 142, 146, 147, 148, 149, 150, 153, 154, 155, 156, 157, 158, 159, 160, 167, 168, 169, 170, 171
norepinephrine, 137, 165
North America, 36, 182
Norway, 6, 7, 8, 10, 12, 111
nucleus, 137, 190
nurses, 161
nutrients, 178
nutritional status, 36, 40, 146

O

obesity, 40, 83, 113
obstructive lung disease, 173
occupational illness, 179
OECD, vii, 3, 4, 5, 6, 7, 8, 9, 10, 11, 12, 13, 15, 16, 19, 20, 98
OECD Countries, v, 3, 5, 7, 9
officials, 81, 86
omission, 12
opportunities, 30, 123
oral cavity, 186
organ(s), 161, 173, 175, 178, 187
osmolality, 177
osseointegration, 135, 151
osteoclastogenesis, 141, 148
osteoporosis, 154
ovarian cancer, 192
ovaries, 187
oxidation, 138, 154, 174, 186, 188
oxygen, 66, 137, 138, 173, 174, 175, 177, 178, 179

P

Pacific, 5
pain, 178
paints, 175
Pakistan, 183
pancreas, 173, 178, 186, 187, 188

pancreatic cancer, 193
paralysis, 178
parathyroid, 153
parents, 23, 80, 86, 89, 98, 99, 110, 111
parity, 79, 85, 86, 91, 92, 93, 94, 95, 96, 99
participants, 27, 75, 86
particle mass, 117
passive smoking, 3, 4, 17, 29, 82, 85, 110, 112, 119, 124, 173
pathogenesis, 169
pathogens, 136, 159, 172
pathophysiology, 122
pathways, 27, 36, 37, 56, 189
patient care, 166
PCR, 142
PDL, 165
peace, 28
penalties, 39
per capita cost, 7
per capita income, 85
perfusion, 178
peri-implant soft tissue, 153
peri-implantitis, 135, 158
perinatal, 80, 111
periodontal, 135, 136, 139, 140, 141, 142, 143, 144, 145, 146, 147, 148, 149, 156, 157, 159, 160, 161, 162, 163, 164, 165, 166, 167, 168, 169, 170, 171, 172
periodontal disease, 135, 136, 139, 142, 143, 145, 146, 147, 148, 149, 156, 159, 162, 163, 165, 166, 168, 171
periodontitis, 135, 136, 139, 142, 145, 146, 147, 154, 155, 156, 157, 159, 161, 163, 165, 166, 167, 168, 169, 170, 171
peripheral blood, 143
peripheral vascular disease, 66, 173, 178
permeability, 158
permission, 79
peroxynitrite, 124
personal stories, 25
personality, 127, 128
personality disorder, 127, 128, 133
pesticide, 175
phagocytosis, 159
pharmacological treatment, 129, 130
pharynx, 186
phenol, 175
phenotype, 186, 189, 190, 191
Philippines, 139
phosphate, 149
phosphorylation, 183
physical activity, 40, 62
physicians, 80, 91

physiology, 110, 140, 147, 153
pilot study, 171
plants, 175
plaque, 146, 147, 148, 158
plasma levels, 110
plasminogen, 152
plasticity, 188
plastics, 180
platelet aggregation, 139, 160, 177
platelets, 179, 182, 183
pneumonia, 179
Poland, 6, 8, 10, 11, 20, 112, 139
policy, vii, viii, 9, 11, 13, 16, 21, 23, 28, 29, 30, 36, 37, 74, 75, 77
policy makers, vii, viii, 9, 13, 16, 37
pollutants, 180
pollution, 37, 58, 138, 173, 174, 180
polycyclic aromatic hydrocarbon, 125
polymorphism, 159
pools, 143
population, vii, 5, 6, 7, 22, 23, 24, 27, 31, 37, 40, 66, 75, 81, 82, 84, 86, 87, 96, 110, 118, 119, 127, 128, 130, 131, 137, 146, 147, 157, 159, 185, 186, 187, 188, 191, 192, 193
population group, vii, 23
Portugal, 6, 8, 10
poverty, 27, 58
pregnancy, vii, 27, 80, 81, 82, 83, 90, 92, 96, 109, 110, 111, 112, 113, 183
premature death, 118, 185
prevalence of smoking, vii, 35, 41, 43, 80, 82, 83, 85, 93, 96, 98, 112
prevention, 124, 193
price changes, 73, 74
private costs, 36
private practice, 167
probability, 40, 46, 47, 48, 49, 50, 51, 52, 53, 54, 55, 58, 93
production technology, 4
professionals, 16, 161
progenitor cells, 193
prognosis, 136, 145, 146, 148, 155, 159, 165, 170, 186, 190
pro-inflammatory, 142
proliferation, 135, 136, 140, 141, 142, 149, 151, 159, 167, 171, 185, 186, 188, 189, 190, 191, 192, 193
propagation, 193, 194
propylene, 175
prosperity, 22
prostaglandins, 142
prostate cancer, 192, 193
prostheses, 167
protection, 135, 136

protective mechanisms, 40
protective role, 54
protein kinase C, 182, 190
proteinase, 167
proteins, 140, 165
prototype, 191, 194
psychiatric disorders, 127, 132
psychiatric illness, 129, 132
psychiatric morbidity, 113
psychopathology, 127
psychotropic medications, 181
public awareness, vii, 92
public concern(s), 82
public education, 73
public health, 4, 27, 81, 85, 111, 112, 135, 136
public policy, viii, 78
publishing, 29
purchasing power, 7
purification, 187
P-value, 69
pyrolysis, 175

Q

quality of life, 16
quantification, 138
questionnaire, 85, 86

R

race, 130
radical hysterectomy, 154
radio, 9, 24
radiography, 159
reactions, 158
reactivity, 182, 184
real time, 142
reasoning, 120
recall, 167, 171
receptors, 177, 183, 193, 194
recession, 146, 147, 148, 150
recognition, 184
recommendations, 133, 171
recovery, 131, 160, 174, 177
red blood cells, 177
reform, 30
regeneration, 142, 143, 144, 145, 152, 169, 170
registry, 111
regression, 37, 50, 87, 88, 156
regression analysis, 88, 156
regression equation, 87
regulations, 3, 4, 10, 11, 12, 15, 18, 19, 20, 78

rehabilitation, 136
relaxation, 177
relevance, 143
reliability, 81
relief, 127, 128, 174
repair, 138, 141, 142, 151, 152, 153, 166
reproduction, 178
researchers, viii, 12, 15, 36, 37, 39, 43, 58, 74, 76, 140, 141, 143
resilience, 29
resistance, 29, 186
resources, 27, 28, 30, 171
respiration, 138
respiratory problems, 174, 180
response, 12, 23, 24, 39, 73, 74, 80, 81, 86, 136, 139, 140, 143, 144, 148, 149, 151, 158, 160, 165, 177
responsiveness, 128, 183
restaurants, 11, 12, 14, 15, 17, 19, 24, 25, 75, 139
restoration, 157
restrictions, vii, 5, 9, 10, 11, 12, 13, 14, 15, 16, 17, 19, 69, 70, 73, 75, 88, 118
restructuring, 130
retail, 9
retinol, 188
rings, 137
risk aversion, 86
risk factors, 22, 26, 31, 63, 79, 87, 154, 155, 162, 165, 173, 174
risk profile, 120
root, 98, 142, 143, 145, 148, 165, 170
rules, 11
rural areas, 23, 27, 29
Russia, 139

S

safety, 37, 77, 124, 163, 178
saliva, 138, 148
sample mean, 81
savings, 27
scaling, 143
schizophrenia, 127, 128, 131, 132
schizophrenic patients, 128, 133
school, 24, 37, 38, 42, 50, 54, 56, 60
schooling, 26, 56, 61
science, 124, 140, 168, 193
scope, 73, 76
second hand smoke, vii, 15, 16, 25, 138, 178, 179, 180
second hand smoking, vii, 92
Second World, 4
secondary education, 58
secretion, 177

sedentary lifestyle, 55
self-reports, 39, 54, 87, 100
sensations, 127, 128
sensitivity, 40, 77
serum, 170, 187
services, 22, 25, 26, 27, 180
SES, 25, 36, 37, 41, 43
sewage, 175
sex, 24, 35, 38, 39, 40, 50, 57, 58, 130, 157
shelter, 28
showing, 25, 141, 143, 145, 146, 147, 148, 151, 160, 174
sibling(s), 37, 85
sickle cell, 178
sickle cell anemia, 178
signaling pathway, 177, 189, 190, 195
signs, 9, 159, 167
sinuses, 156
size-dependent particle counts, 117, 121, 122
skin, 137, 168, 179, 183
smoke exposure, 79, 97, 99, 110, 120
smoking cessation, 21, 24, 25, 27, 28, 29, 30, 36, 92, 96, 99, 109, 111, 113, 119, 123, 124, 128, 129, 130, 131, 132, 133, 135, 136, 138, 145, 149, 160, 161, 162, 164, 165, 167, 181
Smoking Cessation and Reduction, v, 127
smoking during pregnancy, 27, 80, 82, 91, 112, 113
smoking related diseases, 36, 118, 119
smoking restrictions, vii, 9, 10, 14, 15, 16, 17, 73, 75
smooth muscle, 194
smooth muscle cells, 194
smuggling, 20, 77
SNAP, 25, 31
social change, 109
social class, 78
social context, 28
social determinants of health, 21, 22
social environment, 28, 79, 87
social justice, 28
social norms, 13, 15
Social Security, 62
society, 15, 16, 21, 25, 174
socioeconomic status, 28, 35, 36, 37, 39, 56, 57, 62, 110, 111
software, 87
solid tumors, 187
solution, 16, 153
South Asia, 176
South Korea, 109
Spain, 6, 8, 10, 12, 16
specialists, 97
species, 148
spending, 13, 14, 20

spinal fusion, 160, 165, 170
sponsorship bans on smoking, 4
spontaneous abortion, 80
Spring, 132
squamous cell, 189, 195
squamous cell carcinoma, 189, 195
stability, 148, 154, 170
standard deviation, 82
standard error, 82, 83
state(s), 4, 9, 11, 14, 15, 17, 19, 23, 36, 82, 109, 132, 153, 177, 181, 184, 192, 193
statistics, 40, 41, 43, 57, 62, 79, 81, 83, 87, 88, 100, 119, 123
stem cells, vii, 142, 185, 187, 188, 189, 192, 193, 194, 195
stimulant, 137, 151
stimulation, 140, 141, 152, 189
stomach, 98, 137, 186
stress, 38, 62, 127, 128, 129, 131, 173, 174, 177, 180
striatum, 181
stroke, 23, 39, 66, 119, 133, 139, 173, 178
structure, 177
style, 36, 51, 52, 53, 54, 58
subcutaneous injection, 153
subgroups, 30
submicron, v, 117
substance abuse, 127, 128, 133, 137
substance use, 23
substitutes, 99
success rate, 155, 158
sudden infant death syndrome, 83
suicidal ideation, 129
suppression, 183
surface area, 120, 125
surface treatment, 153, 164
survival, 22, 146, 153, 154, 155, 156, 157, 158, 160, 164
survival rate, 22, 153, 154, 155, 160
susceptibility, 169, 182
sustainable development, 28
Sweden, 6, 8, 10, 112
swelling, 177
Switzerland, 6, 8, 10, 20
symptoms, 86, 128, 129, 133, 174, 179
synergistic effect, 160
synthesis, 140, 142, 149, 151, 159, 169
systolic blood pressure, 177

T

T cell(s), 159
tar, vii, 12, 65, 71, 117, 118, 120, 121, 122, 124, 125, 175, 176, 182

target, 75, 169, 186, 189
target organs, 186
tartrate-resistant acid phosphatase, 140
tax increase, 29
tax rates, 74
tax reform(s), 31
tax system, 73
taxation, 20, 23, 25
taxes, vii, 13, 14, 16, 17, 20, 73, 74, 75, 76, 77, 78
techniques, 6, 37, 159, 161
teeth, 135, 136, 139, 142, 145, 146, 147, 156, 166
television advertisements, 25
temperature, 140
tension, 83, 174
territory, 11
tertiary education, 23
test statistic, 69
testing, 117, 118, 120, 124, 125, 143
Thailand, 139, 182
therapeutics, 194
therapy, 24, 128, 130, 145, 146, 148, 149, 154, 157, 160, 161, 164, 165, 166, 168, 169
thoughts, 130
threats, 78
thrombosis, 179, 182
time preferences, 36
time series, 19
time-frame, 37
TIMP, 152
tissue, 121, 137, 138, 140, 141, 142, 143, 144, 145, 148, 149, 152, 153, 157, 165, 170, 171, 179
titanium, 149, 152, 153, 154, 157, 161, 164, 166, 168
TNF-α, 171
tobacco consumption, 3, 4, 5, 7, 9, 12, 13, 15, 16, 19, 20, 173, 176
tobacco smoke, 66, 75, 112, 125, 138, 139, 146, 149, 169, 171, 176, 177, 178, 179, 181, 184
tobacco smoking, 22, 63, 80, 127, 128, 131, 132, 137, 148, 163, 170, 183, 191
tooth, 146, 147, 150, 161, 162, 164, 166, 167, 168
toxic effect, 120, 140
toxic substances, 137
toxicity, vi, 117, 120, 122, 124, 141, 143, 163, 171, 181, 185
toxicology, 125
trade, 38
training, 27
transcription, 142, 190
transcription factors, 142
transformation, 188
transmission, 177
transplantation, 194
transport, 24, 139

transportation, 14, 97
trauma, 144, 145, 161, 163, 168
treatment, 25, 77, 128, 129, 130, 131, 132, 133, 141, 146, 148, 149, 152, 153, 155, 157, 159, 160, 161, 164, 165, 166, 168, 169, 170, 174, 175
trial, 27, 123, 131, 132, 168, 169
tumor, 147, 148, 158, 165, 185, 187, 189, 192, 193, 194, 195
tumor cells, 187, 189
tumor growth, 193, 195
tumor necrosis factor (TNF), 147, 148, 158, 165, 171
tumor progression, 189
tumorigenesis, 191
tumors, 185, 187, 188, 190, 192, 195
tumour growth, 194
Turkey, 3, 6, 7, 8, 10, 139
turnover, 141, 152
twins, 61

U

Ukraine, 139
uniform, 82
united, 6, 8, 10, 61, 62, 63, 73, 77, 110, 119, 123, 128, 133, 184
United Kingdom (UK), 5, 6, 7, 8, 10, 19, 25, 123
United States (USA), 6, 8, 10, 20, 61, 62, 63, 73, 110, 119, 123, 128, 131, 133, 137, 161, 192
urban, 15, 18, 21, 23, 28, 84, 85, 110
urban areas, 15, 18, 85
urban population, 28
urinary bladder, 173, 178
urine, 112, 113, 138, 139
urokinase, 152
Uruguay, 139
US Department of Health and Human Services, 165

V

validation, 112
vapor, 124
variables, 35, 40, 50, 56, 86, 87, 88, 91, 154
variations, 9, 11, 81
varieties, 123
vasculature, 147
vasoconstriction, 139, 160
vasopressin, 177
vehicles, 75

Vietnam, 139
viscosity, 173, 178, 179
vomiting, 91, 179
vulnerability, 37, 128

W

Washington, 19, 20, 63, 162, 165, 168, 184
waste, 175, 183
waste water, 175
water, 27, 137, 173, 180
water quality, 180
weakness, 179
web, 66
Western Europe, 7, 83
white blood cells, 159
withdrawal, 129, 130, 132, 177, 183
withdrawal symptoms, 129, 130, 132, 177
wood, 180
workers, 25, 27, 62, 75, 97, 170, 176, 181
workforce, 22
working hours, 85
working memory, 184
workplace, 11, 15, 18, 25, 75, 139
World Bank, 4, 168
World Health Organization (WHO), 4, 5, 7, 9, 10, 11, 20, 23, 29, 31, 35, 63, 124, 136, 137, 138, 139, 171, 185, 191, 195
World War I, 138
worldwide, 35, 122, 132, 135, 136, 139, 174, 185
wound healing, 166, 170

X

X-axis, 119, 122
xenotransplantation, 187

Y

Y-axis, 119, 122
yield, 124, 125
young adults, 17, 35, 77, 78, 132, 168, 169, 170
young people, 25, 70, 73, 74, 75, 76, 78
youth smoking, 17, 20, 25, 65, 66, 69, 73, 74, 75, 77, 78